Insights into Clinical Neurology

Insights into Clinical Neurology

Robert Laureno
Georgetown University

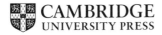

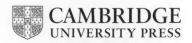

Shaftesbury Road, Cambridge CB2 8EA, United Kingdom

One Liberty Plaza, 20th Floor, New York, NY 10006, USA

477 Williamstown Road, Port Melbourne, VIC 3207, Australia

314–321, 3rd Floor, Plot 3, Splendor Forum, Jasola District Centre, New Delhi – 110025, India

103 Penang Road, #05–06/07, Visioncrest Commercial, Singapore 238467

Cambridge University Press is part of Cambridge University Press & Assessment, a department of the University of Cambridge.

We share the University's mission to contribute to society through the pursuit of education, learning and research at the highest international levels of excellence.

www.cambridge.org
Information on this title: www.cambridge.org/9781009234979

DOI: 10.1017/9781009234986

First published 2023

Printed in the United Kingdom by TJ Books Limited, Padstow Cornwall

A catalogue record for this publication is available from the British Library.

A Cataloging-in-Publication data record for this book is available from the Library of Congress.

ISBN 978-1-009-23497-9 Hardback

For Mark M. Lin, MD, PhD

Contents

Preface

In this volume I discuss 20 neurological topics. My purpose is to add to the existing literature on these subjects by way of simplification, synthesis, or original information. In some chapters I rely heavily on personal experience, for example, in the discussions of asterixis and amnesia. In other chapters I summarize and put in perspective older, less accessible literature, for example, writings on the upper motor neuron syndrome and vibration sensing. In the discussions of the limbic system and progressive multifocal leukoencephalopathy, I make use of information from interviews which I have undertaken over the years. Previously unpublished data are included, especially in the chapters on the grasp reflex and Wernicke disease.

This book is not typical. It is neither a comprehensive text nor is it a volume focused on a single aspect of neurology. Instead, this collection of writings is presented in the hope of providing some insight into a variety of neurological topics. It orients the clinician to some challenging and confusing areas of neurology. It offers the experienced neurologist discussion of some controversial subjects and some little discussed phenomena. Finally, it provides some historical perspectives not readily available elsewhere.

Acknowledgments

I appreciate the assistance of many colleagues. Dr. Lee H. Monsein provided essential help in finding CT and MRI images of cases, which were "buried" in an old system. He and other neuroradiologists, Louis O. Smith, Anette Virta-Paras, and April Farley, provided and analyzed images. Mark Lin, MD, PhD, devoted many hours to helping me format images for publication.

At the William B. Glew Medical Library, Ms. Jory Barone provided invaluable help organizing references. Also essential in finding literature were Ms. Layla Heimlich, Mr. Fred King, and Ms. Sharon Williams-Martinez.

Mrs. Louella Baterna patiently prepared the manuscript in innumerable versions. Ms. Jennifer Wood helped obtain needed medical literature.

Drs. Louis Smith, Guillaume Lamotte, Alexander T. Lalos, and Gianluca DiMaria helpfully reviewed individual chapters. Special thanks to Dr. William W. Campbell who read the entire manuscript and made helpful corrections and suggestions.

I thank the departed Walsh McDermott, MD, Michael A. Petti, MD, Efraim Racker, MD, and Robert Aronson, PhD, who were kind to a young student.

The Amnesic Syndrome

A neurologist does not forget his first encounter with the amnesic syndrome. The patient is normal in so many ways that a conscientious doctor can be embarrassed by his failure to recognize that a patient has a profound problem. The person is alert, aware, responsive, and fluent. He has lost none of his social graces. He can calculate and reason. He does not complain of memory difficulty. Only if the physician does a simple bedside test of word retention will he recognize that his patient is severely disabled. Although the patient can register information, he cannot recall it minutes or sometimes seconds later. In other words, the patient has lost the ability to learn and remember (anterograde amnesia). Further investigation will then reveal that the patient has to some extent also lost memories for events preceding the onset of the amnesia. When the retrograde amnesia is severe, years of memories can be erased. If there is cognitive abnormality other than amnesia, it is minimal compared to the memory disorder.

By and large the amnesic syndrome is due to damage to one of four brain regions: the medial portions of the temporal lobes, the medial aspects of the thalamus, the fornices, or the basal forebrain. In certain diseases more than one of these regions can be affected. Severe and persistent amnesia usually indicates that there is bilateral disease.

1.1 Inferomedial Temporal Lobe (Hippocampal Region)

In an attempt to treat patients with intractable epilepsy and schizophrenia, Scoville performed bilateral resection of the inferomedial temporal lobes. The surgery left 10 of his patients with an amnesic syndrome. The patients who had developed the amnesic syndrome were among those who had undergone bilateral resection of the hippocampus and parahippocampal gyrus. Those patients, who had undergone hippocampal sparing removal of the amygdala and the uncus, had not developed amnesia. The idea that the hippocampus plays an important role in memory developed from study of these neuro-surgical patients.

The association of the amnesic syndrome with bilateral damage to the hippocampal region has subsequently been confirmed in patients with herpes simplex encephalitis, auto-immune encephalitis and cerebral infarction [1,2]. We have seen the amnesic syndrome result from a global ischemic process affecting the hippocampi (Figure 1.1), One carefully studied amnesic patient had survived for two and a half years after having suffered generalized status epilepticus. At autopsy the anoxic injury severely affected the hippocampi but largely spared the rest of the temporal lobes [3]. This and similar cases demonstrate that lesions, which are restricted to the hippocampi proper, suffice to cause the amnesic syndrome.

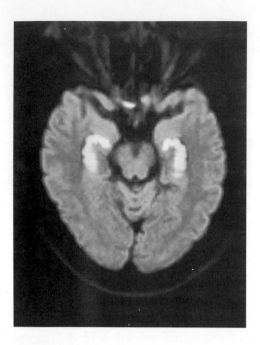

Figure 1.1 Bilateral hippocampal infarction after a hypoxic ischemic event. (Diffusion weighted MRI)

Study of transient global amnesia (TGA) provides additional information about the relationship of the hippocampus to memory function. Many patients during or after TGA show restricted diffusion in the hippocampus on magnetic resonance imaging. The typically punctate abnormality may be on either the right or the left. It occurs most often in the CA1 region of the hippocampus. Although TGA is a diagnosis made clinically, the presence of the imaging abnormality may support the diagnosis when the history is not clear [4,5,6]. The pathophysiology of TGA is unknown. Nevertheless, the location of the imaging finding provides further evidence that a hippocampal disorder can interfere with memory function.

Degenerative brain diseases, which eventually cause global cognitive impairment, can begin with a relatively isolated loss of memory. In such cases the amnesic syndrome can last for years before other cognitive problems, personality change, and aphasia emerge. Although imaging in such cases eventually shows prominent medial temporal lobe atrophy, the scans can be unimpressive early in the course of the disease, when amnesia is already prominent (Figure 1.2).

The evidence amassed from these varied conditions shows that the hippocampus is a critical region for memory function.

1.2 Medial Thalamus

Victor and colleagues studied brains of patients with Wernicke disease [7]. Those whose clinical manifestations had included amnesia (Korsakoff psychosis) always had bilaterally symmetric medial thalamic lesions, mainly in the dorsomedial nucleus. In some patients a single artery supplies the medial thalamus bilaterally. Embolism to or occlusive disease of that vessel can cause bilateral thalamic infarctions with a persistent amnesic syndrome (Figure 1.3).

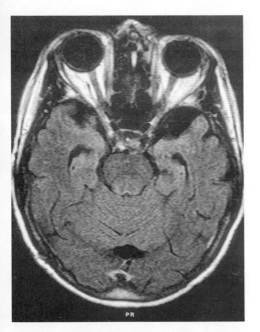

Figure 1.2 Brain MRI of a patient who had isolated amnesia as a manifestation of bitemporal atrophy. Over the years she gradually developed profound global dementia and severe generalized cerebral atrophy.

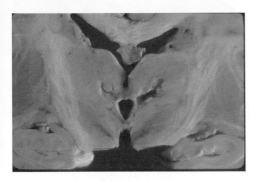

Figure 1.3 Symmetric thalamic infarcts which caused the amnesic syndrome.

This association of medial thalamic lesions with loss of memory in cerebrovascular disease supports the conclusions drawn from study of Wernicke–Korsakoff patients, namely that the medial thalamus is important for memory function.

1.3 Fornix

Because diseases which damage the fornix often affect other parts of the brain, it had long been uncertain whether isolated fornix lesions can cause amnesia. When a tumor affects the fornix, nearby areas are often affected by infiltration and/or edema. Trauma disrupting the fornix ordinarily affects neighboring structures. Infarction of the fornix is often accompanied by infarction of the genu of the corpus callosum. Involvement of the fornix in Wernicke disease is always accompanied by other forebrain lesions. Since nearby structures are involved in these various diseases, one could not know whether fornix damage alone can cause the memory trouble.

However, we now have MRI case reports in which simultaneous infarctions limited to the columns of the fornix have been shown to be the cause of the amnesic syndrome [8]. It is believed that occlusion of a single subcallosal artery, which supplies the right and left columns of the fornix, causes these symmetric infarctions. Although they often lack clinical and/or radiologic detail, accumulating reports of such cases strongly suggest that fornix lesions can severely disrupt one's ability to learn and remember [8].

1.4 Basal Forebrain

Many investigators have recognized that patients with an anterior communicating artery aneurysm can develop an amnesic syndrome as a result of rupture or surgery. The underlying injury is in the basal forebrain [9,10]. This region includes the area of the septal nuclei, the olfactory tubercle, the sub-commissural regions, and parts of the amygdala. Non-aneurysmal cases with a discrete basal forebrain lesion can also leave a patient amnesic (Figure 1.4).

(a)   (b)

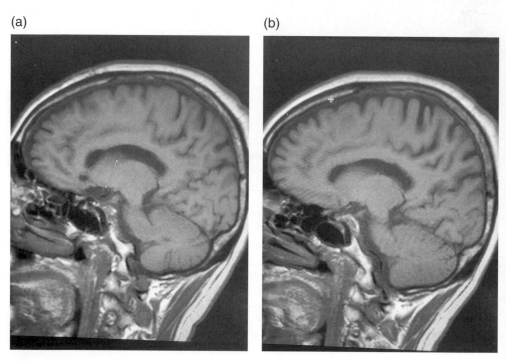

Figure 1.4a Amnesic syndrome due to left basal forebrain damage subsequent to surgery for an anterior communicating artery aneurysm.
Figure 1.4b The paracentral area on the right side is normal.

1.5 Multiple Territories

A permanent amnesic syndrome is typically due to bilateral lesions which are more or less symmetric. There are exceptions:

An 85-year-old physician had suffered a right posterior cerebral artery distribution infarction affecting the medial temporal and occipital lobes. Four years later he developed the amnesic

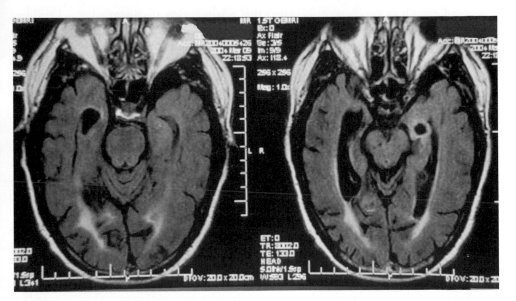

Figure 1.5 Recent left amygdala-anterior hippocampal hemorrhage superimposed on an old right posterior cerebral artery distribution infarction. This combination of lesions caused an incomplete amnesic syndrome.

syndrome when hemorrhage occurred in the area of the left amygdala. On an office visit one month after the hemorrhage he stated: "I hope that I'm not seeing patients." By the time of this visit he was frustrated by his memory trouble: "My memory is shot." His wife explained that, since his hospital discharge, he had been the honored guest at a special lecture attended by many of his former residents and fellows. He had no recollection of this occasion at all.

In this patient the amnesic syndrome resulted from the superimposition of an amygdala/anterior hippocampal hemorrhage on a preexisting, contralateral, inferomedial temporal lobe lesion (Figure 1.5). This case demonstrates that, although the lesions causing lasting amnesia are bilateral, the identical territory need not be affected on each side. Another example would be the emergence of amnesia when a new hippocampal lesion is superimposed on an old contralateral thalamic lesion. When amnesia does occur after sequential damage to differing territories of right and left brain, the cause is not always cerebrovascular disease. In one of Penfield's surgical cases, unilateral removal of the medial temporal lobe resulted in the amnesic syndrome. Autopsy revealed the contralateral lesion, hippocampal sclerosis [11].

1.6 Anatomy and Memory

At first one may be surprised that the amnesic syndrome can result from lesions in so many different regions of the brain. Actually, developmental and evolutionary relationships show that the territories under discussion are closely related. For example, the great arch of the human fornix is less of a puzzle when one looks at a platypus brain. In this mammalian brain (with a relatively smooth cortical surface) the hippocampus is a dorsomedial structure [12]. It gives rise to the fornix, which projects directly ventrally to septal gray, adjacent to which are the thalamus and hypothalamus. In the human embryo one can likewise confirm the proximity of the hippocampus, fornix, thalamus, and basal forebrain. It is only with the expansive growth of neocortex (isocortex) that relationships are distorted. Sulci and gyri develop. The hippocampus is pushed back from the dorsomedial position above the corpus callosum to the inferomedial temporal lobe. The fornix follows as it is similarly forced back and thus elongated. Hence, in higher mammals the fornix has to run a long path forward from the medial temporal lobe to the basal forebrain and diencephalon. Exactly why normal memory function requires these regions to be intact we do not know. However, embryology and comparative anatomy show that these structures are intimately associated.

1.7 Unilateral Lesions

Occasionally, amnesia develops after unilateral damage to an appropriate region, most often the hippocampus or medial thalamus. In such cases there was always the possibility that there were bilateral lesions, that there had been a preexisting lesion contralaterally. In the era of magnetic resonance imaging, however, a preexisting, sizable, contralateral lesion can be excluded. Compared to amnesia caused by bilateral lesions, amnesia following unilateral stroke is likely to be incomplete and is likely to improve over days to months. Some have suggested that unilateral stroke on the left side of the brain is more likely to cause amnesia than is stroke on the right [13].

1.8 The Mammillary Bodies

Lesions of the mammillary bodies commonly occur in Wernicke disease. Early writing about this disease suggested that these conspicuous lesions were the cause of the memory deficit of the Wernicke–Korsakoff syndrome. Careful study of Wernicke disease eventually showed that mammillary body lesions occur in the absence of the amnesic state and that profound memory loss can occur when there are no mammillary body lesions [7]. In that series of patients, the consistent association of Korsakoff psychosis with symmetric medial thalamic lesions indicated that it was bilateral diencephalic damage that caused the amnesia. It is noteworthy that animal experiments provide no convincing evidence that mammillary body lesions cause an amnesic syndrome comparable to that observed in humans. In sum, mamillary body lesions are irrelevant to the amnesic syndrome [14,15].

1.9 Memory and Amnesia

Amnesia is most evident on tests of memory for personal events or memory for facts. The former type of memory is referred to as episodic memory and the latter as factual ("semantic") memory [16]. If one cannot remember that he was the honoree at an annual lecture a month earlier or that his daughter visited him yesterday, the patient is said to have a problem with episodic memory. If a patient cannot remember that Tokyo is in Japan, he has a problem with factual memory. If he remembers Laureno, with whom he has worked for decades but cannot remember that Laureno is a neurologist, the patient also has a problem with factual memory. Since many facts are learned in a biographical context there can be ambiguity as to whether a memory is "episodic" or "factual."

Additional comment on memory for facts is appropriate. Because we usually do not know what facts a patient has learned in the hours, days, or weeks prior to development of amnesia, it is hard to know whether very recently acquired facts have been forgotten. Certainly, factual memory is affected in anterograde amnesia. In severe cases the patient will not remember anything (including facts) which you discussed with him 30 seconds earlier. Much of one's store of facts is "overlearned" information that has been stored for decades. This kind of information seems more resistant to loss in retrograde amnesia.

A remarkable aspect of the fully developed amnesic syndrome is the patient's failure to complain of memory trouble. This lack of insight is striking because the disability is severe. As with other neurologic abnormalities there can be a partial defect. There can be a partial impairment of memory and there can be a partial impairment of insight into the amnesia. (Note the case of the physician presented above.) Insight is less impaired when amnesia is caused by a unilateral lesion than it is when the disease is bilateral. With amnesia due to bilateral lesions, loss of insight is more consistently seen in thalamic than in hippocampal disease

1.10 Terminology

When Korsakoff described the amnesic syndrome, often referred to as Korsakoff psychosis, it was clear that he was describing a syndrome, a clinical constellation, not a manifestation of a specific disease. Thus, from a historic point of view, Korsakoff would be a perfectly appropriate label for the amnesic syndrome regardless of cause. Although Korsakoff wrote that his patients were not all alcoholic, today the eponym carries the connotation of alcoholism and malnutrition for many physicians. Hence, it is best to use the adjective Korsakoff only when the memory disorder is due to Wernicke disease and to use the term amnesic syndrome in other situations. Some have used the alternative term "amnestic syndrome." This usage would be appropriate. However, it should be avoided because the word "amnestic" carries special meaning in the field of immunology. To lessen the chance of confusion and for that reason alone the word "amnesic" is preferable to the alternative adjectives, "amnestic" and "Korsakoff."

References

1. M. Victor, J. B. Angevine, E. L. Mancall et al. Memory loss with lesions of hippocampal formation. Report of a case with some remarks on the anatomical basis of memory. *Arch Neurol* 1961; 5: 244–263.

2. G. Franck, B. Sadzot, E. Salmon et al. [Paraneoplastic limbic encephalopathy, inappropriate ADH secretion and recurrent subclinical epileptic seizures. Clinical, anatomo-pathological and metabolic correlations by positron emission tomography]. [French]. *Revue Neurologique* 1987; 143: 657–669.

3. M. Victor, D. Agamanolis. Amnesia due to lesions confined to the hippocampus: a clinical-pathologic study. *J Cogn Neurosci* 1990; 2: 246–257.

4. H. Y. Lee, J. H. Kim, Y. C. Weon et al. Diffusion-weighted imaging in transient global amnesia exposes the CA1 region of the hippocampus. *Neuroradiology* 2007; 49: 481–487.

5. O. Sedlaczek, J. G. Hirsch, E. Grips et al. Detection of delayed focal MR changes in the lateral hippocampus in transient global amnesia. *Neurology* 2004; 62: 2165–2170.

6. K. Szabo, C. Hoyer, L. R. Caplan et al. Diffusion-weighted MRI in transient global amnesia and its diagnostic implications. *Neurology* 2020; 95: e206–212.

7. M. Victor, R. D. Adams, G. H. Collins. *The Wernicke-Korsakoff Syndrome and Related Neurologic Disorders Due to Alcoholism and Malnutrition*. Philadelphia, F.A. Davis Co., 1989.

8. Q. Y. Zhu, H. C. Zhu, C. R. Song. Acute amnesia associated with damaged fiber tracts following anterior fornix infarction. *Neurology* 2018; 90: 706–707.

9. S. Phillips, V. Sangalang, G. Sterns. Basal forebrain infarction. A clinicopathologic correlation. *Arch Neurol* 1987; 44: 1134–1138.

10. M. K. Morris, D. Bowers, A. Chatterjee A et al. Amnesia following a discrete basal forebrain lesion. *Brain* 1992; **115**: 1827–1847.

11. P. Gloor. *The Temporal Lobe and Limbic System*. New York, Oxford University Press, 1997.

12. L. H. Hyman. *Comparative Vertebrate Anatomy*. Chicago, The University of Chicago Press, 1942.

13. B. R. Ott, J. L. Saver. Unilateral amnesic stroke. Six new cases and a review of the literature. *Stroke* 1993; **24**: 1033–1042.

14. M. Victor. The amnesic syndrome and its anatomical basis. *Can Med Assoc J* 1969; **100**: 1115–1125.

15. M. Victor. The irrelevance of mammillary body lesions in the causation of the Korsakoff amnesic state. *Int J Neurol* 1987; **21–22**: 51–57.

16. M. Mesulam. *Principles of Behavioral and Cognitive Neurology*. Oxford, Oxford University Press, 2000.

Aphasia, Apraxia, and Agnosia

Early in his career the neurologist has the impression that the terms aphasia, apraxia, and agnosia denote totally different phenomena. It is true that separate authors put forth these words, each intended to indicate a group of disorders with a common theme. The term aphasia was utilized by Armand Trousseau for disorders of language comprehension and/ or language expression. The term apraxia was used by Hugo Liepmann to denote the inability to perform certain purposeful movements when mental, sensory, motor, and coordinative functions are intact. It was Sigmund Freud who applied the term agnosia to disorders of recognition which cannot be attributed to a loss of primary sensation. Although one often separates these three categories of disorder for the sake of exposition, aphasia, apraxia, and agnosia are not always distinct. A given phenomenon may be appropriately described by more than one of these terms. The following discussion emphasizes the relationships of these terms and of the neurologic problems to which these terms are applied.

2.1 Aphasia

Distinctions between aphasias have served two purposes. First of all, they have assisted clinicians in localizing lesions. Secondly, clinico-pathologic patterns of aphasia have stimulated thought about the cerebral mechanism of language.

In the West, aphasia classifications have centered on the dichotomy, which has been variously termed Broca/Wernicke, motor/sensory, expressive/receptive, nonfluent/fluent, or simply anterior/posterior. For a century this dichotomy helped doctors determine the sites of strokes and tumors. However, we have gradually learned that language localization is a complex subject. Investigators have abandoned the idea that there is a consistently located Wernicke area or Broca area [1, 2]. Aphasia can occur with lesions of the left or right hemisphere. It can occur with lesions of the thalamus or striatum. Thus, for purposes of localization of a disease, MRI scanning has supplanted distinctions between aphasic syndromes.

In addition to its clinical use for localization, study of aphasias has stimulated thought about the cerebral mechanism of language. Knowledge of aphasia syndromes and their associated lesions, however, does not provide a clear or simple explanation for the working of language in the brain. The clinical features of an aphasia demonstrate the residual capacities of the damaged brain but do not reveal the normal language mechanism. As John Hughlings Jackson explained, it is more difficult to localize functions than it is to localize lesions.

2.2 Apraxia

When a neurological patient would misuse an object, such as holding a fork by the prongs, the anomalous behavior became known as apraxia. Before the writings of Liepmann it was believed that patients made mistakes of this type because they did not recognize objects. In other words, agnosia was assumed to be the basis of apraxia.

Hugo Liepmann approached apraxia differently. He analyzed it as a problem with higher control of movement, not a problem of recognition. Liepmann's approach to the word apraxia has been the basis of all subsequent definitions. He used the term only for a patient who "cannot properly perform a movement which he is verbally ordered to do, or which is appropriate for the circumstances" when he has sufficient sensorimotor and mental function to do so. He applied the word to loss of purposeful movements, which had been learned through "experience, example or instruction." [3]

Modern writers about apraxia offer variations on the definition. Some refer to apraxia as a deficiency in purposeful movement, others in learned movement and others in learned skilled movement. All exclude disorders of fundamentally innate movement like crawling. Although a child develops coordinated crawling through experience (repetitive attempts), the ability to crawl, once there is adequate myelination, is inborn.

Since the time of Liepmann the term apraxia has been strongly associated with bilateral impairment of skilled, purposeful movement of the upper limbs and with lesions of the left hemisphere. However, we now know that a right hemisphere lesion can cause apraxia [4].

Classifications of apraxia are more varied than those of aphasia. Liepmann classified apraxia into three types: ideational (trouble with the concept of movement), ideomotor (difficulty accomplishing an intended movement which one has clearly in mind), and limb kinetic (poor performance of the movement rather than failed performance). Not only does Heilman accept Liepmann's categories but also he adds types, which he terms dissociation, conduction, and conceptual apraxias [5]. Brain, on the other hand, challenges Liepmann's categories, doubting that limb kinetic apraxia is truly apraxia and arguing that one cannot distinguish ideomotor and ideational apraxias [6]. Goldenberg agrees that there is no clear way to distinguish Liepmann's categories. He classifies most apraxias by observed clinical deficits not by psychological concepts. His three types are apraxia for communicative gestures, apraxia for tool use, and apraxia for imitating gestures [7].

Restricting the use of the term apraxia to Goldenberg's three categories would leave us in need for words to refer to dressing apraxia, constructional apraxia, gaze apraxia, eye opening apraxia, truncal apraxia, and gait apraxia. Certainly, experts on dementia do apply the word apraxia to these diverse phenomena [8].

If one uses the term apraxia in this wider sense, one encounters fascinating combinations of disability and ability. I remember a patient who could not figure out how to take his pants off (dressing apraxia). He was able, however, to use scissors to cut them off (no tool use apraxia).

The literature on apraxia is replete with discussion of putative circuits to explain psychological concepts. However, it is very much in need of more case documentation with careful clinico-radiologic study. Even when the word apraxia is used in the limited sense of manual apraxia, Goldenberg states that "apraxia is not a unitary disorder" and that "there is no single locus of the brain responsible for all manifestations of apraxia" [7].

2.3 Agnosia

Agnosia is a failure in recognition, which cannot be attributed to an impairment of primary sensation, alertness, cognitive function, or language. Most authors classify agnosia by the sensory modality via which the recognition problem is manifest. Thus, there are visual agnosias, auditory agnosias, and tactile agnosias. The are many varieties. The deficit in visual agnosia, for example, may be for recognition of objects, faces, colors, and/or the meaning of a complex scene.

Often regarded as an agnosia is a hemiplegic's failure to recognize his own paralyzed arm and hand and/or his inability to recognize that his limbs are paralyzed [9]. Frequently, after an acute right hemisphere infarction, the disorder will evolve. At first the patient will not recognize his own hand; later he will recognize his hand but will not recognize that it is paralyzed; and later he will recognize the paralysis but not its importance. Denny-Brown and colleagues have suggested that this striking disorder is not a problem of higher recognition function (agnosia) but that it is simply the result of one having lost all primary sensory input from the affected side of the body, a problem of severely impaired somesthesis [10].

Whether failing to recognize one's own body part should be regarded as an agnosia is part of a more general issue. Bender believes that there is no such a thing as visual agnosia absent a deficit in primary sensation [11]. Brain explained that agnosia is strictly a term which is useful to the observing physician. "If, . . . we analyze the process of recognition it becomes clear that though the term agnosia is of practical convenience in clinical neurology it does not correspond in psychophysiological terms to the loss of any functions which can be clearly isolated and defined" [6]. Thus, when an infarction, such as the one shown in Figure 2.1 causes homonymous hemianopsia, prosopagnosia, and other types of visual agnosia, Bender would say that the loss of visual field, decreased visual acuity (20/200 OD, 20/80 OS) and the mild memory abnormality should exclude this case from being regarded as a higher disorder of recognition separate from the combined effects of impaired vision and cognition.

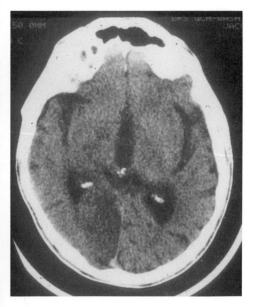

Figure 2.1 Right posterior cerebral artery distribution infarction in a 75-year-old law professor. He could recognize his wife by her clothing not her face. He could recognize his doctor by his voice but not by face. By sight he could name a paper clip or a key. He could identify scissors or staples by touch but not by sight.

2.4 Summary

Aphasia, agnosia, and apraxia are the terms we use to denote the loss of synthetic function of the parietal lobes. The parietal cortex is bordered by areas related to vision, hearing, and tactile/kinesthetic sensation, and the parietal lobe allows association of information related to these different senses. This integration allows us to recognize the meanings of spoken or written words. It enables us to recognize a shirt, how to put it on and button it. It helps us recognize familiar footsteps and associate them with a name. With this higher integrative ability, we can recognize the face of a person and greet him by name. These many abilities can be impaired in various combinations. At times more than one of our three terms is applicable.

There is complexity in the relationship of apraxia and agnosia and of their relationship to aphasia. Distinguishing apraxia and agnosia are problematic for several reasons. First of all, Liepmann pointed out that apraxia and agnosia often occur together. Secondly, as mentioned above, some have attributed apraxia for the use of a tool to failure to recognize the tool, that is an agnosia, as opposed to Liepmann, who attributed apraxia to a loss of a higher cortical engram for skilled movement. Uncertainty about these concepts has led some to use the term apractagnosia. Dressing apraxia, for example, could be viewed as a lack of recognition of the parts of a garment and/or the parts of one's body and the relationship of the garment to the body. However, not all forms of apraxia can be attributed to agnosia.

The phenomena of aphasia can be viewed as apraxia and agnosia. It is appropriate to consider some of the speech difficulty in Broca aphasia and other motor aphasias as an apraxia for speech. The difficulties in language comprehension in posterior aphasias, on the other hand, are agnosias for the symbols which we call words. Nielsen sums this subject up: "Aphasia includes all agnosias and apraxias which have to do with language." [12]

In sum apraxia, agnosia, and aphasia are clinical terms. Each term is applied to a variety of neurologic disorders. In a given case more than one of the terms could be appropriate to describe the clinical deficit. The conditions to which these words are applied, have no uniform patho-anatomic basis.

References

1. J. R. Binder. The Wernicke area: modern evidence and a reinterpretation. *Neurology* 2015; **85**: 2170–2175.

2. N. F. Dronkers, O. Plaisant, M. T. Iba-Zizen et al. Paul Broca's historic cases: high resolution MR imaging of the brains of Leborgne and Lelong. *Brain* 2007; **130**: 1432–1441.

3. J. W. Brown, ed. *Agnosia and Apraxia: Selected Papers of Liepmann, Lange, and Pötzl*. Hillsdale, L. Erlbaum Associates, 1988.

4. R. B. Mani, D. N. Levine. Crossed buccofacial apraxia. *Arch Neurol* 1988; **45**: 581–584.

5. K. M. Heilman. Apraxia. *Continuum (Minneapolis, Minn)* 2010; **16**: 86–98.

6. R. Brain. *Speech Disorders: Aphasia, Apraxia, and Agnosia*. London, Butterworth, 1961.

7. G. Goldenberg. Apraxia. *Handb Clin Neurol* 2008; **88**: 323–338.

8. J. Cummings, D. F. Benson. *Dementia: A Clinical Approach*. Boston, Butterworth-Heinemann, 1992.

9. J. C. Adair, D. L. Na, R. L. Schwartz et al. Anosognosia for hemiplegia: test of the personal neglect hypothesis. *Neurology* 1995; **45**: 2195–2199.

10. D. Denny-Brown, B. Q. Banker. Amorphosynthesis from left parietal lesion. *AMA Arch Neurol Psychiatry* 1954; **71**: 302–313.

11. M. Bender, M. Feldman. The so-called "Visual Agnosias." *Brain* 1972; **95**: 173–186.

12. J. M. Nielsen. *A Textbook of Clinical Neurology*. New York, Hoeber, 1951.

Spurious Symptoms and Behaviors

Frequently neurologists encounter quasi-neurological problems. These spurious "disorders" are products of the mind or emotions. (Spurious is a nonpejorative term defined as "superficially resembling or simulating something but lacking its genuine character or qualities" [1].) It is the neurologist's responsibility to determine whether a given syndrome is directly due to disease of the nervous system or whether it is a spurious condition for which there is no material basis. I have chosen the word "spurious" to avoid the conceptual and terminological difficulties that can be associated with many more commonly used terms. (See Section 3.8.)

3.1 Neurologic Diagnosis

Use of the systematic neurological method is perhaps more important in recognizing spurious disease than it is in diagnosing genuine disease. Through collection of historical information and by careful observation of a patient the neurologist must demonstrate a "discrepancy between symptoms and the anatomical and physiological arrangements in the body" [2].

3.1.1 History

History taking is particularly useful when observations by friends or relatives show that the neurologic problem is grossly inconsistent. For example, a family member may report that the patient has been unable to move his legs for two weeks, but she has twice seen him walk naturally to the lavatory during this time of paralysis. Such an observation may support the diagnosis of spurious paraplegia.

The patient will not necessarily volunteer that there are legal proceedings related to his symptoms. Well into the course of an empathic evaluation Maurice Victor would say, "So tell me about the accident . . . is it pretty much behind you?" In response the patient would often spill out details about his lawsuit or application for disability benefits. This information can be illuminating.

Of course, a complete history includes tracking down old medical records and speaking to prior doctors, relatives, friends, and coworkers. Finding that a patient has had spurious symptoms in the past may shed light on current symptoms.

3.1.2 Exam

Although history can be helpful, the diagnosis of neurological symptoms as nonneurologic depends on the neurologic examination disclosing "normally preserved functional capacities" in a person with "superficial appearance of incapacity" [3]. It is important to do repeat examinations to avoid precipitously drawing wrong conclusions. If necessary, the repeat exam may be done under special conditions like sedation.

Spurious findings may be so florid that a single exam is diagnostic. If a patient in his bed is unable to plantar flex his foot but a moment later can walk on his toes, there is no possible neurophysiologic explanation for the inconsistency. If a patient cannot adduct a leg but can forcefully adduct both legs when asked to press the legs together, there can be no physiologic explanation for the weakness.

If a patient, eyes closed, is asked to tell the examiner whether he feels a pin stick or not and then repeatedly says "No" when the "anesthetic" area is pricked, there can be no neurologic explanation. Also unphysiological is a circumferentially demarcated area of distal anesthesia on a forearm or a leg. If, on position sense testing, the patient consistently gives the wrong answer (up for down and down for up) it is clear that the problem is not one of neuropathology.

Near miss answers can be suggestive. I once asked an educated, nonaphasic woman to remember three items: "Dr. Laureno, house, 3pm." Her answers: "Captain Lero, hoose, 3pm." Another patient I asked to remember: "Dr. Victor, Saturday, 8 o'clock." Her answers: "Dr. Vincent, Monday, 10 o'clock." Such answers, which mimic the pattern of the test words, are unlikely to be due to brain disease.

Inter-examination inconsistencies that cannot be readily explained by evolving or fluctuating nervous system disease may point to a spurious condition. Variation from one exam to another is sometimes the natural history of the disease. In Guillain–Barré syndrome, for example, the exam can vary from one visit to the next. Thus, one must not rush to the diagnosis of spurious disease. Only the most gross inconsistency should be weighed heavily.

The neuro-ophthalmic examination provides many opportunities to demonstrate that symptoms violate principles of anatomy and physiology [4]. One can sequentially check the visual field of the right eye, left eye, right eye, left eye, etc. When the visual field of one eye or the other changes from moment to moment, it is clear that the problem is not a simple impairment of vision. A blind person with intact kinesthetic sense can, on command, look at his left hand or touch his two index fingertips together or sign his name on a paper. When a patient cannot do these things, the problem is not blindness. If visual acuity is measured at 20 feet from the chart and then the patient is moved 10 feet closer, he should be able to read a smaller line of letters. If he continues to be able to read only the same line that he read at 20 feet, the result is spurious. When one eye has a normal confrontation visual field and the other hemianopsia, persistence of hemianopsia when both eyes are open is spurious. (The eye with the full field should largely compensate for the monocular field defect of the other eye.) When the visual field is constricted, doubling the distance between the examiner and the patient should result in an increased visual angle and an expansion of the field. If there is no enlargement, the deficit is not biological. These are only a few of the many ways ophthalmologists can show that a complaint is spurious. Analogous to these neuro-ophthalmic tests, there are methods used to reveal spurious disease in movement disorders, gait disorders, etc.

Surveillance may reveal inconsistency. A person claiming an unsteady gait may walk perfectly well after she leaves the doctor's office. Keen, Mitchell, and Morehouse established a "system of espionage" during the American Civil War [5]. They arranged for nonmedical personnel to spy on "disabled" soldiers whom they suspected of faking. In the modern hospital environment, one can enlist the aid of nurses and physical therapists who may report and even document by video patient behaviors inconsistent with the abnormalities found by the neurologist.

Sedation can facilitate evaluation. If anything, it will worsen most deficits due to neurologic disease. The spurious nature of a hemiparesis, for example, can be confirmed if the patient, with encouragement during sedation (e.g., sodium amytal), is able to move the paretic limb(s) well [6]. S. Weir Mitchell and colleagues relied heavily on this method during the American Civil War. In that prebarbiturate era, he used ether to prove complaints of blindness, deafness, paralysis, etc. as spurious. Others have successfully administered opium, alcohol, or benzodiazepines to sedate patients for examination.

Causing a patient pain or putting him in danger can reveal functional capacity not demonstrated under standard examination circumstances:

> There is also the story, among many others, of the Weir Mitchell room in the Providence Hospital in Washington. In this room lay a paralyzed lady patient, the diagnosis of whose case had puzzled Washington and Baltimore physicians. Dr. Mitchell was sent for. A careful examination was made by him during the consultation. When he had finished Dr. Mitchell asked the other doctors to step out in the hall a minute. Dr. Mitchell soon joined them. "Will she ever be able to walk?" asked one of the doctors. "Yes, in a moment," said Dr. Mitchell. Then the door of the room flew open and the paralyzed patient in her night gown rushed out and down the hall. Smoke exuded from the room. "What on earth is the matter?" asked someone. "I set the bedclothes on fire," said Dr. Mitchell. After this incident the room was named the Weir Mitchell room [7].

Imaginative doctors have used many methods for causing a patient pain to help in diagnosis and therapy (see Section 3.5). A century ago, however, such methods were already being condemned as cruel, inhuman, and not permissible [8]. Because contemporary sensibilities are compatible with this view, it is best to rely on neurologic analysis for diagnosis without resorting to punitive measures.

Electrophysiologic study is an extension of the neurologic exam, which can solidify the diagnosis of spurious disorder. Continuous electroencephalographic and video recording can document that a spell of unresponsiveness and generalized shaking is not electrocerebral in origin. Electromyographic recording of continuous motor unit potentials from the tibialis posterior can raise the possibility that a "disabling" fixed inversion of the foot is due to active contraction rather than contracture; in contracture there would be electrical silence [4].

Doctors are on more solid ground when they have the opportunity to observe patients over time. Evaluating a patient after some time has elapsed is a great advantage. If a patient with isolated pure mutism but no abnormality on brain MRI or EEG recovers fully over weeks or months, it becomes obvious that the disorder was spurious. Caution in diagnosis is particularly necessary when one evaluates an isolated symptom on a single occasion. Experienced movement disorders specialists can find it challenging to determine on a single exam whether isolated tremor or dystonia is spurious. When there is doubt, neurologists should state their uncertainty and withhold judgment.

Having concluded that neurologic symptoms are spurious, the doctor can document an analysis in the medical report. Harold Stevens would often write, "There is no evidence of disease of the central nervous system or peripheral nervous system."[1] Jones and Llewellyn

---

[1] Personal communication, c. 1979.

favored the expression, "The troubles complained of do not correspond with the objective facts" [8].

3.2 Neurologic Misdiagnosis

When doctors perform incomplete examinations or lack knowledge, they are more likely to misdiagnose a complaint as spurious. The doctor may document 20/20 vision, normal fundi, pupils, and extraocular movements in an overdramatic patient who reports "blurred" vision. However, diagnosing his problem as spurious without examining the visual fields is careless. A doctor may correctly recognize that a psychiatric patient thrashing about in bed is not having a seizure or a movement disorder. However, one must consider the possibility that the patient is delirious before concluding that he is seeing spurious movements.

There is always a risk that doctors will misdiagnose disorders as spurious when they describe conditions as "bizarre." This is a poor basis for concluding that signs or symptoms are spurious. In fact, when the word "bizarre" comes to mind, the neurologist must stop and take a fresh look at the case. If one cannot better articulate why the problem is spurious than to label it "bizarre," one must reassess. One may view a phenomenon as bizarre simply because it is unfamiliar. Apraxia of eye opening is an example. Unfamiliar is not unphysiological. Caution is the master word. Less than 50 years ago some neurologists would diagnose torticollis, writer's cramp, acute dystonic reaction, or essential blepharospasm as psychogenic. Today, although there is no known structural basis for these conditions, they are universally recognized as forms of dystonia. No doubt the development of effective non-psychiatric therapies has helped shift mainstream attitudes on these disorders.

Abnormalities on the neurological exam are not usually specific for spurious disorder. Although give away weakness can be seen in spurious weakness, it can also be seen in amyotrophic lateral sclerosis, Guillain–Barré syndrome, and fatigue. Likewise, inconsistency does not necessarily indicate a spurious problem. For example, one may have a positive straight leg raising test which seems to disappear when the patient is seated. This "inconsistency" may only be apparent; the explanation may simply be that, when seated, the patient may be leaning back a bit to decrease the stretch on the sciatic nerve. Strange patterns of sensory loss are not always spurious. Morris Bender saw a patient with vibration sense absent at the elbow but retained at the distal ulna; there was definitely an organic cerebral lesion as the cause.[2]

When the history reveals that the neurologic problem appeared in the setting of an emotionally charged situation, one must be cautious about connecting the symptom to the context. Special circumstances of ambivalence or stress (e.g., therapeutic abortion, delivery of a baby, tubal ligation, or certain sexual encounters) are sometimes related to the symptoms but often they are not. Thus, one should not use onset situations as a major strut for diagnosis [9].

Stress-triggered symptoms are not necessarily simple symptom reactions. In some patients, the physiologic response to interpersonal stress can trigger epileptic seizures. I evaluated one patient, a Las Vegas gambler, whose face twitched whenever he had a good poker hand. His problem was early hemifacial spasm, which was accentuated by

---

[2] Personal communication, c. 1977.

his excitement. What hormonal or other physiological mechanism is responsible for such effects is worthy of investigation.

Furthermore, improvement with suggestion does not necessarily mean that a problem is purely spurious. I recall a patient with a wild reeling gait who improved partially when encouragement was offered. The abnormal gait, it turned out, had been due partly to ataxia of phenytoin intoxication and partly to exaggeration of it.

The physician can be misled by the analysis or description of a symptom offered by a patient or family. A patient may report "triple vision" when he the problem is simply mild unilateral sixth nerve palsy. A schizophrenic patient with early spinal cord compression may report that "my legs can't walk" due to static from the television. A family may emphasize that the patient has always had trouble walking rather than that it has worsened recently, as it may have when a superimposed problem has developed. In sum, input from the patient or family cannot be given so much weight as to interfere with careful neurologic evaluation.

We, in the twenty-first century, have advantages which great nineteenth-century diagnosticians did not. Modern diagnostic tests can help us to avoid mistakenly labeling a condition as spurious. An abnormal EEG can help the neurologist recognize the neurologic basis of an unusual cognitive or psychiatric symptom. One may suspect that a complaint of weakness is spurious but, in this era, the neurologist will recognize the presence of Eaton–Lambert syndrome by using nerve conduction studies [4]. Magnetic resonance imaging is a sensitive test that can demonstrate brain or spinal cord lesions when the physician expects that none will be found. Of course, the physician cannot benefit from such tests unless care is taken to order them or to direct them to the proper part of the neuraxis.

One is inclined to abandon the suspicion that a behavior is spurious when the patient hurts himself. However, a patient can bite his tongue during a nonepileptic episode.[3] I have examined a patient with a spurious gait disorder during resident rounds. Confident of my diagnosis, I allowed the patient to continue without my support. After a few steps, she hurtled into the floor. I was humbled and the residents were horrified. Later in the day, I happened to observe her strolling down a long corridor. My diagnosis had been correct. Her gait had been an act, but she could have easily hurt herself by crashing into the floor.

3.3 Patients with Both Spurious and Genuine Neurologic Disease

When a spurious disorder is superimposed on a true neurologic problem, diagnosis is challenging. A patient who once had transverse myelitis may have a residual Babinski sign. If he presents with spurious paraplegia, the physician, unaware of the prior illness, may have difficulty in dissecting the findings. Furthermore, a patient with an active neurologic disorder can exaggerate or elaborate abnormality. For example, Keane has described a patient with Bell's palsy who manifested an associated "hemiparesis" [10]. The previously mentioned patient with phenytoin intoxication is another example of such elaboration.

When serious neurologic disease alters a person's personality, the patient may secondarily develop a spurious neurologic condition. I have seen spurious episodes of loss of consciousness occur in a woman depressed by Wilson disease. Likewise, I have observed nonepileptic attacks of unresponsiveness, chanting, and hyperventilation in a patient with

---

[3] Cary Suter, personal communication, c. 1980.

glioblastoma. Steroid medication can affect a patient's personality and thinking. Such a patient, for example, can report blindness. On examination, the patient may report inability to see the visual acuity chart. Careful observation may reveal that the patient is not at all blind. The claims of blindness end when the dose of the steroid medication is tapered. In another case, resolution of hypophonia by suggestion/hypnosis showed the problem to be spurious. That the spurious hypophonia was due to personality change from Creutzfeldt–Jakob disease was revealed only when progressive dementia developed [11].

One patient may experience both epileptic seizures and nonepileptic episodes. Occasionally, an epileptic patient may habitually develop spurious seizures that bring the same attention and/or "benefit" as the epileptic ones. Such spurious seizures can erroneously be assumed to be epileptic when the coexisting diagnosis of epilepsy is firm. On the other hand, a clinician may correctly diagnose spurious seizures on first encountering a patient. The doctor may not know that there is also true epilepsy because that history has not been provided and because no neurologist has had the opportunity to witness one of the epileptic fits. In such circumstances one may understandably conclude that all of the patient's episodes are spurious. As a rule, in the case of a patient who has both epileptic and nonepileptic seizures, the two types of episodes are temporally distinct. However, a partial seizure can affect occasional patients in such a way that a secondary nonepileptic seizure will immediately appear [12]. The reverse sequence can also occur. When hyperventilation is a part of a nonepileptic episode, the overbreathing can elicit an absence seizure in a susceptible individual [13].

Mistaking nonepileptic seizures as epileptic can have serious consequences for the patient. Medication administered for suspected "status epilepticus" has caused the death of a patient with nonepileptic "seizures" [14]. Obviously, misdiagnosing epileptic seizures as spurious can also have negative consequences.

3.4 Psychological Classification

Persons who manifest spurious neurologic conditions elude simple classification. However, we can consider four major categories. In one group, depression is the fundamental problem. In other cases, intense emotion, or psychosocial stress, triggers neurological symptoms. In a third group, the patients purposefully produce the symptoms and/or signs for which they come to medical attention. This deception brings them financial gain or other benefit. Finally, some patients do not fit into any of these three groups. They have nothing obvious to gain from their spurious neurologic symptoms. They do not seem to be depressed or emotionally overcome. These patients are for one reason or another inclined to play the role of patient.

Those with clear cut mood disorders comprise the first group of patients with spurious neurologic disorders. It is most important for the neurologist to recognize depression because it can so often be treated successfully. When in doubt about the diagnosis of depression, it is best to begin treatment. The response to therapy may help with diagnosis. (See Section 3.5.)

The second group of patients are those overwhelmed by emotion. Many of these patients are highly anxious and histrionic by nature. Hence, on witnessing a relative lose consciousness the patient may herself fall to the ground with spurious hemiparesis. One of our patients, when her boyfriend found her with another man in flagrante delicto, fell to the floor unresponsive with right arm shaking. Some patients, by imitation, may collapse into a state of unresponsiveness and generalized shaking during an emotional gathering of a religious sect. Ambivalence, such as that experienced by a patient after or during a therapeutic abortion, can result in a nonepileptic seizure.

Category three consists of malingerers. These are patients who try to simulate neurological disease for their own benefit. With a medical diagnosis one may escape the battlefront. Others, following an accident, may be able to retire from an unpleasant job by gaining a formal declaration of disability or a financial award in a civil suit.

To consider a patient a malingerer, one must recognize that there is obvious benefit like obtaining money and/or escaping from a situation. For example, a malingerer can gain transfer from the jail to a hospital. In fact, one can avoid going to jail altogether by malingering. There was once a trespasser who was found wandering in the resident physicians' sleeping quarters. While being questioned by hospital security guards, he slid to the ground and became unresponsive. The security guards brought the man to the emergency room, where the consulting neurologist determined that the episode had not been medically based. The emergency room doctor released the patient from the hospital without calling the security department.

Why do the patients in the fourth group present with spurious symptoms when they have no obvious money, safety, or comfort to gain thereby? The literature is full of speculation. One idea is that such patients interact with the doctor as a form of game [15]. Another idea is that such persons are gratified by the attention they get in the process of being patients. Walshe believed that these patients initially simulate consciously (i.e., as actors) but after a time end up in the audience (believing in their own ailments). This Walshe concept can only be applied to a chronic persistent neurologic problem. Certainly, the Walshe theory cannot explain the psychology of patients who episodically present to emergency rooms with stroke-like manifestations, for which urgent diagnostic tests and treatment with tissue plasminogen activator are provided [16]. Some of these patients have underlying psychiatric conditions.

The four categories of persons with spurious neurological presentations are not mutually exclusive. A depressive can also be a malingerer. An anxious patient under acute stress may have background depression. A patient who does not qualify as a malingerer may with time evolve into one when, after a time, he seeks disability payments. An impostor, having never intended to seek financial gain, may find herself the beneficiary of a fundraising dinner, which others have conceived and promoted.

3.5 Treatment

Having determined that symptoms are very likely spurious, one approach is to reassure the patient that there is no neurologic disease, that some people's bodies respond to stress with somatic symptoms and that he or she will make a fine recovery. At the same time, one invokes the aid of all nursing and physical therapy staff in encouraging the patient to "practice moving his legs." Raymond Adams would tell a patient that she had a "constitutional nervous weakness" that caused her symptoms and would refer her to an empathic internist for long-term management.[4]

---

[4] Personal communication, Raymond Adams, 2006.

A more active approach was advocated by Harold Stevens, who considered spurious neurologic symptoms of acute onset to be a medical emergency. He, concerned that symptoms would congeal and become irreversible, admitted patients to the hospital for intravenous amobarbital hypnosis with suggestion.[5] As noted previously, Weir Mitchell and colleagues used ether for this purpose in the prebarbiturate era. The use of sedation in this way is not in vogue today.

In the past, doctors have been less gentle. Injection of iced water into the external ear has been an important method of testing extraocular movements in comatose patients. The resulting pain can "awaken" a person with spurious coma. In the 1940s, at the University of Utah, crushed ice would be packed into a patient's rectum to awaken him from "coma".[6] At Boston City Hospital, as late as the 1960s, orderlies would inject calcium chloride into muscle; the injection was so painful that it would immediately terminate a spurious convulsion and cause the patient to sit up and curse.[7] The irritation of inhaled anhydrous ammonia can terminate "dystonic" posturing or nonepileptic seizures [17]. Such procedures carry risk for medical personnel; I have seen punches thrown by a "comatose" patient aroused by a doctor's attempt to insert an uncomfortably large-bore nasogastric tube. The "old country surgeon approach" to mobilize such a patient was to pull on the patient's pubic hair. [8]

In the setting of war, there is less tolerance for spurious disorders. Painful electric shock was commonly used during World War I [18]. "As a remedial measure for exaggerators and malingerers, a very strong, faradic current is the most generally useful of all remedies . . . It is almost infallible. The malingerer may stand one or two applications, but he cannot stand the prospect of a daily repetition, and so he quickly gets well. Several strong men are required to hold the patient during the treatment.!!" [19].

Proving that a patient's neurologic complaint is spurious may be sufficient for military and emergency doctors. However, getting the patient suddenly upright and aroused is not a solution for a depressed patient, who needs long-term treatment of the underlying psychiatric problem. When the diagnosis of depression is clear, one should prescribe antidepressant medication in addition to physical therapy. In some patients, modern medications such as selective serotonin reuptake inhibitors (SSRIs) show evident (not maximal) benefit in days. A good response to the medication strengthens the diagnosis. When one suspects or even wonders about the diagnosis of depression, one should also treat.

Perhaps the best approach in the modern litigious era is a compassionate one like that of Maurice-Williams:

> Judging from our experience, the clue to successful treatment, at any rate in the short term, is somehow to convey to the patient that the nature of his behavior is clearly understood. Success is more likely if this can be done with sympathy without any hint of disapprobation. At the same time the patient must be given some excuse for escaping from the situation he has created without humiliation, or loss of face. Such maneuvers as hypnosis, amytal abreaction and injections of sterile saline may serve as reasons, in the patient's eyes, for a "cure" which would otherwise be difficult for him to explain. In some of the cases of short duration, firm and sympathetic reassurance was enough to lead to a rapid recovery. The

---

[5] Personal communication, Harold S. Stevens, c. 1979.
[6] Personal communication, Maurice Victor, 1982.
[7] Personal communication, Steven Shapiro, c. 1980.   [8] Personal communication, Cary Suter, 1980.

usual approach was to tell the patient that his paralysis was due to "nervous shock" and that it would soon clear up [20].

In the context of litigation, symptoms seldom resolve until a verdict or settlement is reached.

3.6 Deception

Deceit helps animal species to survive. Humans deceive by spoken lies and by pretending behaviors. A teenager once described how her brother would fall and pretend to convulse on the floor of a crowded subway train. When passengers jumped to his aid, his sister would be able to find a place to sit down with their schoolbooks.

Charcot knew that people were often deceptive:

In fact, we all know that the desire to deceive, even without concrete benefit, but with a kind of disinterested worship of art for its own sake [*culte de l'art pour l'art*] or admittedly with the idea of provocation to excite pity or another emotion is a common enough occurrence [21].

Nevertheless, Charcot believed some patients were unconscious of their spurious behaviors. He thought these patients had a brain disease that rendered them vulnerable to having manifestations which they did not know to be spurious. Freud abandoned the idea that such patients had brain disease and postulated a psychological mechanism. He believed life events led to mental conflicts that were unconsciously converted to bodily symptoms. Babinski denied both the brain disease and the psychological mechanism. He considered spurious symptoms a phenomenon of suggestible persons who could be cured by persuasion.

The conversion concept of Freud has been so pervasive that doctors focus much of their energy trying to distinguish malingered spurious symptoms (faking) from nonmalingered spurious symptoms (unconscious mechanism, conversion reaction, symptom reaction). This distinction between patients who are lying from those who are not has never been validated. In fact, "nothing resembles malingering more than hysteria, nothing hysteria more than malingering" [7]. As an empirical matter, the liars (malingerers) certainly include those who gain money, comfort, safety, protection of reputation, etc. through their spurious symptoms.

3.7 Conclusion

With the ideas of the doctors so varied and the psychology of patients so diverse, the neurologist should focus on analyzing the symptoms and signs and determining whether they are neurological or spurious. When the patient is depressed, the neurologist should not hesitate to begin treatment. The doctor should explain to the patient that there is no neurologic disease, that some bodies develop such symptoms in the absence of disease and that a full recovery is expected. The possibility of emotional stress, a situational trigger, or depression should be raised. When necessary a psychiatrist can assume responsibility for management, or an internist can provide continuity of care.

3.8 Terminology

I have chosen "spurious" as an umbrella term for neurologic symptoms which are not truly caused by neurological disease. By and large I have avoided the following terms:

Briquet syndrome – A polysymptomatic condition of young women which leads to frequent medical encounters including surgeries. Some of the symptoms can be neurologic but there is no neurologic disease. There is nothing wrong with this concept as operationally defined.

Hysteria – Over millennia this term has been used in many ways. In the latter part of the nineteenth century and much of the twentieth century its use for neurological symptoms implied a subconscious cause. It is often used as an adjective, for example, hysterical seizure. The term has fallen into disfavor because it is considered pejorative.

Conversion – This Freudian term implies that there is a recognizable subconscious psychological mechanism behind the spurious neurological symptom. The term is often used as an adjective, for example, conversion reaction.

Psychogenic – This term implies that there is a psychological (subconscious) mechanism responsible for a symptom. The opposite term "organic" implies that there is a clear neurological disease as the basis of a neurological symptom. This term psychogenic (nonorganic) should not be considered pejorative [22]. However, for many patients it has a negative connotation and therefore interferes with a person accepting a diagnosis [23].

Functional – This term indicates that there is no objective structural or chemical disease of the nervous system as the basis of a spurious symptom, for example, functional paralysis. The problem with the word is that there are many functional disorders which are not spurious. Migraine and essential blepharospasm are examples. Nevertheless, authorities consider the term equivalent to "psychogenic" when used in the appropriate context [24].

Factitious – This term explicitly identifies false intent, that a patient is purposely giving the impression of disease where there is none. For example, repeated episodic loss of consciousness with convulsions can be epileptic but factitious in the sense that the patient has caused the seizures by recurrently taking a convulsive dose of medication like amitriptyline [25]. A nurse patient may present with headache and a fixed, dilated pupil which she has purposefully caused by instilling anticholinergic drops into the eye. Not all factitious disorders are neurological. When factitious symptoms benefit the patient in an evident way they are considered as a form of malingering not a factitious disorder.

Malingerer – This word is not a medical term. It implies that there is no medical problem, that the patient hopes to benefit by pretending to have a medical condition. In Poland during World War I, malingering was taught in special schools to help men avoid military service. Tremors and Babinski signs could be taught but nystagmus could not.[9]

Munchausen syndrome – This label is applied to malingerers and others with feigned conditions who wander from one medical facility to another seeking medical attention.

Munchausen by proxy – In this variant of Munchausen syndrome, an adult takes a child from facility to facility either reporting a neurologic disorder or producing one. I remember a mother who took her child from hospital to hospital for CSF rhinorrhea which she tried to mimic with vinegar. Some people have similarly abused their pets by traveling from one veterinarian to another.

The terms listed above are not mutually exclusive. Hysterical symptoms and conversion reactions are psychogenic by definition. The illness of a Munchausen patient or a malingerer is factitious. A Munchausen patient can be a malingerer but is not necessarily one.

---

[9] Personal communication, Paul Yakovlev, c. 1980.

References

1. *The Shorter Oxford English Dictionary. Volumes 1–2.* Oxford, Oxford University Press, 2002.

2. F. M. R. Walshe. *Diseases of the Nervous System Described for Practitioners and Students.* London, E&S Livingston, 1947.

3. E. Slater. Diagnosis of "hysteria". *Br Med J* 1965; **1**: 1395–1399.

4. M. I. Weintraub, ed. Malingering and conversion reactions. *Neurol Clin* 1995; **13**: 229–450.

5. W. W. Keen, S. W. Mitchell, G. R. Morehouse. On malingering, especially in regard to simulation of disease in the nervous system. *Am J Med Sci* 1864; **48**: 367–394.

6. H. Stevens. Conversion hysteria: a neurologic emergency. *Mayo Clin Proc* 1968; **43**: 54–64.

7. B. R. Tucker. Speaking of Weir Mitchell. *Am J Psychiatry* 1936; **93**: 341–346.

8. A. B. Jones, L. J. Llewellyn. *Malingering or the Simulation of Disease.* Philadelphia, P. Blakiston's Son and Co., 1918.

9. L. Davis. Treachery of the hysterical diagnosis. *West J Med* 1994; **161**: 431.

10. J. R. Keane. Hysterical hemiparesis accompanying Bell's palsy. *Neurology* 1993; **43**: 1619.

11. E. M. Stevens, R. Lament. Psychiatric presentation of Jakob–Creutzfeldt disease. *J Clin Psychiatry* 1979; **40**: 445–446.

12. O. Devinsky, E. Gordon. Epileptic seizures progressing into nonepileptic conversion seizures. *Neurology* 1998; **51**: 1293–1296.

13. B. Vlcek, D. Olson, A. Wilensky et al. Do pseudoseizures beget epileptic seizures? *Neurology* 1987; **37** (suppl 1): 98–99.

14. M. Reuber, G. B. Baker, R. Gill et al. Failure to recognize psychogenic nonepileptic seizures may cause death. *Neurology* 2004; **62**: 834–835.

15. J. Naish. Problems of deception in medical practice. *Lancet* 1979; **2**: 139–142.

16. R. Willenberg, B. Leung, S. Song et al. Munchausen syndrome by tissue plasminogen activator: patients seeking thrombolytic administration. *Neurol Clin Pract* 2021; **11**: 64–68.

17. W. R. LeVine, C. Ramirez. Identifying pseudoseizures with anhydrous ammonia. *Am J Psychiatry* 1980; **137**: 995.

18. L. Tatu, J. Bogousslavsky, T. Moulin et al. The "torpillage" neurologists of World War I: electric therapy to send hysterics back to the front. *Neurology* 2010; **75**: 279–283.

19. J. Collie. *Malingering and Feigned Illness.* London, Edward Arnold, 1917.

20. R. S. Maurice-Williams, H. Marsh. Simulated paraplegia: an occasional problem for the neurosurgeon. *J Neurol Neurosurg Psychiatry* 1985; **48**: 826–831.

21. C. G. Goetz. J.-M. Charcot and simulated neurologic disease: attitudes and diagnostic strategies. *Neurology* 2007; **69**: 103–109.

22. J. D. Sapira. Is "psychogenic" pejorative? *New Engl J Med* 1973; **288**: 1129.

23. J. Nonnekes, E. Ruzicka, T. Serranova et al. Functional gait disorders: a sign-based approach. *Neurology* 2020; **94**: 1093–1099.

24. J. F. Baizabal-Carvallo, M. Hallett, J. Jankovic. Pathogenesis and pathophysiology of functional (psychogenic) movement disorders. *Neurobiol Dis* 2019; **127**: 32–44.

25. S. O'Rahilly, T. H. Turner, J. A. Wass. Factitious epilepsy due to amitriptyline abuse. *Ir Med J* 1985; **78**: 166–167.

Hallucinations

With systematic analysis the clinician can determine the nature of hallucinations. One must note the temporal profile and the complexity of the hallucinations and the sensory modality involved. When these false perceptions are recurrent, stereotypy or lack thereof is important. By attending to these features, the clinical context, and any associated signs and symptoms, the neurologist can usually make a diagnosis. One must consider as possible causes various encephalopathies and cerebral degenerations, focal brain lesions, neurophysiologic disorders, abnormalities of sensory systems, and psychiatric conditions.

4.1 Cerebral Degeneration

Hallucinations may be associated with degenerative disease of the brain. Their prevalence is said to depend on the type of degenerative disease: Alzheimer's disease (11–17%), fronto-temporal dementia (1.2–13%), and Lewy body disease (55–58%) [1]. It is hard to interpret this reported difference in prevalence because these entities are not distinct. The diseases overlap in pathology and clinical manifestations [1]. In addition, the presence of hallucinations predisposes the clinician to diagnose a dementia as being due to Lewy body disease rather than Alzheimer's disease or some other type of dementia.

4.2 Encephalopathies

Hallucinations can occur during encephalopathies due to systemic disorders such as derangements of blood chemistry, the presence or withdrawal of exogenous toxins, effects of medications, septicemia, or fever. Patients experience visual, auditory and/or tactile hallucinations. Olfactory and gustatory hallucinations are seldom recognized in the context of these systemic problems.

In my experience, staphylococcal sepsis is particularly prone to cause hallucinations. I have encountered a patient who saw a pumpkin near his bed, another who saw silent, colorful movies and another who saw normal images of his children and dogs. In these cases, there was no gross pathology detected on MRI scans of the brain.

Acute severe arterial hypertension can cause reversible subcortical/cortical areas of edema, which can be seen on MRI scans. A common site for this phenomenon is the occipital lobe. Central visual loss and visual hallucinations can be manifest until the blood pressure has been lowered. These hallucinations are typically geometric patterns and lights. As a rule, the MRI abnormality clears after the blood pressure has been normalized. However, there can be small areas of residual ischemic change. Occipital ictal hallucinations sometimes occur in these cases.

Visual and auditory hallucinations can occur in acute alcohol withdrawal. Similar withdrawal hallucinations occur on cessation of intake of other depressant substances, especially barbiturates and benzodiazepines. They are typically visual and/or auditory. When a patient is brushing spiders off his legs, it is hard to know whether the hallucinations are purely visual or whether they are tactile as well. Olfactory hallucinations are the least common type of withdrawal hallucination. The visual hallucinations can be natural looking or distorted and frightening. In the florid form of alcohol withdrawal there is profound confusion and autonomic hyperactivity. In this state, delirium tremens, the hallucinations are particularly vivid. The relationship to withdrawal was not always obvious. An excellent observer like Mark Twain portrayed alcohol intoxication as the cause of hallucinations in Huckleberry Finn. Only after systematic study did the medical community as a whole recognize alcohol withdrawal to be the cause.

Usually, hallucinations in abstinence states are a transient phenomenon. Acute auditory hallucinosis is a distinctive form of withdrawal hallucination in the alcoholic. Despite the presence of a clear sensorium, the patient perceives of the hallucinated voices as real. (See Section 4.3.)

4.3 Medications

Medications used to treat Parkinson's disease can be hallucinogenic. L-dopa hallucinations are dose related. The wife of one of my patients found him punching an invisible intruder on the bedroom floor. When she tried to pull him up, he pushed her away saying, "I'm winning … I'm winning." Dopaminergic drugs likewise cause hallucinations. Amantadine is another cause. One patient saw boys riding bicycles through her house. Another saw people who were not present and also heard people at her door when nobody was there. Trihexyphenidyl and benztropine and other anticholinergic drugs can also cause hallucinations. Fisher published a wonderfully detailed description of a patient's experience while taking the antimuscarinic drug atropine [2].

Many other medications can cause encephalopathy with hallucinations. Ciprofloxacin and other fluoroquinolone antibiotics can cause encephalopathy with visual hallucinations. Other anti-infective agents including penicillin, cephalosporins, and acyclovir can also cause hallucinations. Although vincristine is best known for its toxicity to the peripheral nervous system, it occasionally causes formed or unformed visual hallucinations. Codeine and other narcotics may be responsible for hallucinations. Codeine caused one of my patients to see a gray mouse silently scamper on her desk. Tricyclic antidepressants can cause dose related hallucinations with or without an associated confusional state. Amitriptyline, for example, caused one of my patients to see a distorted face emerge from her desk. Anti-inflammatory medications can surprise a patient with hallucinations. One patient, who had recently started taking prednisolone for Bell's palsy, fleetingly saw a Native American, black hair in a headband. He was seated on her bedroom floor, where he was cutting the hair of a child who was on his lap. Indomethacin and salicylates can also cause hallucinations.

Hallucinogenic cardiovascular medications include beta adrenergic blockers, disopyramide, ephedrine, calcium channel blockers, and ACE inhibitors. While receiving an infusion of Abciximab, a clear-minded man saw horses in the room and recognized them as hallucinations. Clonidine, as another example, caused a patient to see hands reaching out for her from her closet [3]. Lidocaine in one instance, caused four hours of visual hallucinations in an alert physician who described them to his doctors. His neurologist made detailed notes:

> The visual hallucinations consisted of four main topics: books and other printed material, street scenes, snowy landscapes, and animals of many kinds. The images followed one another in quick succession, "nonstop with no rhyme or reason," each one lasting 2 or 3 seconds. When he opened his eyes, the visions disappeared. Although he was wide awake and apparently clear mentally, it was for some reason difficult to keep his eyes open. "It was as if they were being forced shut." He was not frightened or alarmed but was restless and unduly excited; he attributed this to a feeling of being out of control and helpless. The images were colored and projected into the center of space before him, without lateralization. They were silent, and figures showed no facial movements to suggest that they were speaking. The individual hallucinations were entirely unrelated to one another, with no recognizable narrative connection. It was broad daylight, and the room was brightly lit.
>
> The printed matter consisted of books and pages; in addition, handwritten material was present. The colored street scenes were not recognized as being in any particular city; many people about 1 m tall were rushing across the street from side to side at great speed, dashing hither and thither, creating a bewildering confusion. The streets were lined with buildings on each side. The people seemed to be further away than the surroundings, creating the appearance of miniaturization. There were no autos. The snow scenes stretched for miles over low hills. As the hospitalization was in the wintertime, when there was snow, this may have been a determining factor; but a snow scene could quickly be followed by one without snow. There were no trees. The animals were deformed and repugnant; for example, there were ugly, one-eyed Picasso-like monsters, or, grotesque, nongeometrical shapes that were everchanging. The animals were stationary, as in a picture. There were no recognizable normal animals, such as dogs, cats, horses, or rodents. The coloring was mostly of watercolors and pastels, except for white, which was quite bright, and orange, which was vivid [4].

4.4 Ictal Hallucinations and Migraine

Penfield and colleagues have documented that seizures can cause episodic hallucinations [5]. When these hallucinations are accompanied by other obvious manifestations of seizure, the diagnosis is less difficult than when they are an isolated symptom. The classic ictal hallucinations are olfactory but auditory, visual, somatic, and visceral hallucinations can be epileptic. Gustatory hallucinations and vestibular hallucinations (ictal vertigo) in the absence of other seizure features must be quite rare [6]. The key to the diagnosis of ictal hallucinations is that they are episodic and stereotyped.

Ictal olfactory hallucinations tend to be simple and unpleasant. Smelling something burning is a typical manifestation. The odor can be so real that a patient traveling on a train may seek out the conductor to report that someone has been smoking in the lavatory.

Ictal auditory hallucinations are often complex. One patient may hear simple tunes, another orchestral music. The music can be familiar or unfamiliar, instrumental, or vocal. Typically, but not always, ictal auditory hallucinations are stereotyped, that is, the same music heard on each occasion.

Visual hallucinations can be ictal. Usually they are elementary, flashing lights, or black and white patterns. They can occur in a homonymous field distribution, or they can

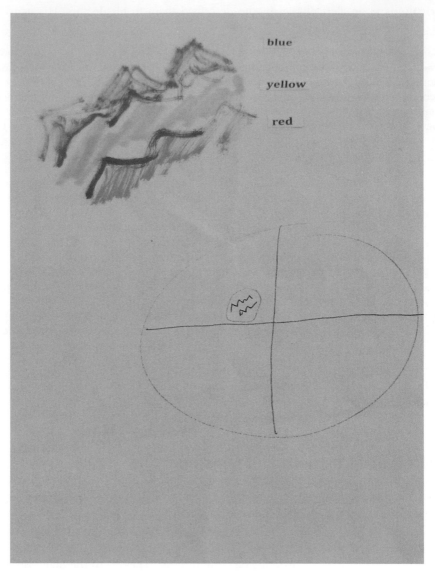

Figure 4.1 Patient's drawings of his homonymous epileptic hallucination of a flashing light. The patient's drawings indicate the light's coloration and its location in the visual field.

involve the entire field of vision. Less often, visual seizures can take the form of people, numerals, or other images. The flashing lights of occipital seizures are typically multicolored and rounded. They terminate abruptly (Figure 4.1).

In migraine, on the other hand, one typically perceives the flickering light as a zigzag line which enlarges over minutes ("fortification") pattern [7]. The migrainous hallucination evolves in a characteristic manner and it ends more gradually than an ictal event. Typically white, it can be multicolored. Although the patterns are stereotyped in temporal profile and general character, they are not identical on each occurrence.

4.5 "Peduncular" Hallucinosis

Lesions affecting the midbrain and thalamus can cause hallucinations. Intrinsic disease or external compression may be responsible. The hallucinations are usually formed, complex, nonstereotyped, and colorful. They are often in motion. Although the patient recognizes that the hallucinations are unreal, he is not disturbed by them. In fact, they may be so untroubling that the patient may not mention them. He may enjoy watching floral arrays or dancing cartoon-like figures.

Unfortunately, the term peduncular hallucinosis has been applied to this phenomenon. It is true that the disordered brain is near the cerebral peduncles, but the peduncles are irrelevant. The cause is deep to the peduncles. The most carefully studied clinicopathologic case showed bilateral infarction of the medial portions of the substantia nigra to be the cause of these hallucinations [8]. Clinico-radiologic study indicates that thalamic hemorrhage without midbrain involvement can also cause peduncular hallucinosis. Many authors have commented that the mesencephalic-diencephalic region contains sleep arousal circuitry which may be related to dreaming. Thus, disease in this region could easily be a cause of "visions" of the sort under discussion here.

There are complexities to this subject. Patients with preexisting visual impairment seem more likely to develop peduncular hallucinosis in the presence of an appropriate focal lesion. For example, a patient with one blind eye may be more likely to have hallucinations after a midbrain thalamic stroke than a patient with perfect vision. In the case of a craniopharyngioma there can be compression of both the anterior visual pathway and the cerebral peduncles. The combined dysfunction of these adjacent areas may result in hallucinations, which can sometimes be terminated by decompression of the cystic component of the tumor.

4.6 Hallucinations with Impaired Vision (Charles Bonnet Syndrome)

Hallucinations due to impaired vision are strictly visual. They have no associated auditory or other features. The patients are alert and awake. Even when the hallucinations look real, patients recognize them as hallucinations and find them undisturbing. In fact, patients commonly find the hallucinations entertaining [9]. These hallucinations come and go. Hallucinatory episodes can last from seconds to days. The images can be still or moving [10].

In Charles Bonnet syndrome the pathology can be anywhere in the visual system. Unilateral enucleation, corneal disease, cataracts, glaucoma, retinal disease, optic neuropathy, and brain lesions all can be responsible for these hallucinations. In one series of patients with macular degeneration, for example, 13% of patients had visual hallucinations [11]. The loss of acuity in cataract or diabetic retinopathy need not be severe for hallucinations to result. In fact, there are patients whose hallucinations cease as their vision worsens. When hallucinations accompany homonymous hemianopsia, they are initially seen in the blind visual field [12]; sometimes in time they are perceived as involving the entire field of vision. People, animals, or objects can be seen [12]. During a given hour a patient may see fireworks, green fences, and yellow flowers. People or animals may or may not be colorful or mobile.

4.7 Hallucinations with Impaired Hearing or a Disordered Vestibular System

In deafness, as in visual impairment, patients may experience hallucinations. The underlying hearing loss can be conductive (e.g., otosclerosis) or sensorineural (e.g., cochlear degeneration). A hallucination can be as simple as a continuous tone. (If tinnitus results from arterial, venous, or other vibrations in the head it is not hallucinatory.) A complex auditory hallucination is the hearing of voices or music. The voices or music may vary and may or may not be pleasing. Voices may or may not be recognized. Superimposition of a prescribed medication can precipitate or accentuate hallucinations in the deaf. In one hearing impaired patient, pentoxifylline use elicited simple roaring tinnitus, voices in conversation, and a male voice singing various religious songs [13]. The singing was so continuous as to be annoying. Central nervous system disease, especially that of the pontine tegmentum, can also cause hearing impairment with hallucinations [14].

Hallucinations from a disordered vestibular system are less varied than that of the auditory system. It is a hallucination of movement (vertigo) whether the disease is in the labyrinth, eighth cranial nerve, the vestibular nuclei, its projections or connections.

4.8 Miscellaneous Causes of Hallucination

Various deprivation phenomena can cause hallucinations. Elimination of vision by blindfolding [15] or removal of all sensory stimuli (sensory deprivation) can do this [16,17]. When Charles Lindbergh made the first solo transatlantic flight he had nothing to see in front of him because there was no windshield. He had only a periscope to use to look ahead. In effect he was deprived of visual stimuli; eventually he saw a copilot sitting beside him.

Sleep deprivation also can cause hallucinations. For example, James Corbett examined 14 American pilots who had been imprisoned in Hanoi during the Vietnam War.[1] One sheepishly admitted to him that he had experienced hallucinations during torture. He had been seated on a stool with his hands tied behind his back. When he would doze and fall from the stool he would be beaten. Thus, there was prolonged sleep deprivation. Eventually he experienced elaborate visual hallucinations: the curtains would open, and a puppet show would begin. It turned out the puppet show was a ruse. Behind the curtains were cartoon-like US soldiers who would run out to rescue him. This hallucinatory experience was recurrent. I had another patient who, while driving in a sleep deprived state, suddenly swerved his car to avoid a coffin he "saw" on the road.

Patients with narcolepsy experience attacks of sleep, cataplexy, sleep paralysis, and hypnagogic and hypnopompic hallucinations. Fragments of the disorder can occur without the full syndrome being manifest. For example, a person, who has no sleep attacks, may have fleeting visual hallucinations while dozing or awakening. These experiences carry no negative prognosis and require no treatment other than educating the patient about the symptom.

4.9 Psychiatric Hallucinations

Hallucinations can occur in psychiatric patients. In schizophrenics they are usually auditory, characteristically voices heard in conversation about or in running commentary about the patient [18]. Sometimes the patient recognizes the voices. Voices can

---

[1] Personal communication, J. Corbett, 2005.

speak to the patient. "Boy are you sick!" These hallucinations can be associated with delusions, for example, that they are sent through his television set by a neighbor. In affective disorders, hallucinations are coherent with the patient's mood. When a severely depressed person hears a voice telling him that he is worthless, the hallucination's content is "understandable" in the sense that it is fully consistent with and derivative from the patient's mood. Schizophrenic hallucinations are usually not "understandable" in this way [18].

4.10 Final Comments

1. Hallucinations can result from neuropathologic change, neurophysiologic disorder, toxic-metabolic effect, psychiatric condition, sensory deprivation, or sleep deprivation.

2. Hallucinations can result from dysfunction anywhere from the peripheral sensory receptors to the cerebral cortex.

3. For diagnosis, the form of a hallucination is more important than the specific content. The detail of the conversation of hallucinated scornful voices is less important than the fact that the psychiatric patient is hearing them. A driver of an automobile may see a distorted version of a famous cartoon character running on a highway. The occurrence is more important diagnostically than is the recognition of exactly which cartoon character has been seen.

4. Nevertheless, hallucinatory content can be meaningful. One of my patients saw a cartoon animal when he was driving past an amusement park which featured the hallucinated character.

5. Insight that a hallucination is not real indicates that the cause is not a delirium or a psychosis.

6. Persistence of hallucinations after a toxic exposure is not usual. However, chronic hallucinosis can result under special circumstances, namely after repeated bouts of alcohol withdrawal [19], chronic amphetamine use, exposure to hallucinogens, and chronic glue sniffing. Persistent hallucinosis can be auditory (e.g., in alcoholics) or visual (e.g., in glue sniffers). No neuropathologic change has been shown to underlie these forms of chronic hallucinosis.

7. Combined factors can facilitate the occurrence of hallucinosis. A midbrain thalamic infarction is more likely to cause visual hallucinations in a person with preexisting visual impairment than it is in a person with normal vision. A generalized encephalopathy, such as that of active cerebral lupus erythematosus, can cause visual hallucinations in a patient with preexisting visual impairment. Degenerative brain disease (e.g., Lewy body dementia) is more likely to result in hallucinations when there is an unrelated visual impairment. Use of a medication with a tendency to cause encephalopathy is more likely to result in auditory hallucinations if the patient is deaf.

8. Many persons find that decreased ambient light or eye closure makes visual hallucinations more evident. However, some report hallucinations only when their eyes are open [20].

9. Irritative hallucinations (focal seizures) are useful for localizing disease. Released hallucinations, due to decreased sensory input, are less helpful for this purpose [21].

10. One may continue to hear a jingle after he turns off the radio or he may continue to see an image after he looks away from it. Such persistence of a perception, after a stimulus

ceases, I do not consider a hallucination. Because the original perception is correct, I consider these phenomena as perseveration. Visual perseveration is referred to as palinopsia (paliopia) and auditory perseveration as palinacousis. Some authors classify these phenomena as hallucinations.

References

1. J. Cummings, C. Ballard, P. Tariot et al. Pimavanserin: Potential treatment for dementia-related psychosis. *J Prev Alzheimers Dis* 2018; **5**: 253–258.

2. C. M. Fisher. Visual hallucinations on eye closure associated with atropine toxicity. A neurological analysis and comparison with other visual hallucinations. *Can J Neurol Sci* 1991; **18**: 18–27.

3. M. J. Brown, D. Salmon, M. Rendell. Clonidine hallucinations. *Ann Int Med* 1980; **93**: 456–457.

4. C. M. Fisher. Visual hallucinations and racing thoughts on eye closure after minor surgery. *Arch Neurol* 1991; **48**: 1091–1092.

5. W. Penfield, P. Perot. The brain's record of auditory and visual experience. A final summary and discussion. *Brain* 1963; **86**: 595–596.

6. A. A. Tarnutzer, S. H. Lee, K. A. Robinson et al. Clinical and electrographic findings in epileptic vertigo and dizziness: a systematic review. *Neurology* 2015; **84**: 1595–1604.

7. P. Panayiotopoulos. Elementary visual hallucinations in migraine and epilepsy. *J Neurol Neurosurg Psychiatry* 1994; **57**: 1371–1374.

8. A. C. McKee, D. N. Levine, N. W. Kowall et al. Peduncular hallucinosis associated with isolated infarction of the substantia nigra pars reticulata. *Ann Neurol* 1990; **27**: 500–504.

9. F. T. Billings, J. Pitt. Charles Bonnet low visions. *Trans Am Clin Climatol Assoc* 2008; **119**: 225–226.

10. G. Schultz, R. Melzack. The Charles Bonnet syndrome: 'phantom visual images.' *Perception* 1991; **20**: 809–825.

11. S. Holroyd, P. V. Rabins, D. Finkelstein et al. Visual hallucinations in patients with macular degeneration. *Am J Psychiatry* 1992; **149**: 1701–1706.

12. J. W. Lance. Simple formed hallucinations confined to the area of a specific visual field defect. *Brain* 1976; **99**: 719–734.

13. G. J. Gilbert. Pentoxifylline-induced musical hallucinations. *Neurology* 1993; **43**: 1621–1622.

14. G. D. Cascino and R. D. Adams. Brainstem auditory hallucinosis. *Neurology* 1986; **36**: 1042–1047.

15. L. B. Merabet, D. Maguire, A. Warde et al. Visual hallucinations during prolonged blindfolding in sighted subjects. *J Neuroophthalmol* 2004; **24**: 109–113.

16. E. J. Kollar, N. Namerow, R. O. Pasnau et al. Neurological findings during prolonged sleep deprivation. *Neurology* 1968; **18**: 836–840.

17. J. P. Zubek. Effects of prolonged sensory and perceptual deprivation. *Br Med Bull* 1964; **20**: 38–42.

18. M. J. Hamilton, ed. *Fish's Schizophrenia*. Bristol, John Wright and Sons, 1976.

19. M. Victor and J. M. Hope. The phenomenon of auditory hallucinations in chronic alcoholism: a critical evaluation of the status of alcoholic hallucinosis. *J Nerv Ment Dis* 1958; **126**: 451–481.

20. R. J. Teunisse, J. R. Cruysberg, W. H. Hoefnagels et al. Visual hallucinations in psychologically normal people: Charles Bonnet's syndrome. *Lancet* 1996; **347**: 794–797.

21. D. G. Cogan. Visual hallucinations as release phenomena. *Albrecht Von Graefes Archiv Klin Exp Ophthalmol* 1973; **188**: 139–150.

Chapter 5

Grasping and the Grasp Reflex

Grasping is a fundamental human tendency. Involuntary grasping in adults implies forebrain disease. Denny-Brown recognized two types of involuntary grasping, the grasp reflex and the instinctive grasp response. These prehensile phenomena differ in their necessary stimulus, their level of motor integration, and their clinical utility.

The grasp reflex proper requires a combined cutaneous-proprioceptive stimulus. Palm up, the examiner reaches across to the patient's hand which is palm down. The examiner's fingers move distally stroking the patient's palm. When the examiner's moving fingers reach the patient's digits, they cause extension at the metacarpophalangeal joints. That is to say, a proprioceptive stimulus is superimposed on the tactile stimulus. If there is a grasp reflex, the patient's fingers will begin to flex. The proprioceptive stimulus is sustained, as the examiner's fingers and the patient's flexing fingers press against each other. In this phase the patient's fingers are grasping the examiner's fingers. As a part of the reflex the thumb adducts. In its stimulus and response, the grasp reflex is a stereotyped phenomenon.

The presence of a grasp reflex is evidence for disease of the contralateral frontal lobe [1]. A bilateral grasp reflex implies bilateral frontal lobe disease. Typically, it is the supplementary motor area which is involved [2]. A neurologist tests for the reflex when he suspects that the frontal lobes are affected.

The grasp reflex is usually asymptomatic. It is a phenomenon elicited by the doctor for diagnostic purposes. However, there are situations when a grasp reflex is so strong that it becomes a clinical problem. A demented elder can so forcefully grasp his grandchild that the toddler will avoid him. A patient with progressive supranuclear palsy can grasp so strongly that the reflex interferes with eating, dressing, and bathing; he may grasp his caregiver [3].

The grasp reflex occurs in many types of brain disease. One of the early papers about the grasp reflex was a description of frontal lobe tumor patients [1]. Cerebral infarction patients have been the basis of studies of involuntary grasping [4,5]. Advanced degenerative disease such as progressive supranuclear palsy, Lewy body disease, Alzheimer's disease, and corticobasal degeneration often cause bilateral grasp reflexes. Hydrocephalus can do the same. Carbon monoxide poisoning is an example of a toxic/metabolic condition that can cause the grasp reflex to appear.

Denny-Brown found it instructive to compare the grasp reflex to the response to passive movement in spasticity. Unlike spasticity the grasp reflex is not length dependent. The grasp reflex can be elicited when the wrist is extended or when it is flexed. Secondly, eliciting a grasp reflex requires the initial cutaneous stimulus prior to elevation of the fingers whereas spasticity is elicited by passive movement alone. Thirdly, the proprioceptive phase of the grasp reflex differs from spasticity in being self-sustaining [6].

The grasp reflex is not always caused by an irreversible brain lesion. With decompression of hydrocephalus the grasp reflex may disappear. With reversal of a metabolic

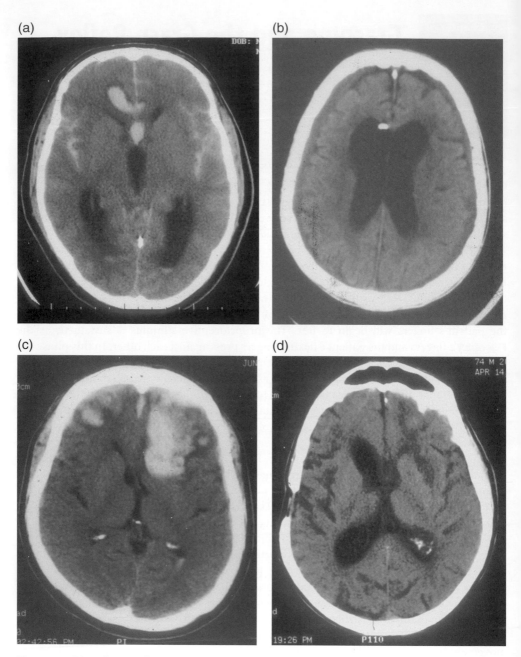

Figure 5.1 Bilateral grasp reflexes in these patients were due to symptomatic hydrocephalus and/or focal lesions.

encephalopathy the grasp reflex can also disappear. Reversibility is an underemphasized aspect of this subject.

Usually, the grasp reflex indicates an active disease (Figures 5.1 and 5.2). Degenerative brain diseases are active in that they are progressive. Glial tumors are active in the same sense. Symptomatic hydrocephalus is also active. Any acute disease such as stroke is active

(a)

(b)

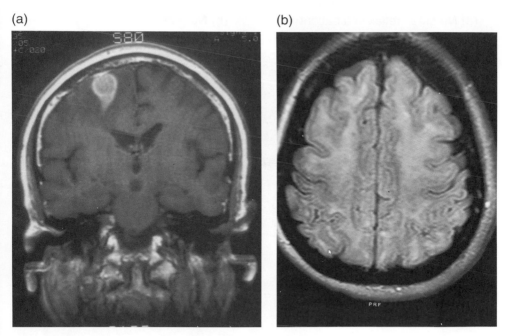

Figure 5.2a Unilateral grasp reflex in a patient due to a contralateral focal lesion.
Figure 5.2b Bilateral grasp reflex in a patient who had days earlier developed delayed post anoxic leukoencephalopathy.

and, if appropriately located, has the potential to cause a grasp reflex. Old traumatic or cerebrovascular lesions are inactive (Figures 5.3, 5.4, and 5.5). Thus, an acute brain injury or stroke may cause a grasp reflex that eventually disappears. A meningioma that has been compressing the brain for many years may be inactive in the sense that the brain has adapted to the mass (Figures 5.3, 5.4, and 5.5).

Not any frontal lobe disorder will cause a grasp reflex. It is dysfunction of the supplementary motor area which is the most consistent correlate of a contralateral grasp reflex. This area is above the cingulate gyrus and anterior to the primary motor cortex, largely but not solely on the medial surface of the frontal lobe. Consistent with this concept one can see that lesions of the undersurface of the frontal lobes or frontal polar lesions do not seem to be associated with grasp reflexes (Figures 5.3, 5.4, and 5.5).

In sum, the grasp reflex is more likely to occur with active disease affecting or approximating the supplementary motor area. Presumably hydrocephalus is affecting this area when it causes grasp reflexes.

Grasping tendencies are deeply ingrained in the mammalian line. In cats and dogs, Sherrington demonstrated clawing as a localized proprioceptive response equivalent to grasping. In normal humans the grasp reflex is a developmental phenomenon. In the fetus, grasping can appear as early as week 11[3]. After birth the grasp reflex typically can be elicited for only the first three months of extrauterine life. Less than 1% of healthy college students have been reported to have a grasp reflex [7]. In normal older adults the incidence is virtually nil.

In a series of patients with hydranencephaly, there was unusual persistence of the grasp reflex until 6–27 months of age. The forebrain of these patients was inadequate to inhibit the

(a) No grasp reflex in a patient with bifrontal meningioma

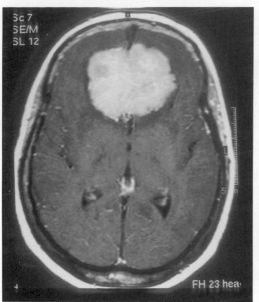

(b) No grasp reflex in a patient with bifrontal contusions

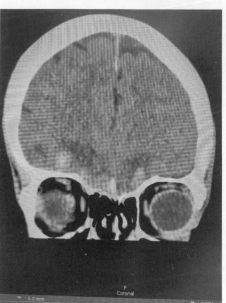

(c) No grasp reflex in a patient with bifrontal traumatic injury

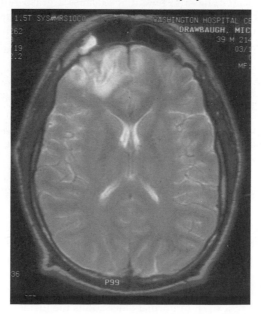

Figure 5.3 No grasp reflex was present in these three patients with bifrontal disease.

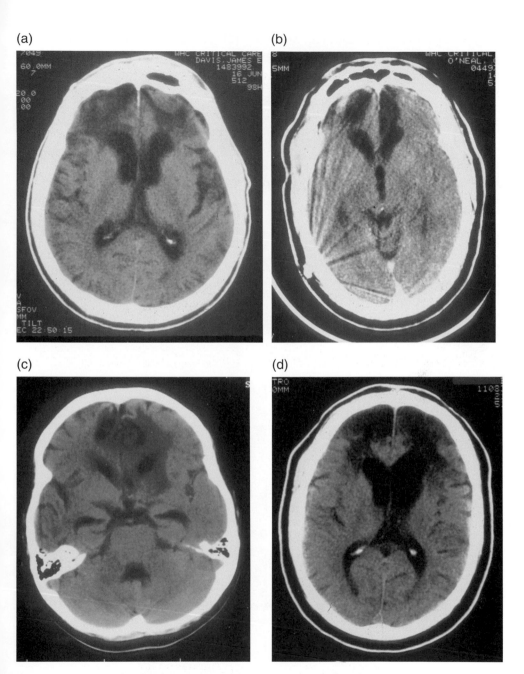

Figure 5.4 No grasp reflex was present in these four patients with old bifrontal lesions.

reflex at three months of age as it normally does. The absence of a grasp reflex in anencephaly indicates that intact mesencephalon and diencephalon are both necessary for reflex grasping to be manifest [8].

Although hydranencephalic patients eventually develop grasp reflexes, they never show an instinctive grasp response. Instinctive grasping, which is a highly integrated motor

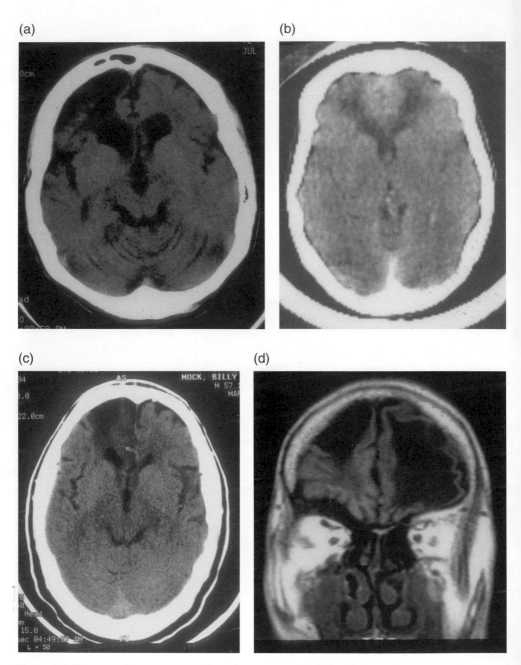

Figure 5.5 No grasp reflex was present in these four patients with old frontal lesions.

behavior, appears later in development than the grasp reflex. As a corollary it is manifest only when there is adequate intact telencephalon [8].

Compared to the stereotyped grasp reflex, the instinctive grasp reaction is a complicated motor behavior in which the limb is projected into the environment (Table 5.1). For this reason,

Table 5.1 Involuntary grasping

Grasp reflex	Stimulus	Instinctive grasp response
Moving palmar cutaneous contact followed by finger proprioceptive	Stimulus	Purely tactile
Stereotyped reflex	Response	Complex, involves groping
Contralateral frontal lobe	Brain disorder	Contralateral or ipsilateral frontal lobe/corpus callosum

it has been referred to as "forced groping." For the instinctive grasp response, the stimulus is purely tactile, light contact to the hand [9]. In response, there are successive flexion-extension movements of the fingers which result in grasping of the stimulating fingers. The instinctive grasp resembles instinctive sucking in that the stimulus is a non-proprioceptive contact. On the one hand Mori relates the instinctive grasp response most often to a lesion of **ipsilateral** perisylvian or subcortical frontal lobe. (He states that this reaction occurs more often in right hemisphere than in left hemisphere lesions [4].) On the other hand Hashimoto attributes the instinctive grasp response to a **contralateral** anterior cingulate gyrus lesion. Clearly there is room for further study of the pathoanatomy underlying the instinctive grasp response [2].

Copresence of the grasp reflex and the instinctive grasp reaction can occur with extensive disease involving both the supplementary motor area and the anterior cingulate gyrus. According to Denny-Brown, both types of response are abolished by total destruction of the primary motor cortex [6].

Abnormal grasping can be seen in the alien hand syndrome. In this condition, a patient's hand can involuntarily grasp "contrary to the patient's stated intention" to such an extent that the "normal hand typically restrains the alien one" [10]. Although the alien hand is often associated with corticobasal degeneration, the relationship is not at all exclusive. In fact, the term was coined in a study of corpus collosum tumors [11]. Some suggest that there are subtypes of alien hand syndrome [10], but others find such distinctions unclear [12]. In any case, when a grasping hand has a "will of its own" [10] it is certainly a phenomenon separate from the instinctive grasp response.

5.1 Conclusion

Grasping is an inborn tendency of human hands. Involuntary grasping behavior is inhibited by the cerebral hemispheres during development. Forebrain disease can release various types of involuntary grasping. The clinically useful grasp reflex occurs with active disease affecting the contralateral supplementary area.

References

1. W. J. Adie, M. Critchley. Forced grasping and groping. *Brain* 1927; **50**: 142–170.

2. R. Hashimoto, Y. Tanaka. Contribution of the supplementary motor area and anterior cingulate gyrus to pathological grasping phenomena. *Eur Neurol* 1998; **40**: 151–158.

3. T. Mestre, A. E. Lang. The grasp reflex: a symptom in need of treatment. *Mov Disord* 2010; **25**: 2479–2485.

4. E. Mori, A. Yamadori. Unilateral hemispheric injury and ipsilateral instinctive grasp reaction. *Arch Neurol* 1985; **42**: 485–488.

5. A. H. Ropper. Self-grasping: a focal neurological sign. *Ann Neurol* 1982; **12**: 575–577.

6. D. Denny-Brown. Disintegration of motor function resulting from cerebral lesions. *J Nerv Ment Dis* 1950; **112**: 1–45.

7. D. L. Brown, T. L. Smith, L. E. Knepper. Evaluation of five primitive reflexes in 240 young adults. *Neurology* 1998; **51**: 322.

8. J. H. Halsey, N. Allen, H. R. Chamberlin. Chronic decerebrate state in infancy. Neurologic observations in long surviving cases of hydranencephaly. *Arch Neurol* 1968; **19**: 339–346.

9. G. Rushworth, D. Denny-Brown. The two components of the grasp reflex after ablation of frontal cortex in monkeys. *J Neurol Neurosurg Psychiatry* 1959; **22**: 91–98.

10. T. E. Feinberg, R. J. Schindler, N. G. Flanagan et al. Two alien hand syndromes. *Neurology* 1992; **42**: 19–24.

11. S. Brion, C. P. Jedynak. [Disorders of interhemispheric transfer (callosal disonnection). Three cases of tumor of the corpus callosum. The strange hand sign.] [French]. *Revue Neurologique* 1972; **126**: 257–266.

12. J. H. Lin, S. Y. Kwan, D. Wu. Mixed alien hand syndrome coexisting with left-sided extinction secondary to a left corpus callosal lesion: a case report. *Mov Disord* 2007; **22**: 248–251.

Asterixis

The clinician usually elicits this sign by asking the patient to hold his wrists in dorsiflexion. Instead of the wrists remaining in dorsiflexion, as is normally the case, irregular, asynchronous flapping of the hands occurs [1,2]. Because gravity accentuates the flapping, dorsiflexion of the hands is a sensitive method to test for asterixis. However, asterixis can be elicited against gravity, which is not fundamental to the phenomenon [3]. Furthermore, asterixis can be elicited in many other parts of the body. The repeated arrhythmic lapses of sustained posture result from episodic cessation of myoelectrical activity.

This movement disorder was recognized as unique by Raymond D. Adams and Joseph M. Foley during their studies of the neurology of liver disease. Asterixis was noted to be an early sign of hepatic encephalopathy, a harbinger of hepatic coma. It was soon recognized that the phenomenon was not specific for liver disease.

Metabolic encephalopathies (Table 6.1) and the effects of medications (Table 6.2) are the usual causes of asterixis. Liver failure, renal failure, and CO_2 retention are commonly responsible. Most medications that can make a patient drowsy or confused can also cause asterixis. Antiepileptic medicine is more likely to cause asterixis when the blood level exceeds the usually therapeutic range or when a loading dose abruptly elevates the blood level. Combinations of metabolic encephalopathies, combinations of medications, or combinations of medication and organ failure may result in asterixis when one factor or another, by itself, would not have been adequate to cause it. In the hospital setting, this combination effect may occur when a new medication is added to those the patient has been taking prior to admission.

It is not only toxic and metabolic disorders that cause asterixis. It can occur in other brain diseases that affect the cerebrum diffusely. Viral encephalitis, Creutzfeldt–Jakob disease, cerebral malaria, and cerebral trypanosomiasis are examples [3].

Table 6.1 Causes of asterixis

Metabolic encephalopathies
Liver disease
Renal disease
Hypercarbia
Hypoxemia
Hyperammonemia
Hypophosphatemia
Hypercalcemia

Table 6.2 Causes of asterixis

Medications
Anticonvulsants
Carbamazepine
Gabapentin
Phenobarbital
Phenytoin
Pregabalin
Valproic acid
Psychotropics
Clozapine
Lithium
Promethazine
Benzodiazepines
Miscellaneous
Narcotics
Anticholinergics
Cephalosporin
Other medications
(Examples are famotidine, ifosfamide, levodopa, metoclopramide, and isoniazid)

Structural brain disease can occasionally cause bilateral asterixis. In these cases, the disorder affects the forebrain bilaterally or the midbrain tegmentum. Specific examples are bilateral subdural hematomas and bilateral thalamic infarctions. Bilateral asterixis can result from unilateral structural disease which, by shifting the brain, causes diencephalic compression.

Although asking a patient to hold his wrists in dorsiflexion is a standard way to test for asterixis, the finding can be elicited in many other parts of the body. One can find asterixis at the shoulders during arm extension, at the hips during hip flexion, and at the ankles during dorsiflexion. Inability to maintain contraction can also occur on sustained tongue protrusion or prolonged facial contraction (forced grimace). Facial and lingual asterixis, however, are not common. When a patient cannot cooperate well enough to maintain a requested muscular contraction, one can try to set limbs in a position and watch to see whether the patient maintains the posture. For example, one can set the legs of a supine patient in a hip flexion–knee flexion position. While firmly holding the feet together with the soles on the bed, the doctor can then watch for flapping abduction–adduction movements of the legs.

Asterixis is typically noticed in the upper extremities. In a given patient, however, asterixis may be easier to elicit in the lower extremities. The trouble detecting asterixis at the wrists in such cases can be due to poor attention from encephalopathy or to limited range of motion. Drowsiness may make it difficult for a patient to attend to maintaining muscle contraction in the upper extremities. Limited range of motion (e.g., scleroderma) may prevent wrist dorsiflexion. However, there are some individuals, absent any such difficulty, in whom asterixis is simply easier to elicit in the lower extremities.

Focal cerebral disease can cause contralateral asterixis, typically when mild to moderate hemiparesis is superimposed on mild generalized encephalopathy [4]. In such cases the encephalopathy alone is inadequate to cause asterixis. The encephalopathy can be secondary to any of the usual metabolic derangements or medication effects or even the metabolic effect of subarachnoid blood on the cerebrum. If the metabolic problem is severe enough, the asterixis may be bilateral but more prominent on the side of the mild hemiparesis.

Asterixis is typically asymptomatic. It is primarily a sign that can alert the doctor to the presence of an encephalopathy. It is also useful for monitoring an encephalopathy for worsening or improvement.

Occasionally, however, asterixis can be the presenting complaint. A patient may report episodes of falling or near falling from the legs "giving out." This symptom is due to a pause in contraction of lower limb extensor muscles. In the upper limbs a chief complaint can be "dropping things." Another patient may be concerned by trouble writing with one hand on a pad which he is holding with the other. A patient may think a bilateral problem is unilateral because he notices the difficulty in the dominant hand, the one using chopsticks or typing on a mobile telephone.

Preexisting disability can make a patient more vulnerable to asterixis. For example, preexisting blindness will render a person with upper extremity asterixis more likely to drop things. Similarly, preexisting leg weakness can make the lower extremity asterixis symptomatic.

The sudden flap of asterixis has reminded some neurologists of the sudden movement of myoclonus. On electromyography the two movement disorders are quite different. A sudden burst of muscle activation is the correlate of myoclonus; a sudden electrical silence is the basis of asterixis. Because the phenomena are electrically "opposite" some authors use the term "negative myoclonus" for asterixis. Myoclonus, however, is not a uniform kind of movement. It is a term that comprises a rich variety of phenomena generated by the cerebrum, brainstem, cerebellum, and spinal cord. Asterixis is a more specific phenomenon in which bursts of electrical silence occur in the flexor and extensor muscles simultaneously. Also, asterixis is elicited by a sustained contraction, which is not required for myoclonus. Thus, we discourage referring to asterixis as "negative myoclonus."

6.1 Summary

Asterixis is typically an asymptomatic clinical sign of metabolic or toxic encephalopathy. As a rule, it occurs symmetrically but asynchronously on the two sides of the body. The varieties and presentations of asterixis have been well described. The underlying central nervous system physiology of the phenomenon is not well understood.

References

1. R. D. Adams, J. M. Foley. The disorder of movement in more common varieties of liver disease. *Electroenceph Clin Neurophysiol* 1953; Supp 3:51.

2. R. D. Adams, J. M. Foley. The neurological disorder associated with liver disease. *Res Publ Assoc Res Nerv Ment Dis* 1953; **32**: 198–237.

3. G. Pal, M. M. Lin, R. Laureno. Asterixis: a study of 103 patients. *Metab Brain Dis* 2014; **29**: 813–824.

4. D. Goldblatt, R. C. Griggs. Unilateral asterixis in a paretic limb: an involuntary movement accentuated by upper motor neuron lesion. *Neurology* 1979; **29**: 541.

Discussion of the Upper Motor Neuron Syndrome

Damage to the upper motor neuron pathways causes a constellation of neurological manifestations familiar to all neurologists. Hemiplegic stroke typifies the upper motor neuron syndrome (UMNS) with its hyperactive stretch reflexes and increased muscle tone. The weak limbs assume a characteristic posture due to the dominance of the antigravity muscles (flexors in upper extremities and extensors in the lower extremities) [1].

Disability in the UMNS results from impaired purposeful movement. In the upper extremity, there is clumsiness of fine finger movements and disproportionate weakness of extensors and abductors. In the lower extremities, the leg flexors and foot dorsiflexors are particularly weak. By and large the reflex changes in the UMNS do not accentuate weakness or cause discomfort, the main exception being the flexor spasms of spinal cord disease. To rephrase, the reflex changes accompany but do not add to disability [2].

It is useful to think of the upper motor neuron pathways as inhibiting both muscle stretch reflexes and spinal flexion reflexes. Damage to the descending pathways disinhibits these reflexes. Unlike stretch reflexes and spinal flexion reflexes, cutaneous reflexes are diminished in the UMNS [1].

Disinhibition of the monosynaptic stretch reflex is manifest in several ways. First, of course, the clinician finds increased muscle tone, that is, resistance to passive stretch. On tendon percussion the reflex is lowered in threshold and increased in amplitude and speed. The threshold can be decreased to the extent that a tendon tap on the opposite side can provoke the stretch reflex. This crossed response occurs because the percussion hammer produces enough vibration through the firm body parts to stimulate the spindles of contralateral muscles. We know this reflex irradiation is not due to stimulation of afferents near the percussion site because cutting the dorsal roots contralateral to the tendon tap eliminates the crossed reflex in spinal animals [1].

Also encoded in the spinal cord are polysynaptic flexor reflexes. The brainstem inhibits them via the reticulospinal tract. In the course of development, a child acquires the ability to stand only when myelination of the descending pathway provides this inhibition. The term triple flexion refers to the synergistic flexion at the hip, knee, and ankle, a combination which is manifest in the flexor spasms of spinal cord disease. Recruitment of the toe into the flexion synergy of the lower limb results in the conspicuous dorsiflexion of the great toe at the metatarsophalangeal joint [1] (Table 7.1).

The release of the stretch reflex and the flexor reflex vary with the tempo of the illness and the size of the lesion. Slowly developing upper motor neuron lesions result in hyperreflexia and weakness. An acute lesion often results in weakness with hyporeflexia. Only after days or weeks may hyperreflexia appear. The size of the lesion is relevant; with smaller

Table 7.1 Abnormalities of spinal reflexes in UMNS

Muscle stretch reflex	Cutaneous reflex	Flexion reflex
Increased muscular resistance on brisk passive stretch	_____	Clasp knife phenomenon (melting of muscular resistance during continued passive stretch)
Exaggerated tendon jerks (i.e., lowered threshold for and increased speed and amplitude of response)	Loss of great toe plantar flexion	Great toe dorsiflexion
Clonus can occur		Flexor spasms

lesions the hyperreflexia typically appears earlier and often abates sooner. There is no simple relationship between the recovery of purposeful movement and the normalization of the stretch reflex. Years after a stroke, movement may have returned to normal while stretch reflexes remain hyperactive [3].

In the nineteenth century, John Hughlings Jackson viewed neurologic symptoms as negative and positive. In Jackson's terminology the negative symptoms of the UMNS are those directly due to upper motor system damage, that is weakness and loss of dexterity. The positive symptoms are those produced by the residual intact central nervous system. In the UMNS, these comprise increased stretch reflexes, hypertonicity, and clonus. Jackson induced his classification from clinical observation long before the physiology and anatomy of reflexes had been investigated. The separateness of positive and negative symptoms has been confirmed by experiment; differential spinal or epidural nerve block can eliminate spasticity without affecting strength [4].

In the light of Jackson's analysis, study of these phenomena occupied many neurologists and scientists for a century. Having reviewed the accumulated information and his own research, Lance was able to synthesize an anatomic/physiologic/clinical concept of the UMNS [1]:

1. Hyperexcitability of the stretch reflex (impaired function of corticoreticulospinal tract)

   Increased muscle tone (velocity dependent)
   Exaggerated tendon jerks
   Clonus

2. Release of flexor reflexes in lower limbs (impaired function of dorsal reticulospinal system)

   Clasp knife phenomenon
   Babinski response
   Flexor spasms

3. Weakness and loss of dexterity (impaired function of pyramidal tract)

   Weakness of extensors and abductors of upper limb
   Weakness of flexors in lower limb
   Clumsiness of fine movement

The Lance classification makes it clear that there is no single upper motor neuron system. The junior clinician's concept of the upper motor neuron as the Betz cells whose axons form the corticospinal tract, which courses through the medullary pyramid and lateral column of the spinal cord, is a simplification. Multiple areas of the brain and brainstem give rise to descending upper motor fibers. In sum, the UMNS is not due to damage to the cell bodies or projections of a single group of motor neurons. The heterogeneity of clinical manifestations depends on the exact site and size of the lesion. Commonly a fragment of the syndrome occurs without the other features.

Landau explains that physicians vary in how they use the term spasticity. He lists six different usages of the word [3]. Lance simply defines it as "the increased resistance to muscle stretch experienced by a clinician" in some patients with upper motor neuron disease [1]. Maurice Victor and Raymond Adams define spasticity as a velocity dependent increase in the resistance of muscles to passive stretch [5]. In other words, there may be no increased resistance if the limb is moved slowly. Lance also offers a more comprehensive definition of spasticity as "disinhibition of the stretch reflex, resulting in velocity dependent increase in tonic stretch reflexes and increased tendon jerks" [6]. Other authors use the word spasticity to include clonus. These definitions do not conflict. They vary only in emphasis and broadness.

Adams and Victor detail the unique type of hypertonicity in the UMNS. If a muscle is "briskly stretched, the limb moves freely for a very short distance . . . beyond which there is an abrupt catch and then a rapidly increasing muscular resistance up to a point; then as passive extension of the arm or flexion of the leg continues the resistance melts away" [5]. This melting of resistance has reminded doctors of that experienced when one closes the blade of a pocketknife (clasp knife) into its handle. The melting resistance Lance attributes to the enhanced flexion reflex overcoming the catch of the hyperactive stretch reflex. In other words, "clasp knife rigidity" can be conceived of as a sequence, first the manifestation of the disinhibited muscle stretch reflex followed by that of the disinhibited spinal flexion reflex [1].

The subject is complex. Babinski considered his sign to be a perversion of the normal plantar flexor response. Over decades he came to accept the view of F. M. R. Walshe, Marie and Foix, and others that the normal plantar flexor response and the pathologic dorsiflexor response of the great toe are unrelated! Van Gijn summarizes the subject. The normal plantar flexor response is a cutaneous reflex with a limited receptive field. As do other cutaneous reflexes, it can disappear with an upper motor neuron disorder. Also occurring with the UMNS is recruitment of toe dorsiflexion into the polysynaptic flexor synergy of the lower extremity (triple flexion). Thus, triple flexion can become quadruple flexion. However, there need not be dramatic leg withdrawal for one to note great toe dorsiflexion. The upgoing toe can be the most prominent flexion response on properly calibrated stimulation. Hence it has diagnostic value. (The fanning of the toes which can accompany toe dorsiflexion is not an essential feature [7].) Detection of loss of cutaneous reflex (plantar flexion of the great toe) can be as clinically important as observation of the pathologic spinal flexion reflex (dorsiflexion of the great toe).

There has been much speculation about the teleology and the evolutionary basis of the extensor plantar and flexor plantar responses. For example, Babinski believed that the flexion reflex including toe dorsiflexion stems from a protective withdrawal mechanism seen in quadrupeds, "réflexes de défense" [8]. Wartenberg believed that great toe dorsiflexion was in its phylogenetic origin part of the toe fanning. He commented that the mass flexion reflex, flexion at the hip and knee, dorsiflexion at the ankle and spreading of the toes, involves movements, all useful for running and climbing in primates. In the human, anatomy has evolved to accommodate the erect position. In this evolutionary process, he believed, the changes in the metatarsophalyngeal joint and the dorsiflexor tendon insertion result in a configuration that makes abduction of the great toe difficult but allows dorsiflexion [9]. In other words, instead of fanning, the great toe has to dorsiflex. It is not possible to prove these and other interesting ideas about our reflexes.

References

1. J. W. Lance. The control of muscle tone, reflexes, and movement: Robert Wartenberg Lecture. *Neurology* 1980; **30**: 1303–1313.

2. W. M. Landau. Editorial: Spasticity: the fable of a neurological demon and the emperor's new therapy. *Arch Neurol* 1974; **31**: 217–219.

3. W. M. Landau. Clinical neuromythology II. Parables of palsy pills and PT pedagogy: a spastic dialectic. *Neurology* 1988; **38**: 1496–1499.

4. W. M. Landau, R. A. Weaver, T. F. Hornbein. Fusimotor nerve function in man. Differential nerve block studies in normal subjects and in spasticity and rigidity. *Arch Neurol* 1960; **3**: 10–23.

5. M. R. Victor, A. Ropper, R. Adams. *Adams & Victor's Principles of Neurology.* New York, McGraw-Hill Professional, 2001.

6. J. W. Lance, J. G. McLeod. *A Physiological Approach to Clinical Neurology.* London, Butterworths, 1981.

7. J. van Gijn. *The Babinski Sign: A Centenary.* Utrecht, Universiteit Utrecht, 1996.

8. J. Babinski, J. Froment, *Hysteria or Pithiatism, and Reflex Nervous Disorders in the Neurology of War.* London, University of London Press, 1918.

9. R. Wartenberg. *Diagnostic Tests in Neurology: A Selection for Office Use.* Chicago, Year Book Publishers, 1953.

Some Aspects of the Lower Motor Neuron Syndrome

8

If one thinks about this subject in terms of electrical circuitry, it is easy to understand that disruption of the lower motor neuron can diminish muscle stretch reflexes and strength. However, this wiring metaphor does not explain all of the changes in lower motor neuron disease. With denervation, twitches and structural alterations occur in the muscle itself.

When muscle is experimentally denervated, the bared muscle surface is "rippled by a restless agitation . . . the whole muscle is . . . a confusion of very small twitches" [1]. These barely visible individual twitches are those of single muscle fibers. Thus, they are termed fibrillations. They are too small to be visible through the skin.

There are also gross twitches, which are too large to be originating in single muscle fibers. They result from the contraction of the many muscle fibers of a motor unit (a motor neuron and the muscle fibers it supplies). It is the depolarization of the axon of a motor unit that gives rise to the coordinated contraction of its multiple muscle fibers. These twitches, which we see in the clinic, Denny-Brown named fasciculations [1]. This term has for a century served to distinguish the motor unit phenomenon, fasciculation, from the muscle fiber phenomenon, fibrillation. The term incorrectly suggests that an entire fascicle is twitching. Actually, the twitch involves only part of a fascicle. The fibers of a motor unit are scattered in a fascicle that includes hundreds of muscle fibers belonging to other motor units.

Although both types of spontaneous muscle activity can occur as a result of denervation, they are not identical in meaning. Fasciculations by definition always originate electrically from axons or their cells bodies; they can be the result of disease, or they can be benign. Fibrillations, on the other hand, are not benign. They originate electrically in muscle. Typically, they indicate pathology (Table 8.1).

When these two types of spontaneous potential are seen with some frequency in the same patient, such as occurs in motor neuron disease, the fibrillations (single fiber

Table 8.1 Two types of spontaneous electrical activity in muscle

Fasciculation		Fibrillation
Many muscle fibers of a motor unit	Depolarization/contraction in muscle	Single muscle fiber
Benign or disease in nerve	Meaning	Disease in nerve or necrotizing myopathy
Nerve	Electrical origin	Muscle fiber

depolarizations) indicate disease and the fasciculations (motor unit potentials) indicate origin in nerve.

These forms of spontaneous activity are distinctive on electromyography. Fibrillations are regularly repetitive. On the screen the depolarization is manifest by a small initially positive deflection, followed by a larger negative spike deflection. Sometimes these single muscle fiber depolarizations are recorded in a different configuration as deep positive waves followed by leisurely trailing negativity; they are otherwise similar to fibrillations in their regular repetitiveness, frequency, amplitude, and meaning. They sound like a metronome or a ticking clock. Fasciculations, which are produced by many muscle fibers of a motor unit, naturally have a greater electrical amplitude (often in millivolts) than fibrillations or positive waves (microvolts). Irregular in occurrence, they sound like corn popping.

In clinical neurology, the denervation we encounter usually occurs gradually. Thus, the muscle fibers do not all atrophy together as they do in experimental denervation. Biopsy of muscle shows healthy muscle fibers side by side with atrophic muscle fibers (Figure 8.1). It is abnormal fibers such as these that give rise to fibrillations and positive waves. In gradually developing denervation, a healthy axon can sprout branches to reinnervate the denervated muscle fibers of a dead motor neuron. If that healthy axon in turn dies, another healthy axon can in turn sprout to reinnervate all of the newly denervated fibers. As a result of this continuing process of collateral reinnervation the muscle fibers in a given motor unit, normally scattered in the fascicle, increase in number and come to lie adjacent to each other. Part way into this process, the pathologist can demonstrate the grouped fibers of an enlarged motor unit by using histochemical stains (Figure 8.2). As a consequence of

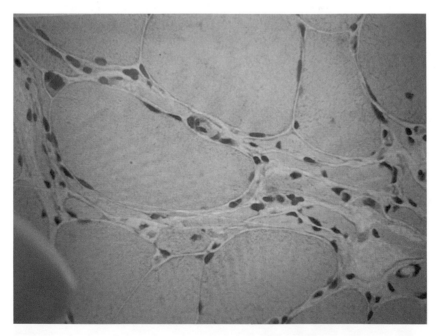

Figure 8.1 Scattered atrophic fibers in denervation. Such isolated atrophic fibers give rise to fibrillations. (Image provided with permission by Dr. Dimitri Agamanolis from his website, Neuropathology an illustrated interactive course for medical students and residents.)

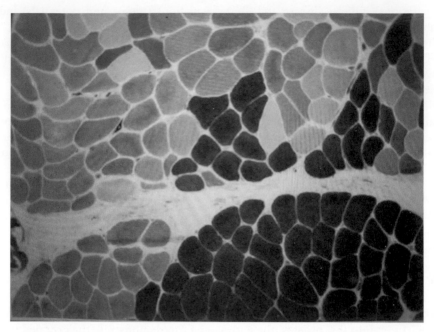

Figure 8.2 Fiber-type grouping (seen by a histochemical stain) is the result of collateral reinnervation causing the fibers of a motor unit to be more numerous and adjacent. The motor unit potentials of these large groups of fibers are increased in amplitude and duration. (Image provided by Dr. Dimitri Agamanolis.)

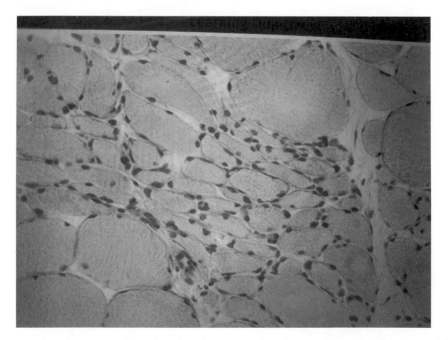

Figure 8.3 When the axon supplying the enlarged motor unit dies, there results atrophy of the grouped fibers. (Image provided by Dr. Dimitri Agamanolis.)

reinnervation bringing more muscle fibers into a motor unit, graded voluntary contraction of muscle reveals motor unit potentials which are increased in amplitude and duration. This increased size of motor unit potentials also can be seen in involuntary motor unit depolarizations (fasciculations). When the process of reinnervation finally fails, the fibers of the enlarged motor unit appear as a group of atrophied fibers. This group atrophy is well seen in Werdnig Hoffman disease (Figure 8.3).

These changes in denervated muscle show that muscle needs its connection to nerve. How nerve maintains muscle in its normal structural and electrical state is not well understood. It is clear that the trophic effect is not simply the result of "propagation and transmission of nerve impulses and the resultant muscle contractions" [2]. One theory is that continuous quantal release of acetylcholine at the neuromuscular junction is responsible. Because axonal transport provides substances to the muscle other than acetylcholine, it is possible that these materials, such as peptides or proteins, are essential for the sustenance of muscle [3]. Support for this idea comes from studies with botulinum toxin [4]. Of course it is possible that a combination of electrical and chemical stimuli may be needed to maintain muscle in a healthy state.

References

1. D. Denny-Brown, J. B. Pennybacker. Fibrillation and fasciculation in voluntary muscle. *Brain* 1938; **61**: 311–312.

2. T. L. Lentz. Trophic functions of the neuron. VI. Other trophic systems. Neurotrophic regulation at the neuromuscular junction. *Ann N Y Acad Sci* 1974; **228**: 323–337.

3. I. M. Korr, P. N. Wilkinson, F. W. Chornock. Axonal delivery of neuroplasmic components to muscle cells. *Science* 1967; **155**: 342–345.

4. J. J. Bray, A. J. Harris. Dissociation between nerve-muscle transmission and nerve trophic effects on rat diaphragm using type D botulinum toxin. *J Physiol* 1975; **253**: 53–77.

The Limbic System

"Limbic system" is ensconced in the medical literature. A PubMed search in 2020 retrieved over 300,000 results for the term. Paul D. MacLean created this term for a forebrain circuit, which he believed to be the basis for emotion. The following account reviews the development of the limbic system as a term and its status as a concept.

MacLean was a fellow at Massachusetts General Hospital [1]. One day he went to the library to search for a journal article. By chance he came across a 10-year-old paper, "A Proposed Mechanism of Emotion" [2]. It fascinated him. His department chairman, Stanley Cobb, could not satisfy MacLean's curiosity about the theory. Hence, Cobb urged him to visit the paper's author. Soon thereafter MacLean traveled to Ithaca, N.Y. where he spent two to three days with James Papez at Cornell University [3].

Papez's now famous paper had proposed that all emotions have a common neuroanatomic substrate. He did not distinguish fear, anger, joy, sadness, or other emotions. His hypothesis was that a circuit from cerebral cortex to hypothalmus/thalamus and from hypothalamus/thalamus to cerebral cortex was the anatomic basis for emotions. Just as the lateral geniculate nucleus of the thalamus projects to the striate cortex for vision, Papez proposed that a thalamic nucleus projects to the cingulate gyrus for emotion. In proposing this circuit Papez mentioned anatomical observations of others, inferences from comparative anatomy, and clinical case reports. (For example, he stated that lesions around the mammillary bodies render patients somnolent. Because such patients are "emotionally inactive" he inferred that the mamillary bodies are a part of the mechanism of emotion.) From these various sources of information Papez synthesized his concept. "It is proposed that the hypothalamus, the anterior thalamic nuclei, the gyrus cinguli, the hippocampus and their interconnections constitute a harmonious mechanism" responsible for emotional experience and emotional expression. These interconnected structures became known as the Papez circuit. This anatomical speculation is remembered largely due to Paul MacLean.

In a sense MacLean had been living in two worlds. On the one hand, his research on temporal lobe epilepsy was electrophysiological. On the other, he was based in Cobb's psychiatry department, the orientation of which was psychoanalytic [4]. When he encountered the concept of Papez, MacLean suddenly saw the possibility of synthesizing biology (neuroanatomy and neurophysiology) and Freudian theory. It was an epiphany.

MacLean devoted himself to Papez's circuit. His first paper on the subject had the subheading "recent developments bearing on the Papez theory of emotion" [5]. In it he summarized Papez's concept, recounted neurophysiologic studies published after the appearance of Papez's article and tried to relate this information to psychosomatic disorders and psychoanalytic theory [5]. Based largely on the animal experiments of others, he modified Papez's anatomic concept by adding to it the amygdala, septum, and prefrontal cortex. He renamed his expanded version of Papez's circuit as the "visceral brain" (the adjective "visceral" was used because it indicates "strong inward feelings") [3].

Physiologists objected to the term "visceral brain" because the word viscera denotes the organs of the body cavities. In response to this criticism MacLean created the term "limbic system" to replace "visceral brain" [6]. He derived this new term from "limbic lobe," Broca's word for much of the medial surface of the cerebral hemisphere. Broca had noticed that in various mammals a sagittal cut between the cerebral hemispheres revealed an oval area of cortex surrounding the corpus callosum. Broca named this region le grand lobe limbique [7]. With his word choice, MacLean took an old, purely anatomic term and converted it to a functional entity, a system.

MacLean's enlarged limbic system "came to subsume a great diversity of neural structures," neocortical, allocortical, and subcortical. It turned out that his limbic structures are involved with functions other than emotion. For example, we now know that the hippocampus is very much involved in memory. We also know that the neocortex is much more involved in emotion than MacLean believed [8, 9]. Although parts of the "limbic system" are implicated in emotional function, experts now believe that the term limbic system is "imprecise and has unwarranted functional (emotional) implications" [10].

The term limbic system has endured in the medical lexicon. Its origin, as noted above, is interesting. However, in a 23-page analysis of the term Kötter and Meyer could find no justification for its continued use [11]. Brodal called for it to be abandoned [12]. Today the term is basically an "anatomical shorthand for areas located in the no-man's land between the hypothalamus and the neocortex" [10]. As a system it does not and never did exist.

When one reads the papers of Papez and MacLean one can sense their affinity. They were imaginative, medical men with wide-ranging interests. Both were knowledgeable to varying extents about medicine, comparative neuroanatomy, brain evolution, and anthropology. Each of them tried to synthesize information from all of these disciplines into a simple scheme to explain the expression and experience of emotions. Their hypotheses intrigued many of us.

9.1 A Note about James W. Papez, MD

In the 1990s I interviewed Eugene Streicher PhD about Dr. Papez (pronounced Pāpes, as one syllable). Streicher was nearing the end of his long career in neurochemistry and administration at the National Institutes of Health. In the 1940s he had been a zoology undergraduate and graduate student of Dr. Papez at Cornell University. The following account is derived from Dr. Streicher's observations unless otherwise specified.

Papez differed from most zoology professors in that he was a neurologist. Although he had made his career as an anatomist, he always continued to do some neurological consulting. When he joined the Cornell faculty, the first two years of instruction of Cornell University Medical College were offered in Ithaca as well as at the main medical facility in Manhattan. Papez taught gross anatomy to medical students at the upstate campus.

When the medical school moved all operations to New York City in 1938, Papez continued to teach anatomy to zoology students in Ithaca. He gave an undergraduate neuroanatomy course. For graduate students he taught seminars on comparative neuroanatomy. To enhance his teaching of neuroanatomy to zoology students he would demonstrate abnormalities on neurological patients.

Papez was often consulted. Patients were referred to him from long distances. Instead of charging a fee for his consultation he would bargain for the patient to commit his brain to

Cornell's collection. Papez also taught a course on physical anthropology in the zoology department. Because of his expertise in this subject, his advice was sought by museum curators about ape and hominid skulls.

Papez was an interesting man. From across a room, he could identify a person by smell alone. He spoke and lectured in a loud whisper. To prepare himself for each academic year Papez would review old, dissected cadavers, reciting aloud the name of each body part. Streicher recalled that Papez "more than made up for his poor lecturing with his effort and interest in teaching." Mettler considered "a certain vagueness" one of Papez's strengths as a teacher [13].

He was available to students on weekdays only. On weekends he and his wife, who was his medical illustrator, put in two solid days of work. No interruptions were allowed.

Streicher stated that Papez was "on the fringe" late in his career, when he asserted that he had found intracellular rickettsia-like organisms in the brains of schizophrenic patients.

Papez's student, Fred Mettler, regarded Papez's major contributions to be his meticulous morphologic observations on the thalamus and his book Comparative Neurology [14]. Papez, however, believed that his most important work was his theoretical formulation on the neuroanatomic substrate of emotion (the Papez circuit) [13].

References

1. P. A. Farley. A theory abandoned but still compelling. *Yale Med* 2008: **Autumn**; 16–17.

2. J. W. Papez. A proposed mechanism of emotion. *Arch Neurol Psychiatry* 1937; **38**: 725–743.

3. P. D. MacLean. Challenges of the Papez heritage. In: K. E. Livingston, O. Hornykiewicz, eds. *Limbic Mechanisms: The Continuing Evolution of the Limbic System Concept.* New York, Plenum Press, 1978; 1–15.

4. R. Laureno. *Raymond Adams: A Life of Mind and Muscle.* New York, Oxford University Press, 2009

5. P. D. MacLean. Psychosomatic disease and the visceral brain; recent developments bearing on the Papez theory of emotion. *Psychosom Med* 1949; **11**: 338–353.

6. P. D. Maclean. Some psychiatric implications of physiological studies on frontotemporal portion of limbic system (visceral brain). *Electroencephalogr Clin Neurophysiol* 1952; **4**: 407–418.

7. P. Broca. Anatomie comparée des circonvolutions cérébrales: le grande lobe limbique et la scissure limbique dans la série des mammifères. *Rev D'Anthropol* 1878; **1**: 385–498.

8. J. LeDoux. *The Deep History of Ourselves: The Four-Billion-Year Story of How We Got Conscious Brains.* New York, Viking, 2019.

9. W. J. H. Nauta. Connection of the frontal lobe with the limbic system. In: L. V. Laitinen, K. E. Livingston, eds. *Surgical Approaches in Psychiatry: Proceedings of the Third International Congress of Psychosurgery.* Baltimore, University Park Press, 1973: 303–314.

10. J. LeDoux. *The Emotional Brain: The Mysterious Underpinnings of Emotional Life.* New York, Simon & Schuster, 1996.

11. R. Kötter, N. Meyer. The limbic system: a review of its empirical foundation. *Behav Brain Res* 1992; 52: 105–127.

12. A. Brodal. *Neurological Anatomy in Relation to Clinical Medicine.* New York, Oxford University Press, 1969.

13. F. A. Mettler. James Wenceslas Papez: August 18, 1883–April 13, 1958. *Anat Rec* 1958; **131**: 279–82.

14. J. W. Papez. *Comparative Neurology: A Manual and Text for the Study of the Nervous System of Vertebrates.* New York, Hafner Publishing Co., 1929.

Chapter 1

Vibration Sensation, the Posterior Columns, and Related Topics

For a century the simple tuning fork has been an essential tool for the clinician. Although we daily test our patients' ability to feel vibration, we don't always remember that there are several issues related to this important part of the neurologic examination. There follows discussion of what we know about sensing vibration, its reception, its pathway in the spinal cord, and its relation to the pathway for sensing position. The relevance of the posterior columns of the spinal cord receives particular attention.

10.1 The Central Pathway

Over a century ago investigators noted the association of posterior column disease and impaired sensation of position and vibration. This correlation led to the concept that the posterior columns of the spinal cord are a pathway for fibers mediating these types of sensation. This concept persists in the twenty-first century [1], perhaps because it appealingly relates methods of bedside sensory testing to a simple anatomic map. In fact, almost all neurologists use this concept in their daily work. However, there is much evidence that the posterior columns are not essential for vibration perception.

The misconception arose from observations on three diseases: tabes dorsalis, subacute combined degeneration of the spinal cord, and Friedreich ataxia. In patients with each of these disorders, position sense and vibration sense were impaired in the lower extremities; in all three diseases there was degeneration of the posterior columns at autopsy. This apparent clinicopathologic pattern was initially considered meaning-ful. However, more thorough neuropathologic observations of these diseases has led to reevaluation.

In tabes dorsalis, Castro showed that posterior column degeneration was caused by the primary lesion, syphilitic inflammation in the dorsal roots of the spinal cord [2]. The radicular disease fully explains the loss of vibration and position sense. There is no need to invoke the secondary posterior column degeneration as the cause.

Unlike tabes, the pathology of subacute combined degeneration is not secondary to disease outside the spinal cord. The lesions are primary to the posterior and lateral columns. The misconception that the posterior column lesions explained the loss of vibration sense came from assuming that the lateral column disease was not relevant, perhaps because other functions for the lateral columns had already been recognized. The lateral columns, however, are not a simple system. They are a region that various systems traverse. It was possible that disease in the lateral columns was the cause of the impaired ability to sense vibration. Furthermore, in vitamin B12 deficiency peripheral neuropathy coexists with the spinal cord disease. The polyneuropathy could easily account for some of the loss of vibration sense. With multifocal lesions of spinal cord and peripheral nerve, one cannot conclude that the posterior column disease is solely or even partially responsible for the loss of vibration sense.

In Friedreich ataxia many parts of the nervous system also degenerate. As opposed to vitamin B12 deficiency, in which there is subacute combined degeneration of **regions**, in Friedreich ataxia, there is degeneration of multiple neural **systems**. The pathology includes degeneration of the posterior columns, corticospinal tracts, spinocerebellar tracts, and posterior roots. Other systems can be affected. In the presence of multifocal disease, one cannot conclude that the posterior column abnormality is the cause of the impaired sensing of vibration in Friedreich ataxia. The root atrophy or disease in some other part of the spinal cord could be responsible.

More careful analysis of these three classical diseases is not the only evidence that throws into question the relationship between posterior column disease and loss of vibration sense. Additional information has emerged from studies of syringomyelia and observations on the effects of cordotomy.

In one of his cases of syringomyelia, Netsky found that loss of vibration sense correlated with extension of the cavity into the medial part of the lateral funiculus. There was no involvement of the posterior columns [3]. In humans, Cook and Browder unilaterally severed the dorsal column to try to relieve limb pain; vibration sensing was not affected [4]. Others have made the same observation [5]. Furthermore, section of the dorsal columns in monkeys who had been trained to respond to vibration, did not impair the animals' ability to detect vibration [6].

If the posterior columns are not important for vibration sense, what pathway in the lateral columns could contribute to vibration sensing? Nathan and Smith studied the spinal cords of 43 cancer patients in whom spinothalamic cordotomy had been performed to treat pain [7]. Although this surgery caused only limited corticospinal tract damage, ascending Wallerian degeneration could be traced through the pyramids and as far as the internal capsule in these patients. This was evidence that afferent fibers are admixed in the corticospinal tract! These fibers are a potential lateral column path for information useful for vibration detection [7]. It is not known whether the lateral column fibers related to the sensing of vibration ascend in one path or more. From one clinicopathologic case, it has been suggested that the dorsal spinocerebellar tract carries information used for sensing position and vibration [8].

Incorrect notions about the posterior columns persist, in part because vibration and position sense are often impaired together. They are thought of as a pair. This combination of deficits occurs in disease of the peripheral nerve in which large, myelinated fibers are affected out of proportion to small, unmyelinated fibers. It also occurs in lesions which spare the spinothalamic tract but damage the medial lemniscus. An appropriately placed lesion in the thalamus can also cause this pattern of sensory loss [9].

One can see the appeal of the notion, a simple path for vibration/position sense from nerve roots through the dorsal columns to the medical lemniscus. The data, however, do not support this neat picture. Evolution has not provided us with distinct pathways for "different qualities (analogous to the differently coloured wires of an electrical circuit)" [10].

That there is no simple relationship between the sensing of vibration and position sense is evident. Thalamic lesions can cause dissociation of deficits in these abilities [11]. Lesions of the cerebral cortex can impair the sensation of position but do not affect vibration sensation [12]. It seems that perception of vibration requires no brain rostral to the thalamus. Furthermore, joint position sense and vibration sense are believed to depend on different receptors [9].

10.2 The Periphery

Considerable disagreement has marked the literature about where vibratory stimuli are received in the periphery. One controversy has centered on whether the vibration is detected in the skin or in the deeper tissue [13, 14]. Whether sensing vibration is an independent sense or whether it is the product of other senses has been another subject of debate.

Early studies indicated that vibration sensation was mediated by deeper receptors in subcutaneous tissue, fascia, muscles, tendons, and periosteum. Later investigators believed that vibration was received by tactile receptors in the skin alone.

The idea that vibration sensation was accomplished through both deep and cutaneous receptors has prevailed among clinical neurologists. Through anesthetized skin, Cosh found residual but reduced vibration sensing. He also anesthetized subcutaneous tissue sparing the skin. Again, vibration sensing was reduced but persistent. The deep tissues were more sensitive to vibration, but vibration could be detected by either skin or deeper structures [13].

Neurologists test vibration and comment on it separately from sensation of pain, light touch, and temperature. Often, they use the term "vibration sense" in referring to their findings. This terminology can suggest that there is a separate vibratory sense. This notion is consistent with the idea that vibration is essentially a distance sense like hearing and is thus unlike other senses. Study of retrogasserian neurectomy patients led Brown and Yacorzynsaki to the conclusion that sensing vibration is unrelated to other somatic senses [14].

Certainly, responsiveness to vibration is important throughout the animal kingdom. Vibration sensing is used for detecting prey and avoiding predators. Vibration is also used for communication [15]. In humans, this phylogenetically ancient vibration sensing is accomplished in the phylogenetically old thalamus; the telencephalon is not involved. Sensing vibration is so pervasive in the animal kingdom that we cannot be surprised if the function, instead of being the result of a distinct sense, can be accomplished in different ways and by different paths.

"The question as to whether there is a separate vibratory sense is really part of a wider question" [16]. When we speak of one modality of sensation or another, the term "modality" could be misleading if it is taken to imply a separateness of different sensations. "The vocabulary of even the most articulate is clearly inadequate to describe the innumerable gradations of sensation" [16], which do not fit into the arbitrary categories of our neurological examination or our classification of sensations. The term modality is problematic in implying anatomical and physiological distinctness, which is not always valid [16].

10.3 Conclusion and Final Comments

1. Vibration sense is not affected by disease in the posterior columns of the spinal cord.
2. Lateral column damage can interfere with vibration sensation.
3. Loss of sensation of vibration and position can occur together, for example, in lesions of the medial lemniscus.
4. Abnormality of sensation of vibration and position can occur separately. The dissociation can be caused by anatomic separation of function, for example, in the

thalamus. Relative dissociation can be due to the tendency of a given disease to affect one function more than another.

5. Vibration sensation is the detection of repetitive tactile and/or pressure variations. Thus, vibratory sense, as we test it with a tuning fork, is analogous to flicker in visual perception [17, 18].

6. Vibration sensing is phylogenetically ancient. Its most rostral representation is in the thalamus. That it is a very basic form of sensation is consistent with it not being perceived in the cerebral cortex. We cannot be surprised if vibration is not sensed by a simple dedicated system.

References

1. H. Blumenfeld. *Neuroanatomy Through Clinical Cases*. Sunderland, Sinauer Associates, 2010.

2. R. Laureno. *Foundations for Clinical Neurology*. New York, Oxford University Press, 2017.

3. M. G. Netsky. Syringomyelia; a clinicopathologic study. *AMA Arch Neurol Psychiatry* 1953; **70**: 741–777.

4. W. Cook, E. J. Browder. Function of posterior columns in man. *Arch Neurol* 1965; **12**: 72–79.

5. P. D. Wall, W. Noordenbos. Sensory functions which remain in man after complete transection of dorsal columns. *Brain* 1977; **100**: 641–653.

6. P. D. Wall. The sensory and motor role of impulses travelling in the dorsal columns towards cerebral cortex. *Brain* 1970; **93**: 505–524.

7. P. W. Nathan, M. C. Smith. Spino-cortical fibres in man. *J Neurol Neurosurg Psychiatry* 1955; **18**: 181–190.

8. E. D. Ross, J. B. Kirkpatrick, A. C. Lastimosa. Position and vibration sensations: functions of the dorsal spinocerebellar tracts? *Ann Neurol* 1979; **5**: 171–176.

9. S. Gilman. Joint position sense and vibration sense: anatomical organisation and assessment. *J Neurol Neurosurg Psychiatry* 2002; **73**: 473–477.

10. R. Melzack, P. D. Wall. On the nature of cutaneous sensory mechanisms. *Brain* 1962; **85**: 331–356.

11. R. L. Sacco, J. A. Bello, R. Traub et al. Selective proprioceptive loss from a thalamic lacunar stroke. *Stroke* 1987; **18**: 1160–1163.

12. R. T. Ross. Dissociated loss of vibration, joint position and discriminatory tactile senses in disease of spinal cord and brain. *Can J Neurol Sci* 1991; **18**: 312–320.

13. J. A. Cosh. Studies on the nature of vibration sense. *Clin Sci* 1953; **12**: 131–151.

14. M. Brown, G. K. Yacorzynski. Studies of the sensation of vibration: II. Vibration sensibility in the face following retrogasserian neurectomy. *Arch Neurol Psychiatry* 1942; **47**: 813–820.

15. E. A. van der Zee. The biology of vibration. In: J. Rittweger, ed. *Manual of Vibration Exercise and Vibration Therapy*. Cham, Springer Nature, 2020; 23–38.

16. D. B. Calne, C. A. Pallis. Vibratory sense: a critical review. *Brain* 1966; **89**: 723–746.

17. J. C. Fox, W. W. Klemperer. Vibratory sensibility: a quantitative study of its thresholds in nervous disorders. *Arch Neurol Psychiatry* 1942; **48**: 622–645.

18. F. A. Geldard. The perception of mechanical vibration: I. History of a controversy. *J Gen Psychology* 1940; **22**: 243–269.

Transneuronal Effects

A brain or spinal cord lesion can cause effects distant from the disease site. The remote manifestation can be physiologic (e.g., in an acute stroke) or pathoanatomic (e.g., in an old stroke). In either case it is via a transneuronal connection that the distant effect is mediated.

Acute clinical changes are primarily detected after stroke or spinal cord injury. For example, with acute stroke there can be initial hypotonia and hyporeflexia on the plegic side. That is to say, there is dysfunction of the stretch reflexes although their anatomic circuitry is intact. Similar distant effects occur in spinal cord injury (spinal shock). Von Monakow created the word "diaschisis" to encompass such acute, typically transient phenomena.

To rephrase, diaschisis is the "sudden inhibition of function produced by an acute focal disturbance in an anatomically intact portion of the brain remote from the original seat of injury but anatomically connected with it through fiber tracts" [1].

Over time this term was applied to distant physiologic abnormalities whether or not clinical symptoms or signs were evident. One example is crossed cerebellar hypometabolism after infarction in the middle cerebral artery distribution. The altered metabolism is inferred from decreased cerebellar blood flow which can be shown by single photon emission computed tomography, MR perfusion imaging, or other methods [2].

In addition to these clinical and physiologic distant effects, there can be pathological effects distant from a primary lesion. Specifically, a stroke can result over time in focal atrophy far from the lesion itself. This transneuronal atrophy can occur in the anterograde or retrograde direction. Anterograde atrophy is due to deafferentation of innervated cells. Retrograde atrophy is due to reaction in the neuron cell body such as that which develops following axon section [3]. The cerebro-cerebellar system and the visual system illustrate these phenomena.

Anterograde transneuronal atrophy is a product of deafferentation (Table 11.1). Loss of afferent input from the descending corticopontine pathway fibers can result in primary transneuronal atrophy of ipsilateral pontine nuclei and secondary transneuronal atrophy in the contralateral cerebellar cortex [4]. Although some have referred to this crossed cerebellar atrophy as crossed cerebellar "diaschisis," I prefer the traditional usage, reserving "diaschisis" for acute, clinical manifestations. Crossed atrophy appears more often when the primary lesion affects the developing brain. However, crossed atrophy sometimes develops after the adult brain is damaged [5]. The neurologist detects no cerebellar manifestation of this atrophy; the hemiparesis of extensive middle cerebral artery territory infarction masks any cerebellar finding.

In the visual system, anterograde transneuronal degeneration also can occur at great distance from the primary lesion. Retinal or optic nerve damage can result in primary anterograde atrophy in the cells of the appropriate layers of the lateral geniculate nuclei.

Table 11.1 Anterograde transneuronal atrophy

System	Visual	Cerebro-cerebellar
Disease site	Anterior visual system	Upper motor neurons
Primary atrophy	Lateral geniculate nuclei	Pontine nuclei
Secondary atrophy	Occipital cortex	Cerebellar cortex

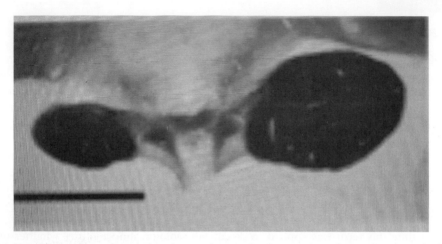

Figure 11.1 Retrograde transneuronal optic tract degeneration in a monkey whose striate cortex had been removed eleven and a half years earlier. Weil myelin stain. (Reproduced by permission from A. Cowey, I. Alexander, P. Stoerig. Transneuronal retrograde degeneration of retinal ganglion cells and optic tract in hemianopic monkeys and humans. Brain 2011; 134: 2149–2157.)

Similarly, enucleation of either eye eventually causes atrophy in the lateral geniculate nucleus bilaterally [6]. Secondary anterograde transneuronal atrophy of the visual cortex occurs after enucleation and other anterior visual pathway lesions. Modern in vivo study has confirmed that secondary anterograde degeneration can occur after optic neuritis. Specifically, quantitative measurement of the optic radiations by MRI reveals the effect of the disease in the anterior visual pathway [7] .

Traditional pathological methods have been used to document retrograde transneuronal atrophy [8]. In humans who have undergone removal of or infarction of visual cortex, one finds primary retrograde transneuronal atrophy of the ipsilateral lateral geniculate nucleus and secondary transneuronal atrophy of both optic nerves [6] and tracts [9]. This retrograde transneuronal degeneration has been replicated in monkeys [9] (Figure 11.1). It can be seen in humans by MRI scanning [9]. Optical coherence tomography shows that thinning of the human retinal nerve fiber layer gradually develops over years after occipital injury [10].

It is primarily in the visual system that modern clinical methods have been successful in demonstrating retrograde transneuronal atrophy. However, retrograde transneuronal atrophy certainly occurs in other "neuronally closed" systems. For example, experimental lesioning in limbic-diencephalic circuitry clearly shows the same phenomenon [3]. In the human, hemicerebellectomy in childhood has been shown to result in retrograde transneuronal atrophy in the contralateral corticopontine tract [7].

A special form of transneuronal atrophy occurs in the inferior olivary nucleus. Seemingly unique is the tendency of this nucleus to becomes hypertrophic before it atrophies. The afferent supply of the inferior olive originates in the dentate nucleus, whose fibers project across to synapse in the red nucleus on the opposite side of the midbrain. The red nucleus projects to the ipsilateral inferior olive via the central tegmental tract. When the lesion is in the central tegmental tract there is primary anterograde degeneration in the inferior olivary nucleus. When the lesion is in the dentatorubral projection or the cerebellum itself there can be secondary anterograde olivary degeneration.

MRI changes can be observed sequentially after damage to the dentatorubral or central tegmental tract [11]. The inferior olive shows increased signal on T_2 weighted or flair images by six months. Enlargement of the inferior olive typically appears by a year after the injury. The olivary hypertrophy lasts for a few years. Postmortem study shows vacuolization of the neuronal cytoplasm. Eventually the inferior olive shrinks. Although the inferior olive becomes atrophic, the increased MRI signal persists. At no time during this sequence of changes is there restricted diffusion or enhancement with gadolinium.

Transneuronal atrophy is more than a pathological curiosity. It carries implications for students of neurologic disease beyond the few examples given. Secondary transneuronal degeneration "must be a commonly occurring process in many regions of cerebral cortex after stroke" and other nervous system lesions [12].

These phenomena demonstrate that systems of neurons have trophic effects directly on their target neurons and on secondarily connected neurons. The mechanism of central nervous system trophism is unknown. The transneuronal effect seems to be more complex than a simple transsynaptic phenomenon because experimental study shows that there is chemical communication along neuronal chains above and beyond that of transmitter release and electrical messaging [13].

11.1 Final Comments

1. Central nervous system lesions have transneuronal distant effects.
2. Acute transneuronal change (diaschisis) is transient and physiologic and often clinically manifest. Neurologists are accustomed to such phenomena.
3. Chronic transneuronal effects are pathoanatomic, progressive, and asymptomatic. This atrophy is well illustrated by the cerebello-cerebral connections and by the visual system. Because this atrophy can be seen on brain MRI scans, it is important for neurologists to recognize the phenomenon.
4. One lesion can but does not necessarily cause both acute and chronic transneuronal effects.
5. Anterograde and retrograde transneuronal atrophy has been useful for tracing neuroanatomic connections after experimental lesioning and in human disease.
6. Retrograde and anterograde transneuronal interactions occur in normal brains [14, 15].
7. Transneuronal transfer of radioactive materials has become a useful tool for tracing normal anatomic connections [14, 15].

References

1. D. K. Nguyen, M. I. Botez. Diaschisis and neurobehavior. *Can J Neurol Sci* 1998; **25**: 5–12.

2. D. D. M. Lin, J. T. Kleinman, R. J. Wityk et al. Crossed cerebellar diaschisis in acute stroke detected by dynamic susceptibility contrast MR perfusion imaging. *AJNR Am J Neuroradiol* 2009; **30**: 710–715.

3. W. M. Cowan. Anterograde and retrograde transneuronal degeneration in the central and peripheral nervous system. In: W. J. H. Nauta, S. O. E. Ebbesson, eds. *Contemporary Research Methods in Neuroanatomy*. New York, Springer, 1970; 217–251.

4. A. M. Strefling, H. Urich. Crossed cerebellar atrophy: an old problem revisited. *Acta Neuropathol* 1982; **57**: 197–202.

5. M. Baudrimont, F. Gray, V. Meininger et al. [Crossed cerebellar atrophy following hemispheric lesions occurring in adulthood]. [French]. *Rev Neurol (Paris)* 1983; **139**: 485–495.

6. R. M. Beatty, A. A. Sadun, L. Smith et al. Direct demonstration of transsynaptic degeneration in the human visual system: a comparison of retrograde and anterograde changes. *J Neurol Neurosurg Psychiatry* 1982; **45**: 143–146.

7. C. Tur, O. Goodkin, D. R. Altmann et al. Longitudinal evidence for anterograde trans-synaptic degeneration after optic neuritis. *Brain* 2016; **139**: 816–828.

8. M. C. Smith. Histological findings after hemicerebellectomy in man: anterograde, retrograde and transneuronal degeneration. *Brain Res* 1975; **95**: 423–442.

9. A. Cowey, I. Alexander, P. Stoerig. Transneuronal retrograde degeneration of retinal ganglion cells and optic tract in hemianopic monkeys and humans. *Brain* 2011; **134**: 2149–2157.

10. P. Jindahra, A. Petrie, G. T. Plant. The time course of retrograde trans-synaptic degeneration following occipital lobe damage in humans. *Brain* 2012; **135**: 534–541.

11. H. Wang, Y. Wang, R. Wang et al. Hypertrophic olivary degeneration: a comprehensive review focusing on etiology. *Brain Res* 2019; **1718**: 53–63.

12. J. C. Horton, E. T. Hedley-Whyte. Mapping of cytochrome oxidase patches and ocular dominance columns in human visual cortex. *Philos Trans R Soc Lond B Biol Sci* 1984; **304**: 255–272.

13. B. Grafstein, R. Laureno. Transport of radioactivity from eye to visual cortex in the mouse. *Exp Neurol* 1973; **39**: 44–57.

14. H. D. Kourouyan, J. C. Horton. Transneuronal retinal input to the primate Edinger-Westphal nucleus. *J Comp Neurol* 1997; **381**: 68–80.

15. R. M. Kelly, P. L. Strick. Rabies as a transneuronal tracer of circuits in the central nervous system. *J Neurosci Methods* 2000; **103**: 63–71.

Spinal Nerve Roots

To diagnose and manage radiculopathy, neurologists must know several points of anatomy. First, they must remember the numeration of the vertebrae, the numbering of the nerve roots, and their relationship. Secondly, they must understand that the dorsal root ganglia (DRG) lie outside of the spinal canal and that their neurons have two axonal processes. In addition, neurologists should be aware that the angulation of the intervertebral foramina in the cervical spine differs from that in the lumbar spine. Furthermore, they must be aware that the territory supplied by a sensory or a motor nerve root varies from one person to another. Finally, they must remember that dermatomes overlap extensively.

Numeration of vertebral bodies and spinal nerve roots do not follow a consistent pattern. By convention, a thoracic or lumbar nerve root exits the spinal canal below the vertebral body of the same number. However, a cervical root exits the spinal canal above the vertebra with the same number. (The C8 root is an exception; it exits above the T1 vertebra [1].)

In the cervical region, the nerve roots exit the spinal canal directly without descending to another level. As a result, a C4–C5 disc herniation or foraminal stenosis affects a C5 root. In the lumbar region, however, the nerve roots do not exit laterally. They pass downward for several segments before reaching the vertebral level with the matching number. As a result of this vertical course, the L5 root, for example, can be affected at many vertebral and disc levels before exiting the spinal canal. The common occurrence is for a lateral disc herniation at L4–L5 to affect the descending L5 nerve root well before it exits at the L5 S1 foramen. Thus, a 4–5-disc herniation is associated with a root 5 radiculopathy in both the cervical and lumbar regions. This is not a meaningful "pattern." It is simply the consequence of the numbering convention and the pathoanatomy described above (Table 12.1).

In radiculopathies, the differences between the motor and sensory axons underlie the differences in the electrophysiologic effects on motor and sensory fibers. The motor fibers of the ventral root arise from monopolar neurons in the anterior horn of the spinal cord. When the motor roots are compromised to the extent that there is axonal degeneration, the peripheral nerve fibers, which are in direct continuity, also degenerate. Thus, in ventral

Table 12.1 Radiculopathy and anatomy

CERVICAL vs LUMBAR COMPARISON		
C5	Root	L5
C4 C5	Typical disc herniation	L4 L5
C4 C5	Exit foramen	L5 S1

root compromise, abnormalities of motor nerve conduction and electromyography can accompany the neurologic symptoms and signs.

The dorsal root differs fundamentally. Its axons arise outside of the spinal cord in the DRG. Each dorsal root ganglion neuron has two processes, one projecting to the spinal cord and one projecting to the periphery. Because the dorsal root ganglia lie in the midzone of the intervertebral foramen, they are distal to the typical spondylotic pathology. Thus, a ganglion and its peripheral process are unaffected by spondylotic compromise of the central process. These facts explain why sensory conduction studies in the limbs are normal when there are sensory symptoms or signs due to compression or irritation of a dorsal root ganglion's central process.

Because magnetic resonance imaging (MRI) is a major tool for the diagnosis of spondylosis and radiculopathy, it is important to be aware of an anatomical difference between the cervical and lumbar vertebral anatomy. In the lumbar region, the nerve roots exit laterally with no anterior or posterior angulation. Because of this anatomic arrangement, sagittal MRI shows superb cross-sectional images of the lumbar inter-vertebral foramina (Figure 12.1). These images are excellent for the diagnosis of foraminal stenosis. The anatomy differs in the cervical region where the intervertebral foramina are angulated anteriorly. For two reasons this obliquity prevents sagittal MRI slices from showing ideal cross-sectional images of the cervical foramina. First of all, the cervical foramina will look more narrow than they are because the plane of the imaging slice is parallel to the midline, not perpendicular to the foramina. Secondly, the angulation of the foramen to the imaging plane results in blending of the signal of bone, soft tissue, and nerve root. In other words, the nerve root cannot always be well distinguished from the surrounding tissue.

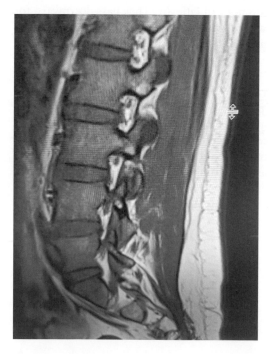

Figure 12.1 Normal lumbar MRI scan. This paracentral slice demonstrates the intervertebral foramina very well because the roots exit nearly perpendicular to the sagittal plane. For some foramina, the oval shape will be better seen on an adjacent sagittal slice.

One important aspect of nerve root anatomy is variability. The segmental innervation of human muscle varies from individual to individual. Thage stimulated individual nerve roots while recording action potentials from lower extremity muscles [2]. When he stimulated L5 and S1 roots in eight patients he found that the extensor digitorum brevis was innervated by L5 but not S1 in two patients, innervated by S1 but not L5 in two patients, by both in three patients, and by neither in one patient. Sensory innervation is similarly variable. Buchthal stimulated fingers 1 to 5 and recorded potentials in the spinal nerves. The cutaneous fibers of digit 5 connected as often to the C8 as to both C7 and C8. Digits 1 and 2 connected as often to C7 as to C6 [3].

A final anatomic point is that dermatomes overlap. In monkeys, Sherrington cut a series of contiguous nerve roots above and below a given preserved nerve root. From the zone of remaining sensibility, he determined the dermatome of the preserved nerve root. By leaving different nerve roots intact in different animals, he showed that the dermatomes of adjacent spinal nerves overlap considerably [4]. Foerster repeated Sherrington's experiments in humans. (He was sectioning nerve roots to relieve chronic pain.) He found that the overlap of dermatomes is so extensive that section of a single root caused no loss of sensation [4].

12.1 Conclusions

1. The dorsal root ganglia is usually distal to the compression of nerve roots due to spondylosis or disc herniation.
2. Since spondylotic pathology is typically proximal to the dorsal root ganglion their axons to the periphery are unaffected by it. Hence, sensory nerve conduction studies are normal in symptomatic radiculopathy.
3. Due to the regional difference in the angulation of the intervertebral foramina, sagittal MRI images are much better for demonstrating stenosis of a lumbar intervertebral foramen than they are for showing stenosis of a cervical foramen.
4. The myotome and dermatome vary among individuals. As a result, the clinical manifestations of compression of a given nerve root will vary from one patient to another.

References

1. W. W. Campbell, R. J. Barohn. *DeJong's The Neurologic Examination.* Philadelphia, Wolters Kluwer, 2019.

2. O. Thage. The myotomes L2–S2 in man. *Acta Neurol Scand Suppl* 1965; **13**: 241–243.

3. Y. Inouye, F. Buchthal. Segmental sensory innervation determined by potentials recorded from cervical spinal nerves. *Brain* 1977; **100**: 731–748.

4. C. S. Sherrington. Experiments in examination of the peripheral distribution of the fibres of the posterior roots of some spinal nerves. *Philos Trans R Soc London B* Part I 1893; **184**: 641–763, Part II 1898: **190**: 45–186.

5. O. Foerster. The dermatomes in man. *Brain* 1933; **56**: 1–39.

Ischemic Hypoxic Encephalopathy

Ischemic hypoxic encephalopathy comprises many clinico-pathologic varieties. Gray matter or white matter can be primarily affected. The distribution of brain injury can be determined by regional vulnerability or vascular supply. Although brain damage is usually acute, it can be delayed. These types of encephalopathy are not mutually exclusive. Regardless of type they tend to be symmetric. Patients with these encephalopathies not only provide doctors challenges in clinical management, they also can involve the physician and the hospital in legal proceedings, both civil and criminal.

In gray matter, cell types and brain territories differ in vulnerability to ischemia hypoxia. Furthermore, regional susceptibility varies from one person to another. For example, cerebral cortex and striatum are more vulnerable than the thalamus in most people. However, there are patients in whom the thalamus is much more affected than the striatum. Ischemic cell change occurs more in neurons than in glial cells. However, not all neurons are equally sensitive. Especially vulnerable are pyramidal cells, Purkinje cells, and striatal neurons.

In the cerebral mantle, ischemia hypoxia affects both the vast neocortex and the hippocampus (archicortex). In the hippocampus, neuronal vulnerability varies from one sector to another. The Vogts believed that the hippocampus is constitutionally vulnerable to ischemia hypoxia. Spielmeyer disagreed. He contended that the particular susceptibility of the hippocampus is due to a poor blood supply rather than to an innate sensitivity of the tissue. Some continue to prefer Vogts' concept of innate sensitivity [1]. The ideas of these pathologists were derived from the study of hippocampal sclerosis in epileptics and others.

In our era, we commonly see ischemic hypoxic injury of the hippocampus in patients who have suffered cardiac arrest. As a rule, the injury is more or less symmetric (Figure 13.1 and Figure 1.1). Occasionally, however, the hippocampal damage is strikingly asymmetric (Figure 13.2). Inherent vulnerability of hippocampal tissue is unlikely to account for such asymmetry. Absence of hippocampal ischemia on one side is likely due to a better ipsilateral arterial supply. (It is well known that patterns of arterial supply can vary from one side of the brain to the other.) Of course, it is possible that there is some truth to both theories, that of the Vogts and that of Spielmeyer. However, asymmetric MRI scans such as this one show that there certainly can be an important vascular factor in hippocampal vulnerability.

Carbon monoxide poisoning is a special form of ischemic hypoxic encephalopathy in which selective vulnerability is conspicuous. Carbon monoxide preferentially binds to hemoglobin thereby preventing it from carrying oxygen to the brain. This "anemic" anoxia (i.e., no red blood cells able to bind oxygen) is associated with disproportionate damage to the globus pallidus. Interestingly, experimental carbon monoxide poisoning reproduces the globus pallidus lesions only when hypotension is superimposed [2].

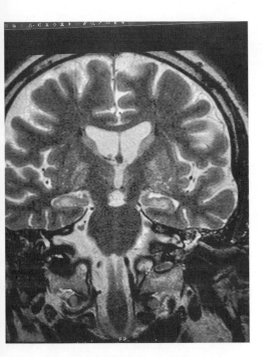

Figure 13.1 Increased signal in the hippocampi due to symmetric ischemic anoxic injury.

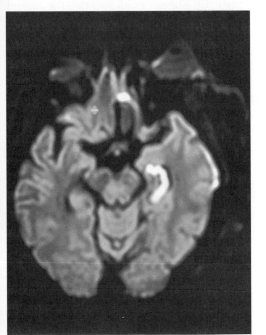

Figure 13.2 Unilateral ischemic hypoxic injury of hippocampus.

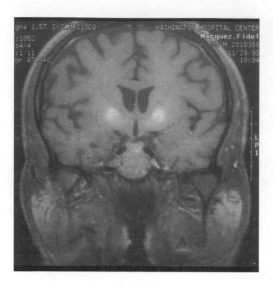

Figure 13.3 Globus pallidus ischemic hypoxic injury caused by hypotension in a patient whose hematocrit was 7. This image resembles the pattern of injury seen in carbon monoxide poisoning.

Combined ischemia hypoxia can occasionally cause identical lesions in the absence of carbon monoxide exposure or profound anemia. Narcotic overdosage and cardiac arrest following myocardial infarction are examples (Figure 13.3). Similar globus pallidus lesions occur in rare survivors of cyanide poisoning, in which the anoxia is "histotoxic" (i.e., the brain tissue is prevented from using oxygen bound to hemoglobin). In sum, prominent symmetric globus pallidus necrosis is characteristic of, but not at all specific, for carbon monoxide poisoning.

In both of these examples of selective vulnerability, the sensitivity of the hippocampus in many patients and the selective vulnerability of the globus pallidus in selected patients, arterial hypotension is essential. The importance of blood flow is evident when one compares the neuropathologic effects of relatively isolated hypoxemia to those of ischemia without hypoxemia. There is little documentation of neuronal change in anoxia without severe hypotension [3]. However, severe hypotension without hypoxemia is enough to cause brain injury, for example, border zone infarction.

Delayed clinical deterioration has occurred days after the initial neurologic recovery in some of the carbon monoxide poisoned patients with bilateral globus pallidus lesions. In other patients, delayed encephalopathy after carbon monoxide poisoning has been associated with symmetric leukoencephalopathy. In some cases, globus pallidus disease and cerebral white matter disease develop in the same patient [4, 5]. Delayed leukoencephalopathy can occur in ischemic hypoxic insults other than carbon monoxide poisoning.

Why is delayed anoxic encephalopathy not uncommon in carbon monoxide poisoning but infrequently observed following resuscitation from cardiac arrest? Differences between these forms of ischemia hypoxia may be pertinent. For example, the former insult is typically longer lasting, whereas the latter is relatively brief if the patient is to survive. Furthermore, delayed neurologic deterioration may not be clinically detectable in a patient who has been comatose ever since the cardiac arrest.

In sum, ischemic hypoxic encephalopathy can be manifest by varied clinical syndromes and neuropathologic features. Duration of ischemia and type of hypoxemia can be factors in these variations. Furthermore, brains differ in their regional vulnerability and in their arterial supply. The importance of poor perfusion cannot be overstated.

13.1 Social and Legal Topics

Pulse oximetry helps prevent hypoxic brain injury during general anesthesia. Exactly when did it become a standard practice to use this simple monitoring device in the operating room? Case 1 brought this subject to my attention.

Case 1

In 1987, a 35-year-old woman was placed under general anesthesia for a therapeutic abortion. The nurse anesthetist had placed the endotracheal tube into the esophagus instead of the trachea. The patient did not regain consciousness after the procedure. Coma evolved into a vegetative state which persisted. The family sued for damages. The anesthesiology group settled out of court. The hospital was alleged to be negligent in not having had pulse oximetry equipment available in all operating rooms. The jury determined that the hospital was negligent and awarded the patient millions of dollars.

The plaintiff's lawyer alleged that the hospital was negligent because the American Society of Anesthesiologists' Standards for Basic Intra-Operative Monitoring, adopted in 1986, one year before the patient's procedure, "encourage" the use of pulse oximetry [6]. Professional acceptance of pulse oximetry was in flux. In 1988, the year following the trial, an editorial in Anesthesiology stated that pulse oximetry "should become part of the routine monitoring of all patients undergoing general anesthesia" [7]. In 1989, another editorial looked forward to a clinical trial which would determine whether pulse oximetry affected outcomes [6]. In other words, the jury in Case 1 had decided that use of a new technology was required before it had been proven beneficial. There is no doubt that verdicts such as this one hasten the adoption of new standards.

In the second half of the twentieth century, improved methods of resuscitation and mechanical ventilation allowed many patients to survive cardiac arrest. In this context, doctors developed the concept of "brain death." In other words, it was decided that a person with a beating heart could be declared dead by neurological criteria. With experience neurologists developed, revised and re-revised neurologic and neurodiagnostic guidelines for such patients. After half a century the experts remain concerned about a lack of uniformity in criteria [8].

Mechanical ventilators also sustain terribly brain damaged patients, who are not dead by neurological criteria. These patients never emerge from a vegetative state or a state of profound dementia. The survival of these "brain dead" and vegetative patients can put great stress on families, clinicians, medical institutions, and the entire social structure.

In case two the issue was whether presumptive brain death should mitigate a charge of murder against a lay person. A more common problem has been the attempt of killers to avoid the homicide charge because a hospital had disconnected a victim from a ventilator after the declaration of "brain death." The criminal's position in such cases has been that the

Case 2

After three months of hospitalization for cardiac amyloidosis an 84-year-old woman suffered cardiac arrest. She was successfully resuscitated and transferred to an intensive care unit. She did not awaken. In view of her severe disease, the intensivist approached the family about removing the patient from the respirator and decreasing other medical efforts.

The family was bitterly divided, unable to agree on a plan. Some of her children felt that her illness had already caused her many months of suffering, that she had suffered enough. Others viewed the situation differently. They felt that she had been comatose for only a day or two. They viewed the coma as a very new development from which she needed time to awaken.

In this context I was consulted one Friday evening. The patient could not tolerate the apnea test. Thus, full evaluation of brainstem function could not be made. I suggested a nuclear brain scan. Expecting there to be no evidence of cerebral flow, I thought that the information might help the family understand the hopelessness of the brain injury. The nuclear study could not be performed immediately on the weekend.

Late the following night her 29-year-old grandson came to visit. A sudden change in the electrocardiogram alerted nurses who rushed to investigate. They found a butcher knife stuck in the patient's chest. She was taken for emergency surgery but died one and a half hours later. The grandson surrendered himself to the police. The stabbing was widely viewed as a mercy killing.

When two detectives came to discuss the case with me, they explained that they had shown the medical records to another neurologist, who believed the patient to have been "brain dead" at the time of my examination. Since the grandmother was "dead" when he stabbed her, the detectives implied that the prisoner could not have killed her. I explained that the patient had been awaiting another study, that she had never been declared dead. In the end the police did not charge the grandson with homicide. Instead, they charged him with desecrating a corpse.

patient, with a beating heart, had been alive until the medical staff had taken away the respirator, that is to say, the patient had been killed by medical personnel. The problem of homicide and "brain dead" patients has been contentious to the extent that the legislatures and courts have disagreed about the subject [9].

Case 3

After resuscitation from cardiac arrest, a woman was left in a vegetative state. A mechanical ventilator was needed for adequate respiration. After many months she remained in a vegetative state. She continued to need a respirator. Still on a ventilator, she was transferred from the intensive care unit to a bed on an internal medicine ward.

Eventually her medical insurance company refused to accept responsibility for further hospital and physician bills. The position of the insurer was that the patient no longer needed hospitalization, that she could be transferred to a chronic care facility. The hospital asked the patient's husband to enroll her in Medicaid (a government program which pays for chronic care of patients without resources). The husband refused, believing that the patient was receiving better care in the hospital than she would elsewhere.

After nearly three years she remained both vegetative and ventilator dependent. The husband continued to refuse to apply for Medicaid. Nursing facilities would not accept her without her having insurance. The hospital proceeded to petition the Commission on Mental Health, alleging that the patient was mentally ill and a danger to herself and others. The patient's attorney stated that the hospital was claiming mental illness in order to "kick the patient out of the hospital" to a government facility. After hearing testimony from several neurologists and psychiatrists the commission ruled that her "chronic organic brain syndrome" made her a danger to herself (i.e., mentally ill) and that she be committed to a skilled nursing facility at government expense.

In cases 2 and 3, governmental agencies contorted themselves to do what they thought was right. Today case 3 would not have lingered for years. Nowadays there are in place various discharge procedures to deal with noncompliant families. For example, when a spouse is noncompliant, a hospital can go to court to seek a Guardian and Conservator who can, in turn, submit a Medicaid application. As for case 2, most hospitals do not require visitors to go through metal detectors. Thus, it is still possible for a distraught relative to bring a weapon into a hospital to terminate a patient's existence.

References

1. W. W. Boling, S. Ettl, K. Sano. Professor Uchimura, Ammon's horn sclerosis, and the German influence on Japanese neuroscience. *J Hist Neurosci* 2010; **19**: 182–194.

2. R. Okeda, N. Funata, S. J. Song et al. Comparative study on pathogenesis of selective cerebral lesions in carbon monoxide poisoning and nitrogen hypoxia in cats. *Acta Neuropathol* 1982; **56**: 265–272.

3. W. Blackwood, J. A. N. Corsellis. *Greenfield's Neuropathology*. London, Edward Arnold, 1976.

4. M. E. Sharp, J. B. Chew, M. K. S. Heran et al. Delayed restricted diffusion in carbon monoxide leukoencephalopathy. *Can J Neurol Sci* 2012; **39**: 393–394.

5. A. K. Thacker, A. B. Asthana, N. B. Sarkari. Delayed post-anoxic encephalopathy. *Postgrad Med J* 1995; **71**: 373–374.

6. F. K. Orkin. Practice standards: the Midas touch or the emperor's new clothes? *Anesthesiology* 1989; **70**: 567–571.

7. D. E. Cohen, J. J. Downes, R. C. Raphaely. What difference does pulse oximetry make? *Anesthesiology* 1988; **68**: 181–183.

8. D. M. Greer, S. D. Shemie, A. Lewis et al. Determination of brain death/death by neurologic criteria: The World Brain Death Project. *JAMA* 2020; **324**: 1078–1097.

9. L. P. Poppe. People v. Eulo: New York adopts the brain death standard for homicide cases. *Catholic Lawyer* 1984; **29**: 375–389.

The Liver–Brain Relationship in Wilson Disease

Hepatologists often assume that copper neurotoxicity is the cause of the brain lesions of Wilson disease [1]. Actually Wilson disease is one type of hepatocerebral degeneration. That is to say, the liver disease causes the brain disease. Two modern developments, MRI scanning and liver transplantation, have made it easier for the clinician to see the connection between liver and brain in Wilson disease.

Although the hepatic encephalopathy of acquired (non-Wilsonian) liver disease is typically a reversible neurologic condition, occasional patients have neurologic residua. Dysarthria, dementia, ataxia, choreoathetosis, tremor, and/or corticospinal tract signs can occur in this permanent hepatocerebral degeneration [2]. This chronic hepatocerebral disease typically develops in patients who have had overt hepatic encephalopathy, especially repeated bouts of hepatic coma. However, it can occur in patients with liver disease and portal hypertension who have never experienced acute encephalopathy [2].

Brains of such patients show hepatocerebral degeneration with more or less symmetrical, patchy neuronal loss, and protoplasmic astrocytosis. These abnormalities are typically maximal in the putamen and caudate and/or the cerebral cortex and subcortical white matter, where there is polymicrocavitation and pseudolaminar necrosis. The globus pallidus is often affected as is the cerebellum [2]. These lesions are visible on MRI scans as symmetric areas of increased signal on T2 weighted images. MRI study shows that the thalamus and other structures can be affected in a given patient.

The neuropathological and cerebral imaging features of Wilson disease resemble those of the acquired, chronic hepatocerebral degeneration described above. There is considerable resemblance of the clinical features as well. This striking similarity of familial (Wilsonian) and acquired hepatocerebral degeneration imply a common pathogenesis. Somehow the liver disease, whether genetic or not, causes the brain disease [3, 4].

Three possible ways of explaining the association of the liver pathology and the brain degeneration were considered [3]. One view was that the brain and the liver were both affected by a primary process. A second view, Wilson's own suspicion, was that the diseased liver led to disease of the brain. A third theory was that the brain disease, by affecting autonomic centers, caused the liver disease; this idea never attracted support.

We now know that the fundamental problem in Wilson disease is the liver's inability to normally excrete copper into the bile. Underlying this failure to excrete copper is a wide array of genetic mutations affecting carrier proteins. Accumulating copper damages hepatocytes. These cells leak, causing increased copper levels in the blood and consequent deposition of copper in other organs. In fully developed cases, the excess liver copper causes cirrhosis and/or liver failure [1].

Some authorities assume that copper deposition in the brain is responsible for the brain disease because copper chelation can be beneficial to the neurologic disorder. However, the idea that copper is neurotoxic does not account for the neurologic worsening that not infrequently occurs with chelation. In addition, the amount of copper in the brains of patients with acquired hepatocerebral degeneration is far below that seen in the Wilson disease [4]. Furthermore, copper toxicity has not been shown to experimentally reproduce the neurologic disease. In sum, the idea that copper causes hepatocerebral disease is not supported by evidence the way the role of ammonia in acute hepatic encephalopathy is [4]. Nevertheless, many continue to view copper toxicity as the cause of the brain lesions in Wilson disease [1, 5, 6, 7].

Liver transplantation has provided new information about the neurology of Wilson disease. Transplanting the liver essentially cures the liver disease by restoring a non-cirrhotic liver, relieving portal hypertension, and eliminating the effect of the mutation that prevents copper excretion into the bile. Two-thirds of patients bedridden with neurologic handicap experienced major or moderate neurologic improvement after liver transplantation [6]. Highly significant improvement in brain MRI abnormalities also followed liver transplantation in these disabled patients, all of whom had experienced continued neurologic worsening despite copper chelation therapy and all of whom lacked a hepatic indication for liver transplantation. In sum, curing Wilsonian liver disease helps the brain disease. Similarly, liver transplantation can improve the neurologic disorder and brain MRI abnormalities in non-Wilsonian hepatocerebral disease[8,9].

Because the neurological disorder and brain MRI abnormality often improve following liver transplantation, it is now easy to visualize that the neurologic and neuropathologic aspects of Wilson disease are due to liver disease. Hepatologists favor the view that the liver cure eliminates copper leakage and thereby benefits the nervous system. Another possibility is that the liver cure helps the brain disease by normalizing some function of the liver and/or by relieving portal hypertension. We favor the latter explanation because of the neuropathologic analysis noted previously [2, 4]. Furthermore, copper deposition abnormalities occur commonly in advanced cholestatic liver disease, in which there is no cerebral degeneration. Also, there are other copper-associated liver diseases in humans and dogs in which plasma free copper is elevated but the brain is not affected [10, 11]. It remains unproven that copper plays any role in causing the brain lesions of Wilson disease or for that matter of acquired hepatocerebral disease. However, the sequential clinical and radiological observations noted here support the substantial neuropathologic evidence that in Wilson disease the liver disorder somehow causes the brain lesions, as it does in acquired hepatocerebral degeneration.

14.1 Summary and Comments

1. Wilson disease is a hereditary disease of the liver, in which the liver fails to excrete copper into bile. The consequent copper accumulation damages the liver and results in leakage of copper into the blood.
2. This liver disease is associated with a chronic cerebral disease, which Wilson referred to as hepatolenticular degeneration.
3. The neurological and neuropathological features of Wilson disease resemble those seen in nonfamilial (acquired) hepatocerebral degeneration.

4. Liver transplantation cures the liver disease and can markedly improve the brain disorder in both Wilson disease and acquired hepatocerebral degeneration.

5. It has not been shown that copper toxicity contributes to producing the neuropathology in familial or acquired hepatocerebral disease.

6. With chelation for Wilson disease neurological improvement occurs in only some of the patients. It is possible that chelation is beneficial through its effect on the liver.

7. To summarize, in Wilson disease there occur liver disease, elevated free copper in the blood, and neurologic disease. The liver disease causes both the neurologic abnormality and the leakage of copper into the blood. The association of the elevated serum copper and the brain disease is likely not causal.

References

1. E. R. Schiff, M. F. Sorrell, W. C. Maddrey. *Schiff's Diseases of the Liver*. Chichester, John Wiley & Sons, 2012.

2. M. Victor, R. D. Adams, M. Cole. The acquired (non-Wilsonian) type of chronic hepatocerebral degeneration. *Medicine (Baltimore)*1965; **44**: 345–396.

3. R. W. Waggoner, N. Malamud. Wilson's disease in the light of cerebral changes following ordinary acquired liver disorders. *J Nerv Ment Dis* 1942; **96**: 410–423.

4. M. Victor. Neurologic changes in liver disease. *Res Publ Assoc Res Nerv Ment Dis* 1974; **53**: 1–12.

5. P. Dusek, T. Litwin, A. Czlonkowska. Neurologic impairment in Wilson disease. *Ann Transl Med* 2019; 7: S64.

6. A. Poujois, R. Sobesky, W. G. Meissner et al. Liver transplantation as a rescue therapy for severe neurologic forms of Wilson disease. *Neurology* 2020; **94**: e2189–e2202.

7. A. Compston. Progressive lenticular degeneration: a familial nervous disease associated with cirrhosis of the liver, by S. A. Kinnier Wilson (from the National Hospital, and the Laboratory of the National Hospital, Queen Square, London) Brain 1912: 34; 295–509. *Brain* 2009; **132**: 1997–2001.

8. L. M. Shulman, A. Minagar, W. J. Weiner. Reversal of parkinsonism following liver transplantation. *Neurology* 2003; **60**: 519.

9. T. Naegele, W. Grodd, R. Viebahn et al. MR imaging and (1)H spectroscopy of brain metabolites in hepatic encephalopathy: time-course of renormalization after liver transplantation. *Radiology* 2000; **216**: 683–691.

10. M. S. Tanner. Indian childhood cirrhosis and Tyrolean childhood cirrhosis. Disorders of a copper transport gene? *Adv Exp Med Biol* 1999; **448**: 127–137.

11. I. C. Fuentealba, E. M. Aburto. Animal models of copper-associated liver disease. *Comp Hepatol* 2003; **2**: 5.

Chapter 15

Wernicke Disease

It seemed that nothing could be added to the classic monograph, *The Wernicke-Korsakoff Syndrome* [1]. It succinctly summarized that Wernicke disease is a thiamine deficiency condition manifest by acute or subacute ocular palsies, nystagmus, gait ataxia, decreased alertness, and confusion. Often a partial syndrome occurs. Resolution with treatment is often but not always complete. If there is a residual cognitive problem, it takes the form of a Korsakoff amnesic state. The symmetric pathological change is largely in the paraventricular regions of the third and fourth ventricles.

The purpose of this chapter is to point out newer information that was not available when Victor et al. published the landmark volume on Wernicke disease. First of all, the patients in their study were collected before the era of magnetic resonance imaging. This sensitive scanning method is now widely employed; many hundreds of patients with Wernicke disease have been examined with it. This enlarged sample of patients has revealed some previously unknown facts about disease topography. Also, included here is previously unpublished epidemiologic information related to the midline cerebellar lesion. In addition, we note here new details about the clinical manifestations of Wernicke disease. Finally, recently promulgated ideas about thiamine dosing receive comment.

15.1 MRI

Widespread availability of MRI has revealed that the disease can involve territories other than those previously well-known to be affected. It is not surprising that the studies by Victor et al. did not recognize every area of the brain that can be affected. On slices of formalin-fixed brains, lesions are recognized when they are visible or palpable. If there is not necrosis, gross softening, petechial hemorrhage, or other discoloration the pathologist will not see the disease. Standard sampling with small sections for microscopic examination may not include every area of disease. By displaying the entire organ on multiple imaging sequences and in multiple planes, MRI makes the topography of lesions more obvious. One can confidently know that lesions in atypical territories are due to Wernicke disease because of their symmetry, because they appear at the same time as typical Wernicke symptoms and/or signs, and because they match the well-known Wernicke lesions in their MRI signal and in their response to therapy.

Victor and colleagues made no mention of basal ganglia lesions in their own material or their review of the human literature. However, modern imaging now has shown caudate and putamen lesions in several cases [2]. In most cases the caudate head was the primary site of basal ganglia disease. In another report, the putamen was disproportionately affected [3]. These neostriatal lesions on MRI can occur in isolation or they can accompany

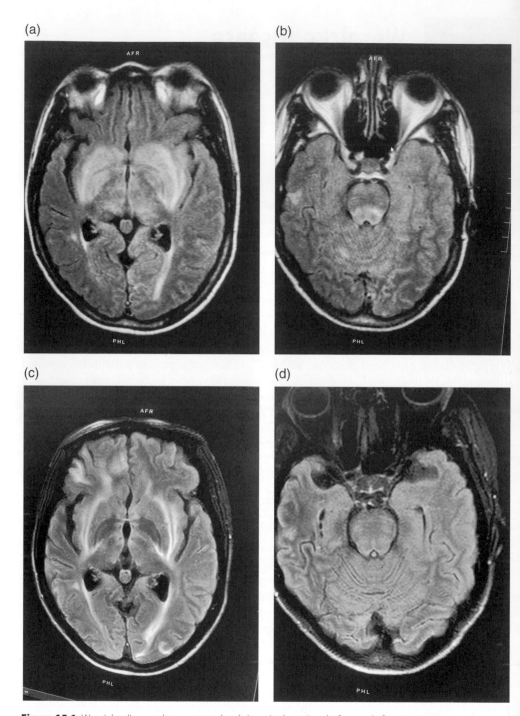

Figure 15.1 Wernicke disease shown at two levels in a single patient before and after treatment.
a. Striatal disease, acute.
b. Pontine tegmental disease, acute.
c. Striatal disease after treatment with thiamine.
d. Pontine tegmental disease after treatment with thiamine.

(a) (b)

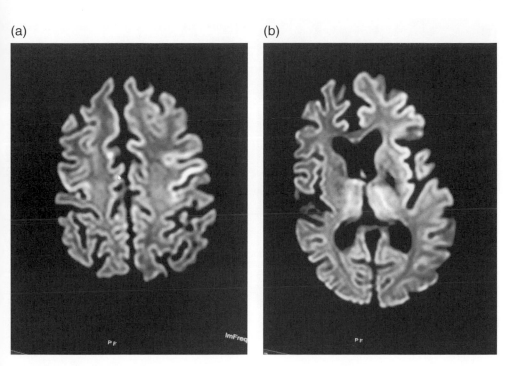

Figure 15.2 MRI of a single patient.
a. Cortical Wernicke disease, acute.
b. Thalamic Wernicke disease, acute.

(a) (b)

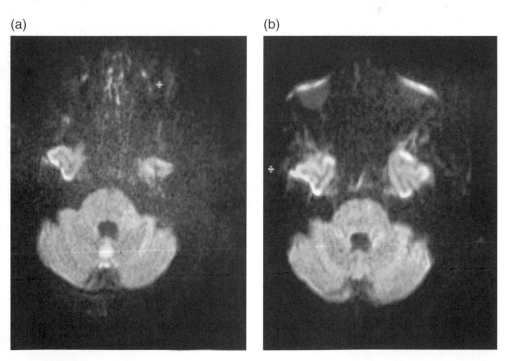

Figure 15.3 Sequential MRI of a single patient.
a. Midline cerebellar Wernicke disease before treatment.
b. Midline cerebellar Wernicke disease after treatment with thiamine 500 mg daily.

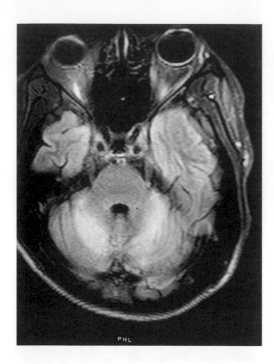

Figure 15.4 Lateral cerebellar disease, an atypical topography for Wernicke disease.

abnormalities in regions typical of Wernicke disease (Figure 15.1a). The occurrence of caudate and putamen involvement is not surprising because basal ganglia lesions occur in other species. Thiamine deficient rhesus monkeys are the best example [4].

In one of the cases with basal ganglia involvement, there was disease in the cerebral cortex [2]. Such cases continue to be recorded [5]. As one might expect, cortical involvement has now been shown to occasionally occur without basal ganglia lesions. The published cases with cortical lesions have been reviewed [6]. The images show more or less symmetric frontal and parietal peri-Rolandic disease (Figure 15.2).

In addition to revealing that Wernicke disease can affect territories not previously recognized to be involved, MRI has improved our ability to display some of the well-established areas of disease. FLAIR sequence MRI of the midline cerebellum demonstrates the typical lesions (Figure 15.3). Although the cerebellar lesion of Wernicke disease is known for its predilection for the midline, in occasional patients the lesion can extend far laterally into the cerebellar hemispheres. Victor et al. knew of this, but only by MRI axial brain sections can bilateral involvement be so well displayed [7] (Figure 15.4). The neuropathologists also knew that the floccular lobes could be affected but only the axial MRI slice demonstrates the symmetrical increased signal so clearly [8].

15.2 Epidemiology

Midline cerebellar degeneration in the alcoholic has been suspected to be caused by malnutrition ever since it was first reported. The relationship of midline cerebellar disease to malnutrition is supported by the following previously unpublished analysis of the autopsy series referred to in a prior publication [9]. Over a three-year period at Cleveland

Metropolitan General Hospital, careful study of the sagittal slice revealed that the prevalence of midline cerebellar degeneration varied with the underlying systemic disease (Table 15.1). The disproportionate representation of the cerebellar disease in oropharyngeal/esophageal cancer cannot be explained by alcoholism alone because the cirrhotics showed only an 18% prevalence. Inability to ingest food is the likely explanation. This data strengthens the concept that the midline cerebellar lesion is a nutritional disease. Originally considered an independent entity, midline cerebellar degeneration has, in time, come to be recognized as the cerebellar lesion of Wernicke disease [10] (Figure 15.3).

Table 15.1 Midline cerebellar degeneration (3-year autopsy series)

	Prevalence	Percentage
Cancer (colon)	1/15	7%
Cancer (lung)	1/16	6%
Alcoholic cirrhosis	5/28	18%
Cancer (oropharynx/ esophagus)	9/10	90%

15.3 Clinical Features

In recent decades, certain neuro-otologic phenomena have been recognized as clinical manifestations of Wernicke disease. Most of the literature on vestibular signs and all of the information on hearing loss in Wernicke disease have been reported since the publication of the monographs of Victor, Adams, and Collins [1,11].

In full-blown Wernicke disease, vestibular dysfunction may be masked by encephalopathy and cerebellar involvement. Thus, clinical recognition of its manifestations was delayed. Kattah and colleagues, however, have demonstrated a series of patients in whom vestibular signs appeared early in the course of Wernicke disease; chief complaints were acute vertigo, unsteadiness and/or oscillopsia [12]. In these patients, they demonstrated that there was not only nystagmus but also an abnormal head impulse test. They attributed the findings to disease of the vestibular nuclei, involvement of which have been well documented at autopsy and by MRI scans.

Hearing loss in Wernicke disease was reviewed in 2014 [13]. That report added another patient to the eight previously published cases. Treatment with thiamine led to improvement in these patients. The MRI scans showed symmetric lesions of the inferior colliculi in some of the patients. Inferior colliculus dysfunction without imaging abnormality may have been responsible in the other cases.

15.4 Treatment

Although 2–3 mg of thiamine are sometimes enough to reverse or improve the ocular signs of Wernicke disease, Victor and Adams always felt it prudent to administer a megadose of thiamine for this medical emergency. They would prescribe thiamine 50 mg intravenously and 50 mg intramuscularly. They recommended continuing the intramuscular dose daily until the patient resumed eating a normal diet. Subsequently, all have agreed that the parenteral route is preferred to avoid the risk of poor absorption of orally administered thiamine. However, recommendations about dosage and frequency of administration have varied in recent decades.

Evidence that the half-life of thiamine is short has led to three-time daily regimens [14,15]. It has not been proven that it is important to avoid pulsatile blood levels of thiamine as one does when prescribing an anticonvulsant. However, one cannot take issue with a thrice daily regimen.

Of course, not all treated patients recover fully. For this reason, there has been a recurring concern that a patient with a residual amnesic syndrome had not received enough thiamine. Hence, some authors have escalated their dose recommendation to 200 mg tid or 500 mg tid initially with varied dose schedules on subsequent days. One author has referred to such discussions about thiamine as "how much and how long?" [16]. The real question is "how soon?," and the answer is "as early as possible." One should treat for Wernicke disease as soon as one suspects it. If the term passes through a clinician's mind as in, "I doubt this patient has Wernicke disease," one should treat for the possibility. The one hundred milligram doses have been very effective when the prescription is made early. It is doubtful that giving five times the dose makes a big difference if it is given when the affected brain tissue has become necrotic. The European Federation of Neurological Sciences states that, "there is no evidence to support conclusions as to dosage, route of administration and treatment time" [17]. A case such as that shown in Figure 15.3 requires that we keep an open mind about the benefit of higher dose treatment.

Wernicke disease is precipitated when the thiamine store is inadequate for the carbohydrate load. Thus, any doctor can precipitate Wernicke disease in a nutritionally depleted patient by providing carbohydrate. Most often this iatrogenic problem develops when dextrose containing intravenous fluid is administered. Ironically, this has sometimes been done intentionally. The doctor recognizing that the patient has not been eating well may think or feel that it would be good to provide some calories with the intravenous fluid. The resulting elevation of the blood sugar brings on the symptoms.

Alcoholics, vegans, and patients who have undergone bariatric surgery are not the only persons vulnerable to nutritional deficiency. A renal dialysis patient who has stopped taking routinely prescribed multivitamins may become thiamine depleted. A cancer patient who has a poor appetite or who has a tumor obstructing food intake may also be at risk. Dementia, depression, and psychoses can sometimes cause a patient not to eat well. Likewise, one need not be emaciated to be malnourished. An extremely obese patient may have become thiamine depleted during a recent intentional 50-pound weight loss. In all such circumstances intravenous dextrose should not be given without providing thiamine.

Elevation of blood sugar by corticosteroid medication can also precipitate Wernicke disease in a nutritionally depleted patient. It is sad to see a nutritionally depleted patient, already stricken with vasculitis, who has secondarily developed Wernicke disease from the medication given for the primary disease.

In sum, any patient who may be malnourished should be provided parenteral thiamine, especially when one prescribes steroid medication or a glucose-containing solution. Thiamine should be provided to any patient with acute or subacute ophthalmoplegia, ataxia, or confusion of uncertain cause. Treatment with higher and more frequent doses, which has been recommended in recent decades, seems to be safe [18].

References

1. M. Victor, R. D. Adams, G. H. Collins. The Wernicke-Korsakoff syndrome. A clinical and pathological study of 245 patients, 82 with post-mortem examinations. *Contemp Neurol Ser* 1971; 7: 1–206.

2. G. Zuccoli, N. Pipitone. Neuroimaging findings in acute Wernicke's encephalopathy: review of the literature. *AJR Am J Roentgenol* 2009; 192: 501–508.

3. O. E. Eren, F. Schöberl, M. Campana et al. A unique MRI-pattern in alcohol-associated Wernicke encephalopathy. *Acta Neurol Belg* 2020; 120: 1439–1441.

4. J. F. Rinehart, M. Friedman, L. D. Greenberg. Effect of experimental thiamine deficiency on the nervous system of the rhesus monkey. *Arch Pathol (Chic)* 1949; 48: 129–139.

5. C. Santos Andrade, L. Tavares Lucato, M. da Graca Morais Martin et al. Non-alcoholic Wernicke's encephalopathy: broadening the clinicoradiological spectrum. *Br J Radiol* 2010; 83: 437–446.

6. L. Wu, D. Jin, X. Sun et al. Cortical damage in Wernicke's encephalopathy with good prognosis: a report of two cases and literature review. *Metab Brain Dis* 2017; 32: 377–384.

7. B. Lapergue, I. Klein, J. M. Olivot et al. Diffusion weighted imaging of cerebellar lesions in Wernicke's encephalopathy. *J Neuroradiol* 2006; 33: 126–128.

8. G. Zuccoli, N. Siddiqui, R. Rizzi et al. Neurological picture. Pendular nystagmus showing involvement of the floccular lobes in an atypical case of Wernicke encephalopathy: MRI findings. *J Neurol Neurosurg Psychiatry* 2010; 81: 858.

9. M. Victor, R. Laureno. Neurologic complications of alcohol abuse: epidemiologic aspects. *Adv Neurol* 1978; 19: 603–617.

10. R. Laureno. Nutritional cerebellar degeneration with comments on its relationship to Wernicke disease and alcoholism. In: S. H. Subramony, A. Dürr, eds. *Handbook of Clinical Neurology, Ataxic Disorders.* Amsterdam, Elsevier, 2011; 103: 175–188.

11. M. Victor, R. D. Adams, G. H. Collins. *The Wernicke-Korsakoff Syndrome and Related Neurological Disorders Due to Alcoholism and Malnutrition.* Philadelphia, F.A. Davis, 1989.

12. J. C. Kattah, S. S. Dhanani, J. H. Pula et al. Vestibular signs of thiamine deficiency during the early phase of suspected Wernicke encephalopathy. *Neurol Clin Pract* 2013; 3: 460–468.

13. M. A. Walker, R. Zepeda, H. A. Afari et al. Hearing loss in Wernicke encephalopathy. *Neurol Clin Pract* 2014; 4: 511–515.

14. C. M. Tallaksen, A. Sande, T. Bohmer et al. Kinetics of thiamin and thiamin phosphate esters in human blood, plasma and urine after 50 mg intravenously or orally. *Eur J Clin Pharmacol* 1993; 44: 73–78.

15. A. D. Thomson, P. R. Ryle, G. K. Shaw. Ethanol, thiamine and brain damage. *Alcohol and Alcoholism* 1983; 18: 27–43.

16. J. Chataway, E. Hardman. Thiamine in Wernicke's syndrome – how much and how long? *Postgrad Med J* 1995; 71: 249.

17. R. Galvin, G. Brathen, A. Ivashynka et al. EFNS guidelines for diagnosis, therapy and prevention of Wernicke encephalopathy. *Eur J Neurol* 2010; 17: 1408–1418.

18. E. Day, P. W. Bentham, R. Callaghan et al. Thiamine for prevention and treatment of Wernicke-Korsakoff Syndrome in people who abuse alcohol. *Cochrane Database Syst Rev* 2013; 7: CD004033.

Delayed Neurologic Disorders after Toxic or Metabolic Insults

Neurologic effects of an acute toxic exposure usually occur promptly. The purpose of this chapter is to draw attention to the exceptional situations in which neurological manifestations appear after a delay. No doubt, the reasons for latency vary. Just as the mechanisms of acute toxic effects are not well understood, the mechanisms of delayed toxic effects are typically not known. Delayed brain disorders can appear not only after toxin exposure but also after certain metabolic insults. I write of these disorders to emphasize that they are an opportune field for investigation.

As mentioned in Chapter 13, a delayed form of anoxic–ischemic encephalopathy can occur. Having awakened from coma after carbon monoxide "poisoning" or other types of ischemic/hypoxic coma, a patient can relapse into coma. This leukoencephalopathy occurs days or weeks after the acute anoxic event. Asymptomatic cases have not been reported. The reason for the lag to manifestations is unknown.

Another metabolic injury that emerges after a latency is myelinolysis [1]. This neurologic syndrome typically occurs a few days after rapid correction of hyponatremia. The likelihood of this iatrogenic disease is greater when the hyponatremia has been prolonged and severe and when the rise in serum sodium is large. Thus, a rise of 20 meq/L over 24 hours is much more likely to cause myelinolysis than is a rise of 10 meq/L over 48 hours. Axons and neurons are relatively spared. Asymptomatic cases can be detected by MRI. The clinical manifestations depend on the regions damaged in a given case. Originally discovered by neuropathological detection of central pontine myelinolysis, the disease is now known to cause extrapontine lesions as well. In fact, it is not rare for extrapontine lesions to occur without a pontine lesion. The disease seems to be caused by the insult of an osmotic increment. Hence, some refer to the disease as "osmotic demyelination syndrome." Why there is a latency until the onset of neurologic symptoms is unknown.

Many toxins can cause delayed neurologic syndromes. Dimethylmercury is interesting in that a minimal exposure can be lethal with a latency of months to onset of symptoms [2]. A chemist, for example, spilled several drops onto her glove; 154 days later she developed initial neurologic symptoms which were cerebellar. Ultimately, there was bilateral cerebral injury with obtundation. Animal experiments have confirmed that a long delay can occur between exposure to organic mercury and onset of the neurologic disorder [3]. The cause of the delay is not known.

Accidental or suicidal drinking of diethylene glycol can cause a fulminant polyneuropathy with quadriplegia. The polyneuropathy occurs several days or a week after the ingestion. Autopsy has shown severe demyelination of peripheral and cranial nerves [4]. Axons are affected to a lesser degree. Central nervous system myelin is not affected. There is inflammation. Initially, motor amplitudes are reduced, and conduction velocities are preserved, but during recovery velocities are markedly reduced [5]. This sequence has been interpreted as indicating an initial axonal injury with demyelination becoming evident during the recovery phase. The cranial nerves show enhancement with gadolinium on MRI scan. The reason for the delay in the onset of polyneuropathy is not known.

Ethylene glycol ingestion can also be followed by a delayed neurological disorder, characteristically multiple cranial neuropathies. Optic neuropathies, fixed pupils, facial diplegia, dysphagia, and dysarthria can occur in various combinations. Facial sensory loss also can occur. The latency is typically days but can be longer than a week. There is no understanding of the cause of the latency.

We partially understand the delay in the onset of the neurologic disorder after methanol ingestion. Methanol itself is nontoxic except for its ability to cause transient inebriation. The neurotoxicity, optic neuropathy and cerebral injury, become evident hours to days after ingestion. Twenty-four hours is typical [6]. The latency is due to the metabolism of methanol to formic acid which is believed to be the critical toxin [7]. Putamen involvement is characteristic as is damage to the cerebral white matter.

Tri-o-cresyl phosphate (TOCP) is an organophosphate compound, which after a single dose can produce a distal axonopathy. The latent period is 8–18 days. The neuropathy begins as a cramping pain in the calves and numbness and tingling in the feet. One or two weeks after onset, the upper limbs can be similarly affected. The reason for the delayed onset of axonopathy is unknown [8].

Thallium sulfate is found in rodenticides and insecticides. Homicidal, suicidal, or accidental ingestion can result in a polyneuropathy of delayed onset. Alopecia is the clinical clue that allows distinction of this disease from Guillain–Barré syndrome. A latent period of several days precedes onset of sensory symptoms. The alopecia does not occur for weeks after ingestion [8].

A latent period after a toxic/metabolic insult is advantageous to the doctor. In an experimental model, the investigator can study tissue at different intervals after the insult but before onset of neurologic disorder. In addition to facilitating study of pathogenesis, the presence of latency until onset allows the physician days in which to administer therapy. In some instances, therapy can minimize neurologic damage. The case of methanol poisoning is the best example. Prescription of ethanol (competes for alcohol dehydrogenase), use of dialysis (removes methanol from the body), and administration of fomepizole (inhibits alcohol dehydrogenase) are all of benefit in the early days. During the latent period of myelinolysis, relowering the serum sodium appears to be beneficial. Other metabolic/toxic brain injuries in which there are latent periods provide the researcher great opportunities to investigate the mechanism and treatment of disease.

References

1. R. Laureno. Central pontine myelinolysis following rapid correction of hyponatremia. *Ann Neurol* 1983; **13**: 232–242.

2. D. W. Nierenberg, R. E. Nordgren, M. B. Chang et al. Delayed cerebellar disease and death after accidental exposure to dimethylmercury. *N Engl J Med* 1998; **338**: 1672–1676.

3. D. C. Rice. Evidence for delayed neurotoxicity produced by methylmercury *Neurotoxicology* 1996; **17**: 583–596.

4. Y. D. Rollins, C. M. Filley, J. T. McNutt et al. Fulminant ascending paralysis as a delayed sequela of diethylene glycol (Sterno) ingestion. *Neurology* 2002; **59**: 1460–1463.

5. M. J. Hasbani, L. H. Sansing, J. Perrone et al. Encephalopathy and peripheral neuropathy following diethylene glycol ingestion. *Neurology* 2005; **64**: 1273–1275.

6. I. L. Bennett, F. H. Cary, G. L. Mitchell et al. Acute methyl alcohol poisoning: a review based on experiences in an outbreak of 323 cases. *Medicine (Baltimore)* 1953; **32**: 431–463.

7. J. A. Kruse. Methanol poisoning. *Intensive Care Med* 1992; **18**: 391–397.

8. P. S. Spencer, H. H. Shaumburg. *Experimental and Clinical Neurotoxicology.* Baltimore, Williams & Wilkins, 1980.

Chapter 17

Transolfactory Spread in the Pathogenesis of Meningoencephalitis

Our topic is the concept that certain infectious agents invade brain and spinal fluid through the olfactory nerves and bulbs. For some pathogens the olfactory pathway to human encephalitis has been well-established. For other organisms the olfactory connection has been suggested but not proven.

17.1 Amoebae

Until mid-twentieth century certain amoebae, ubiquitous in soil and fresh water, were considered to be harmless saprophytes and thus were described as "free living" [1]. At first in experimental animals [2] and later in humans, it became evident that certain strains of these amoebae had the ability to cause meningoencephalitis [3]. In the immunocompetent human, the organisms that most commonly cause primary amoebic meningoencephalitis belong to the genus Naegleria. Epidemiologic, pathologic, and experimental evidence support the concept that these amoebae enter the nose and travel through the fila of the olfactory nerves to the central nervous system.

Review of hundreds of documented cases shows that this disease is usually associated with water recreation [4]. Swimming and diving are most common, but other water sports and simple splashing also have been related. Retrospective review indicates that amoebic meningoencephalitis results from the exposure to warm, untreated fresh water. Lakes, ponds, rivers, streams, canals, and untreated swimming pools have been the typical sites of exposure [5].

Not rarely, however, nasal irrigation with water has been implicated. The nasal irrigation cases indicate that the nose, not the eyes, also is the portal in the water recreation cases.

In addition to this epidemiologic information, pathologic studies have pointed to involvement of the olfactory system. Early autopsy reports showed hemorrhagic softening of the olfactory bulbs with relative sparing of the nearby optic nerves. This neuropathologic pattern led to the idea that the amoebae had traveled along an olfactory pathway to the brain [6, 7]. The definitive pathological study in humans came from the six early Australian cases [3]. In addition to necrotic olfactory bulbs, this report demonstrated "ulcerated and inflamed" nasal mucous membranes, inflamed olfactory nerve bundles, and inflamed olfactory nerves penetrating the cribriform plate. Plentiful amoebae were detected in olfactory nerve filaments in the nasal mucosa, at the cribriform plate, and in the ventral portions of the olfactory bulbs. In the olfactory system the pathology was "most advanced peripherally and decreased in severity in a central direction and there was only the slight involvement of other cranial nerves." The distribution of the pathologic findings indicated centripetal extension, that is, peripheral olfactory inflammation spreading inward to the subarachnoid space and brain [3].

Experimental models actually allow us to see this process with light microscopy. In one study, mice received a 10 µl suspension of Naegleri fowleri intranasally. Animals were sacrificed at 24, 32, and 48 hours after inoculation. The cribriform plate was studied with serial sections. Amoebae and inflammation were seen in the submucosal nerve plexus, in the olfactory fila within the cribriform plate, and in the olfactory bulb [8]. This study showed that amoebae can in fact migrate through the olfactory nervous system before the development of meningitis.

In sum, the epidemiologic, pathologic, and experimental studies demonstrate that amoebae suspended in water, after entering the nose, can migrate through the olfactory system and thereby cause meningoencephalitis in humans.

17.2 Herpes Simplex Virus (HSV)

Whereas amoebic meningoencephalitis is clearly a primary infection, it is not clear whether herpes simplex type 1 encephalitis is due to primary infection of the central nervous system or whether it is due to reactivation of virus which has been latent in the olfactory system or trigeminal ganglion. The two hypothesized routes of infection may not be mutually exclusive [9].

Of the proposed reactivation pathways, there is more evidence for the olfactory connection. The finding that the olfactory bulbs are hemorrhagic and necrotic in some cases of herpes simplex encephalitis led to the idea that olfactory system infection spreads into the orbital surface of the frontal lobes or medial surface of the temporal lobes. This concept fits nicely with those cases in which HSV can be seen in olfactory neuroepithelium, olfactory nerve, and olfactory bulb but not in the trigeminal ganglion [10, 11]. Also consistent with this concept are some patients in whom the immunohistochemical methods show viral antigen in the olfactory tract and cortex but not in the trigeminal pathway [12]. Furthermore, in some cases, the HSV can be seen by electron microscopy in the necrotic olfactory bulbs [13]. Experimental studies also lend support to the olfactory theory. Intranasal inoculation of rats with HSV can cause meningoencephalitis and can cause latent infection in the olfactory bulb and neuroepithelium [12].

Trigeminal origin is also a reasonable proposition because polymerase chain reaction shows HSV in the trigeminal ganglion in nearly 20% of persons dying of nonneurological disease. Davis and Johnson hypothesized that the virus, having been latent in the trigeminal ganglion, spreads to fifth nerve branches supplying the dura of the middle and anterior fossa from which it can somehow enter the adjacent temporal lobe [14]. An alternate trigeminal theory suggests that virus in cranial nerve 5 could be transported to the brainstem from which it could be rostrally projected to the forebrain, where the selectively vulnerable limbic system is disproportionately affected [15]. Neuropathological support for these trigeminal speculations is limited.

The presence of these competing theories indicates that the relationship of the olfactory system to herpes encephalitis is not nearly as straightforward or at least not as consistent as it is in amoebic meningoencephalitis. It may well be that HSV encephalitis can be acquired by different routes [16].

17.3 Other Pathogens

Other pathogens can take the olfactory route to the brain in both humans and animals. In humans, inhalation of rabies virus can cause encephalitis [17]. Experiments have shown that the olfactory system can serve as a pathway for a coronavirus (mouse hepatitis virus) to enter the brain and cause encephalitis. Intranasal injection of the virus causes encephalitis, but unilateral ablation of the olfactory bulb prevents inoculation from causing encephalitis on the operated side [18]. It has also been shown that surgical removal of both olfactory bulbs prevents intranasal inoculation of mouse hepatitis virus from causing encephalitis [19]. Nasal inoculation with influenza A virus also can cause neuroinvasion along the olfactory pathway in experimental animals. Many other viruses including measles and polio can do the same [13, 20]. These results confirm that experimental encephalitis after nasal inoculation develops by the olfactory rather than the trigeminal route [19].

17.4 Anatomical Aspects

Certain aspects of anatomy make the olfactory system's association with encephalitis understandable. Olfactory receptor neurons, unlike the receptors of other sensory systems, are exposed directly to the environment. Thus, the olfactory system has a unique ability to take up exogenous substances and transport them to the brain. The olfactory system connects directly to the cerebrum without thalamic relay. No other sensory system similarly bypasses the diencephalon. Furthermore, no other sensory receptors die and regenerate through adult life as do olfactory receptor neurons [5]. Another special feature of the olfactory system is that the olfactory nerves pass through ensheathing channels as they penetrate the cribriform plate. These channels are a pathway, alternative to an intraneuronal one, for virus to reach the brain.

17.5 Conclusion

The unique anatomy of the olfactory sensory system allows for transfer of infectious agents from the nose to the brain. Clearly, Naegleria causes encephalitis after traversing the olfactory system. It is likely that some cases of herpes simplex encephalitis result from virus in the olfactory bulb making its way to the brain. Animal experiments and human case reports show that many other viruses have the capacity to follow this pathway to the brain.

References

1. D. Patras, J. J. Andujar. Meningoencephalitis due to *Hartmannella* (Acanthamoeba). *Am J Clin Pathol* 1966; **46**: 226–233.

2. C. G. Culbertson, J. W. Smith, H. K. Cohen et al. Experimental infection of mice and monkeys by Acanthamoeba. *Am J Pathol* 1959; **35**: 185–197.

3. R. F. Carter. Primary amoebic meningo-encephalitis: clinical, pathological and epidemiological features of six fatal cases. *J Pathol Bacteriol* 1968; **96**: 1–25.

4. R. Gharpure, J. H. Bliton, A. Goodman et al. Epidemiology and clinical characteristics of primary amebic meningoencephalitis caused by Naegleria fowleri: a global review. *Clin Infect Dis* 2021; **73**: e19–27.

5. I. Mori. Transolfactory neuroinvasion by viruses threatens the human brain. *Acta Virol* 2015; **59**: 338–349.

6. C. G. Butt, C. Baro, R. W. Knorr. *Naegleria* (sp.) identified in amebic encephalitis. *Am J Clin Pathol* 1968; **50**: 568–574.

7. J. H. Callicott, E. C. Nelson, M. M. Jones et al. Meningoencephalitis due to pathogenic free-living amoebae. Report of two cases. *JAMA* 1968; **206**: 579–582.

8. K. L. Jarolim, J. K. McCosh, M. J. Howard et al. A light microscopy study of the migration of Naegleria fowleri from the nasal submucosa to the central nervous system during the early stage of primary amebic meningoencephalitis in mice. *J Parasitol* 2000; **86**: 50–55.

9. A. H. Tomlinson, M. M. Esiri. Herpes simplex encephalitis. Immunohistological demonstration of spread of virus via olfactory pathways in mice. *J Neurol Sci* 1983; **60**: 473–484.

10. V. J. Ojeda, M. Archer, T. A. Robertson et al. Necropsy study of the olfactory portal

of entry in herpes simplex encephalitis. *Med J Aust* 1983; **1**: 79–81.

11. J. A. Twomey, C. M. Barker, G. Robinson et al. Olfactory mucosa in herpes simplex encephalitis. *J Neurol Neurosurg Psychiatry* 1979; **42**: 983–987.

12. J. J. Dinn. Transolfactory spread of virus in herpes simplex encephalitis. *Br Med J* 1980; **281**: 1392.

13. I. Mori, Y. Nishiyama, T. Yokochi et al. Olfactory transmission of neurotropic viruses. *J Neurovirol* 2005; **11**: 129–137.

14. L. E. Davis, R. T. Johnson. An explanation for the localization of herpes simplex encephalitis? *Ann Neurol* 1979; **5**: 2–5.

15. A. R. Damasio, G. W. Van Hoesen. The limbic system and the localisation of herpes simplex encephalitis. *J Neurol Neurosurg Psychiatry* 1985; **48**: 297–301.

16. C. M. Menendez, D. J. Carr. Herpes simplex virus-1 infects the olfactory bulb shortly following ocular infection and exhibits a long-term inflammatory profile in the form of effector and HSV-1-specific T cells. *J Neuroinflammation* 2017; **14**: 124.

17. J. P. Conomy, A. Leibovitz, W. McCombs et al. Airborne rabies encephalitis: demonstration of rabies virus in the human central nervous system. *Neurology* 1977; **27**: 67–69.

18. S. Perlman, G. Evans, A. Afifi. Effect of olfactory bulb ablation on spread of a neurotropic coronavirus into the mouse brain. *J Exp Med* 1990; **172**: 1127–1132.

19. E. M. Barnett, S. Perlman. The olfactory nerve and not the trigeminal nerve is the major site of CNS entry for mouse hepatitis virus, strain JHM. *Virology* 1993; **194**: 185–191.

20. R. T. Johnson. *Viral Infections of the Nervous System*. New York, Raven Press, 1982.

Chapter 18

Neurologic Disorders in Endocarditis

All neurologic complications of endocarditis can be divided into three categories: vascular, infectious, and nonspecific. The cerebrovascular disorders are due to cardiogenic embolism, which can cause bland cerebral infarction, hemorrhagic infarction, and intracranial hemorrhage. Infectious complications, abscess, and meningitis, are much less common. "Nonspecific" is the term used for neurologic problems not due to cerebrovascular disease or central nervous system infection. By and large these signs and symptoms are due to systemic infection. Bacteremia alone can cause fatigue, weakness, confusion, depression, personality change, headache, or myalgias.

Table 18.1 shows the three types of neurologic disorders as they typically occur in two types of endocarditis. Although numerous bacteria and fungi can cause endocarditis, these two archetypal forms serve to illustrate the range of neurologic manifestations that occur in endocarditis. Streptococcus viridans, normal mouth flora, tends to cause endocarditis on an abnormal heart valve. This subacute form of endocarditis can smolder for weeks or months. Staphylococcus aureus, a more virulent organism, can infect normal heart valves and can result in infection of the central nervous system. Nonspecific neurologic complications and cerebrovascular disorders occur in both subacute and acute endocarditis.

The three categories of neurologic complications shown in the table are not strictly separable. First of all, cardiogenic embolism can be the cause of both aneurysm and infectious complications. For example, embolic infarcts can evolve into abscesses. Furthermore, vascular and infectious neurologic problems can be manifest by symptoms which are not overtly those of stroke or infection and can thus appear to be nonspecific. Although the three groups overlap considerably, this tripartite classification is useful to structure the neurologist's thinking about endocarditis.

Embolism from the heart to the brain can be asymptomatic [1]. It is overt when it causes a transient ischemic attack or a cerebral infarction. These events are typically due to occlusion of a medium-sized vessel like a distal middle cerebral or posterior cerebral artery branch. In some cases, multiple small emboli can occlude end vessels and cause infarcts to occur in a border zone distribution. Embolic cerebral infarcts in any context have a tendency to become hemorrhagic, and endocarditis is no exception [2].

Embolism to the distal cerebral arterial branches is also the cause of most mycotic aneurysms. The inflammatory material of the embolus works its way into the thin-walled intracranial vessels. Thereby weakened at the site of the embolus, the artery can dilate [3]. The usual distal location of these aneurysms is distinct from that of berry aneurysms, which are proximal, at arterial branching points on or near the circle of Willis. Like berry aneurysms, mycotic aneurysms can be symptomatic or asymptomatic. They can cause subarachnoid, cerebral, or meningocerebral hemorrhage. Although usually distal, mycotic aneurysms can develop in more

Table 18.1 Neurologic complications of endocarditis

	ARCHETYPES	
	Subacute	Acute
	(e.g., *Streptococcus viridans* on an abnormal heart valve)	(e.g., *Staphylococcus aureus* on a normal heart valve)
Vascular		
Embolic infarction	+	+
Mycotic aneurysm	+	+
Infectious		
Brain abscess	_	+
Microabscesses	_	+
Bacterial meningitis	_	+
Spinal epidural abscess	_	+
Nonspecific	+	+

proximal vessels. If a mycotic aneurysm is detected, one must monitor its size with the radiologic test deemed appropriate. Most mycotic aneurysms, including those as large as 10 mm, disappear with antibiotic therapy. Endovascular or open surgical treatment is appropriate for aneurysms that have ruptured. Intervention should be considered for aneurysms that continue to enlarge despite antibiotic treatment.

Subarachnoid hemorrhage with no demonstrable aneurysm can be explained by the mycotic aneurysm having been destroyed during its rupture. When there are multifocal, sequential subarachnoid hemorrhages, cerebral vasculitis has been suspected to be the cause [4, 5]. As opposed to bacterial meningitis, in which cerebral vasculitis is well known to occur [6], there is not pathologic or radiologic evidence for panvasculitis in endocarditis.[1] The cause of multiple hemorrhages could be rapidly developing aneurysms consequent to small sequential emboli. Anticoagulation needed for an endovascular procedure or cardiac surgery may play a role in cases where a panvasculitis has been proposed as the cause of multiple areas of cerebral bleeding.

There is a little data on how to most effectively use neuroradiologic tests in endocarditis. On the one hand, MRI is very sensitive for showing brain lesions [1]. On the other hand, there is concern that the detection of too many asymptomatic lesions may deter cardiac surgeons from promptly proceeding with necessary replacement of an infected heart valve [6]. Thus, Wijdicks and colleagues recommend that no neuroimaging be done unless there are neurologic symptoms which indicate it. They reserve an MRI scan for a patient whose CT scan fails to explain symptoms. They order a cerebral angiogram only when there is intracranial bleeding [7]. Others are more proactive. In endocarditis, they reason, any cerebral embolus has the potential to cause an aneurysm. Whenever there has been cerebral embolism, they argue, the arteries should be visualized.

---

[1] E. Wijdicks, personal communication, 2021.

One manifestation of the virulence of *Staphylococcus aureus* is its ability to cause infection in the central nervous system. Spinal epidural abscess is not rare. Characteristically multiple microabscesses occur adjacent to the cerebral cortex as a result of embolism to end vessels. Uncommonly, a large brain abscess can develop in a cerebral infarct. Bacterial meningitis can also be associated with staphylococcal endocarditis.

Embolic occlusion of a large artery should suggest the possibility that the endocarditis is noninfectious. This clue can be important because marantic endocarditis can mimic the bacterial type with fever, leukocytosis, and petechiae. Marantic endocarditis should also be suspected when scans show multiple small and large brain infarcts in a wide distribution [8].

After purified heparin became available in the 1930s, it immediately became evident that anticoagulant treatment was treacherous in the endocarditis patient. At Peter Brent Brigham Hospital, four heparin treated endocarditis patients died from cerebral hemorrhage in one year.[2] This experience was widely replicated. The danger with anticoagulation is understandable. First of all, anticoagulation would make hemorrhage from a mycotic aneurysm catastrophic. Secondly, embolic infarcts tend to turn hemorrhagic [2]. Anticoagulation can dangerously accentuate this bleeding. Thus, anticoagulation should be used for endocarditis patients only when it is essential to protect a prosthetic heart valve. Because of the described proclivity to intracranial bleeding, intravenous thrombolytic therapy and oral antiplatelet agents should also be avoided [9].

Not all neurologic manifestations of endocarditis are intracranial. Occasionally a mycotic aneurysm will form in a large artery. A subclavian-axillary artery aneurysm, for example, can cause brachial plexopathy. Emboli can occlude the blood supply to a peripheral nerve or cranial nerve [10]. Loss of vision can result from endophthalmitis or from infarction of the retina or optic nerve. Involvement at the spinal level is typically due to staphylococcal discitis leading to epidural abscess and in turn to spinal cord compression. However, we have seen a prevertebral abscess associated with noncompressive myelopathy, presumably due to ischemic and/or inflammatory effects on the spinal cord. Embolic spinal cord infarction is a rare occurrence.

Any of the neurologic phenomena discussed above can be the presenting manifestation of or a very late occurrence in endocarditis. A patient's initial presentation may be a transient ischemic attack, brain infarction, subarachnoid hemorrhage, meningitis, or myelopathy. A silent cerebrovascular manifestation can come to attention when it causes a seizure. Any of the nonspecific neurologic manifestations can be the presenting complaint. As examples, a patient with undiagnosed endocarditis can be admitted to the hospital for personality change, depression, or confusion. Thus, clinicians must always remember the possibility that occult endocarditis could be the cause of their patients' problems.

Attention to systemic medical symptoms and laboratory results is very important. I remember one patient with recurrent depression who had required psychiatric hospitalization many times over a decade or more. On one admission he again underwent electroshock therapy. During the induced convulsion, he suffered a subarachnoid hemorrhage from a mycotic aneurysm. It was streptococcal endocarditis which had precipitated this latest bout of depression. The psychiatrist had not noticed that the patient's hematocrit was less than 30%. On previous admissions it had been normal. The anemia was the overlooked clue to the presence of systemic medical illness.

Unfortunately, the clinician must also be prepared for neurologic manifestations of endocarditis to become evident after the diagnosis has been made and the treatment has

---

[2] Paul Beeson, personal communication, 1977.

been completed. Weeks or months after a full course of antibiotic therapy an unhealed mycotic aneurysm can rupture or a sterilized fragment of a valvular vegetation can break loose and cause embolic cerebral infarction.

References

1. H. A. Cooper, E. C. Thompson, R. Laureno et al. Subclinical brain embolization in left-sided infective endocarditis: results from the evaluation by MRI of the brains of patients with left-sided intracardiac solid masses (EMBOLISM) pilot study. *Circulation* 2009; **120**: 585–591.

2. R. Laureno, R. W. Shields, T. Narayan. The diagnosis and management of cerebral embolism and haemorrhagic infarction with sequential computerized cranial tomography. *Brain* 1987; **110** (Pt 1): 93–105.

3. G. F. Molinari, L. Smith, M. N. Goldstein et al. Pathogenesis of cerebral mycotic aneurysms. *Neurology* 1973; **23**: 325–332.

4. A. Daneshmand, L. Rangel-Castilla, C. Rydberg et al. Ultra-rapid developing infectious aneurysms. *Neurocrit Care* 2019; **30**: 487–489.

5. D. van de Beek, A. A. Rabinstein, S. G. Peters et al. *Staphylococcus endocarditis* associated with infectious vasculitis and recurrent cerebral hemorrhages. *Neurocrit Care* 2008; **8**: 48–52.

6. R. D. Adams, C. S. Kubik, F. J. Bonner. The clinical and pathological aspects of influenzal meningitis. *Arch Pediatr* 1948; **65**: 408–441.

7. T. Chakraborty, A. Rabinstein, E. Wijdicks. Chapter 11 – Neurologic complications of infective endocarditis. In: J. Biller, ed. *Heart and Neurologic Disease.* Amsterdam, Elsevier, 2021; 125–134.

8. A. B. Singhal, M. A. Topcuoglu, F. S. Buonanno. Acute ischemic stroke patterns in infective and nonbacterial thrombotic endocarditis: a diffusion-weighted magnetic resonance imaging study. *Stroke* 2002; **33**: 1267–1273.

9. N. A. Morris, M. Matiello, J. L. Lyons et al. Neurologic complications in infective endocarditis: identification, management, and impact on cardiac surgery. *Neurohospitalist* 2014; **4**: 213–222.

10. L. Weinstein, J. J. Schlesinger. Pathoanatomic, pathophysiologic and clinical correlations in endocarditis (second of two parts). *N Engl J Med* 1974; **291**: 1122–1126.

Secondary Abscess Formation in Primary Brain Lesions

During my first week as a neurology resident, I assumed care of several patients on the ward. I presented each patient to the attending neurologist, Maurice Victor. I explained that one patient, having been hospitalized for several weeks after suffering a cerebral hemorrhage, had become progressively obtunded. Dr. Victor responded: "This is not the natural history of cerebral hemorrhage." He advised that we have the neurosurgeons see what was going on "in there." We were in an era where clinical analysis guided patient management without the help of cross-sectional imaging. (Our hospital did not yet have a CT scanner. There was only one in the city at that time.) As Victor had predicted, the operative findings were not simple. The surgeon found a hemorrhage, which had become a bacterial abscess. It was concluded that chronic bladder catheterization had caused urinary tract infection. The resulting septicemia had in turn infected the brain hemorrhage.

With this experience I became interested in our topic, infection of preexisting brain lesions. We will not touch on other areas of interface of infection and brain lesions such as a brain abscess being mistaken for tumor, infection after intracranial surgery, or infection predisposing to brain lesions, for example, mycotic aneurysm. We will limit this discussion to infection developing in unoperated tumors, infarctions, and hematomas.

Once CT scanning became widely available, one could visualize the development of an abscess in a hematoma as in the following instance:

Case 1

A 68-year-old woman developed a large right putaminal hemorrhage with intraventricular extension (Figure 19.1a). One and a half months later there developed symptomatic swelling in the area of the hemorrhage where there was now a ring-shaped contrast enhancing lesion (Figure 19.1b). A neurosurgeon drained the abscess. The pus revealed innumerable white blood cells and many gram-negative rods.

Ring-shaped contrast enhancement often develops in the natural evolution of a cerebral hemorrhage. Thus, the diagnosis of abscess in a brain hematoma is not made by imaging features alone. One makes the diagnosis by the clinical information in totality. In this case the late neurologic worsening and the late edema were as important as the ring enhancement.

Cerebral infarction can similarly be the site of development of brain abscess. After cerebral infarction a heavy network of cellular capillaries surrounds the lesion for weeks. This reactive change accounts for the breakdown of the blood brain barrier seen around infarctions on contrast enhanced CT scans or gadolinium enhanced MRI scans. The broken blood brain barrier can allow systemic infection to intrude. It is surprising that such infection does not occur more often [1] as it did in the following case:

Case 2

An 85-year-old diabetic man had been recovering from a right middle cerebral artery distribution infarct at a rehabilitation hospital (Figure 19.2a). Six weeks after his stroke he developed a left arm convulsion; his temperature was 103F. A CT head scan revealed right hemisphere swelling around a ring enhancing lesion in the region of the prior infarction (Figure 19.2b). There was urinary infection. The neurosurgeon drained 50cc of purulent material from the brain lesion. Culture revealed *Citrobacter diversus*. With subsequent antibiotic treatment the abscess was cured. In sum, the urinary infection had led to septicemia with seeding of the healing cerebral infarction. A brain abscess resulted.

Most intracranial tumors have blood brain barrier breakdown as indicated by contrast enhancement on brain imaging. Because the barrier is broken, bacteria can enter a tumor of almost any type. For example, there are reports of abscess forming in craniopharyngioma [2]. Secondary abscess in pituitary adenoma is well known [3, 4]. When hemorrhage occurs in a glioblastoma, a secondary abscess can ensue [5]. A meningioma can first become symptomatic when it is seeded with infection [6]. Abscess can also develop in a brain metastasis. What by imaging appears to be liquefactive necrosis in a brain metastasis can actually be the early stage of an abscess [7, 8]. In one patient, each of two brain metastases was infected with gram positive cocci [8]. In the immunosuppressed patient, mycobacterial infection of a brain metastasis has occurred [7].

(a)   (b)

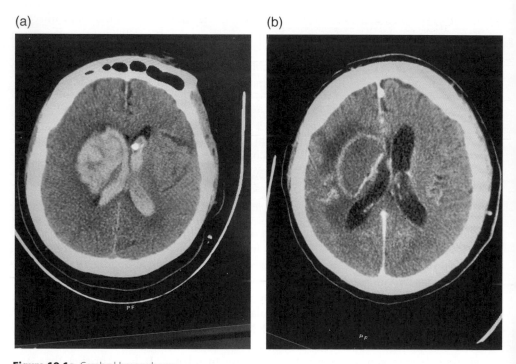

Figure 19.1a Cerebral hemorrhage.
Figure 19.1b Abscess in the area of the hemorrhage discovered 1.5 months after the hemorrhage occurred.

(a)   (b)

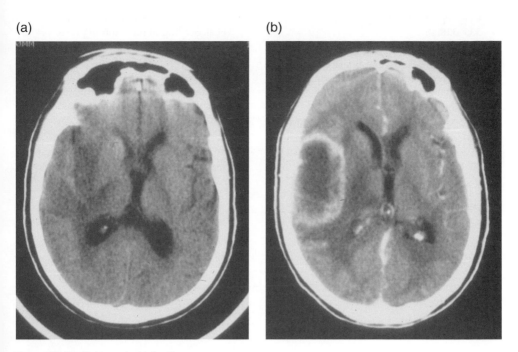

Figure 19.2a Right cerebral infarction.
Figure 19.2b Six weeks after the stroke an abscess has developed in the infarction.

19.1 Final Comments

Although the incidence of secondary abscess formation in primary brain lesions is low, such occurrences are well documented. In infarctions, hemorrhages, and tumors it is septicemia that leads to secondary brain abscess. Bacterial seeding of brain lesions is more likely to occur in diabetic or immunosuppressed patients. Occasionally, a secondary brain abscess may cause the first symptoms of a previously asymptomatic tumor. Recognition of a secondary abscess can be delayed when the symptoms of the infection are mistakenly attributed to a previously diagnosed tumor.

Interpretation of imaging can be challenging. Liquefactive necrosis in a tumor can be mistaken for abscess. Abscess in a tumor can be mistaken for simple necrosis. The possibility of abscess should be strongly considered whenever the lesion has restricted diffusion on the MRI scan. Multiple ring enhancing lesions in the same patient usually are due either to multiple abscesses or to multiple metastases. Only rarely are multiple metastases all infected simultaneously.

References

1. Anonymous. Case records of the Massachusetts General Hospital. Weekly clinicopathological exercises. Case 31–1991. A 67-year-old man with cerebral lesions with ring enhancement demonstrable on a CT scan three months after a myocardial infarct. *N Engl J Med* 1991; **325**: 341–350.

2. K. S. Bhaisora, S. N. Prasad, K. K. Das et al. Abscess inside craniopharyngioma: diagnostic and management implications. *BMJ Case Rep* 2018; **Feb 03**. doi:10.1136/bcr-2017-223040.

3. S. N. Kroppenstedt, T. Liebig, W. Mueller et al. Secondary abscess formation in pituitary adenoma after tooth extraction.

Case report. *J Neurosurg* 2001; **94**: 335–338.

4. A. J. Awad, N. C. Rowland, M. Mian et al. Etiology, prognosis, and management of secondary pituitary abscesses forming in underlying pituitary adenomas. *J Neurooncol* 2014; **117**: 469–476.

5. M. Ichikawa, Y. Shimizu, M. Sato et al. Abscess within a glioblastoma multiforme – case report. *Neurol Med Chir (Tokyo)* 1992; **32**: 829–833.

6. E. Christopher, F. C. Moreton, A. Torgersen et al. Seeding of infection in previously asymptomatic meningioma. *Pract Neurol* 2020; **20**: 247–248.

7. A. A. Little, S. S. Gebarski, M. Blaivas. Nontuberculous mycobacterial infection of a metastatic brain neoplasm in an immunocompromised patient. *Arch Neurol* 2006; **63**: 763–765.

8. W. P. Ng, A. Lozano. Abscess within a brain metastasis. *Can J Neurol Sci* 1996; **23**: 300–302.

Progressive Multifocal Leukoencephalopathy: The Early Years

As I was nearing the end of my neurology residency, I made a mental list of diseases about which I had only read. I wondered whether I would ever encounter them. The list included gumma, adult toxoplasmosis, and progressive multifocal leukoencephalopathy (PML). Within a few years, the AIDS epidemic provided much of what I had been interested to see. Once a rare disease, PML became so common that "PML" would roll off the tongue of a medical student as easily as "UTI" (urinary tract infection). As I became very experienced with PML, I wondered about its history. Over subsequent years, I was able to interview some of the key figures who were involved in recognizing, naming, and understanding this disease.

In 1952 Raymond D. Adams was called to see a patient with a puzzling neurological disorder. Because the patient had chronic lymphocytic leukemia, the internal medicine service at Massachusetts General Hospital suspected that the patient had leukemic infiltration of the central nervous system. Adams doubted this explanation. In his deep experience as a neurologist and neuropathologist, he had never seen a similar case. He believed that the patient had a unique disease [1].

The patient eventually came to autopsy. When the neuropathology fellow, Karl-Erik Astrom brought the slides to Adams, he was "astonished" to see the brain lesions under the microscope [1]. "The pathology was strikingly demyelinative" [1]. In the lesions, many astrocytes were greatly enlarged; their bizarre nuclei showed mitoses. On the periphery of lesions, there were distinctive oligodendrocyte abnormalities; the nuclei were enlarged and basophilic. As Adams had predicted, the brain pathology was unique.

It just so happened that this brain came under study when Adams was investigating neuroimmunologic disease with Byron Waksman. Adams was the neuropathologist and Waksman was the immunologist. They were studying experimental allergic encephalomyelitis, experimental allergic neuritis, and related disorders. Waksman would meet with Adams on Saturday mornings to review the slides from their experimental animals.[1]

These Saturday sessions would last for hours. As Adams, the Bullard Professor of Neuropathology, would teach Waksman microscopic pathology of inflammatory demyelinative disease, he would occasionally slip in a slide to challenge Waksman and to get his thoughts.[2] For example, he might slip in a slide of central pontine myelinolysis, a demyelinative process lacking inflammation. On another occasion he showed Waksman a demyelinative lesion from the leukemia patient described above. Both Waksman and Adams, in separate interviews, stated that Waksman was the first person to notice that there

---

[1] Byron Waksman, personal communication, 2003.
[2] Byron Waksman, personal communication, 2003.

were intranuclear inclusion bodies in abnormal glia [1].[3] From this observation Waksman suspected that he was seeing a viral disease.

Astrom and colleagues worked for months on the paper describing the neuropathology of the leukemia patient and two similar cases [2]. The second case was also from Massachusetts General Hospital. The third case was sent to Boston from Emory University.[4] Coauthors of this classic article were another neuropathology fellow, E. Mancall, and Edward P. Richardson, director of the neuropathology laboratory. (At that time neuropathology was a division of the neurology department headed by Adams.) Adams did not add his name to the paper [1].

In this 1958 paper, the authors named the disease PML to indicate its clinical course and its gross pathology [3] In two of the three case summaries, they described the eosinophilic intranuclear inclusions which Waksman had pointed out. However, in the discussion section of the paper they disregarded the presence of the inclusions, presumably because the other features of the pathology did not resemble that of the known viral encephalitides. In a later article of reminiscence Richardson stated that he had suspected that what he was observing in PML was a demyelinative disease evolving into a malignancy [4].

In 1959 Cavanagh and colleagues speculated about the cause of PML. One of the numerous possibilities they discussed was "viral parasitism." It was the inclusion bodies which led to this suggestion [5]. No proof of the nature of the inclusions would come for several years.

Two years later Richardson again wrote on this subject to offer "some modification" of his 1958 article. He summarized the findings in 10 cases of PML and reviewed the findings in 12 additional cases studied by others. He was able to examine sections from most of the cases in the latter group. He confirmed that perivascular lymphocytic infiltration was absent or minimal. He pointed out that the diseases which appear to predispose to PML share the characteristic of "immunologic hyporeactivity" and suggested that the microscopic pathologic findings in glia were consistent with the cytopathic effect of a virus. He thanked Byron Waksman for "suggesting how viral infection would account for the neuropathologic lesions" [6]. He stated that fresh autopsy material be studied for further progress in understanding PML.

It turned out that fresh brain was not required for the next advance. In 1962 Gabriele Zu Rhein, neuropathologist at the University of Wisconsin, received a brain in consultation from a pathologist at a nearby hospital. She showed the slides to a postdoctoral student, Sam Chou. Having read Astrom's paper, Chou suspected that Zu Rhein's specimen was a case of PML. By chance, soon thereafter another patient with PML was autopsied at University Hospital. Dr. Zu Rhein saved both brains.

Two years later, she was scheduled to leave for a sabbatical in New York. It occurred to her that she could take the PML specimens with her to study during her time away. Sam Chou had recently learned to use the electron microscope (EM), which had been acquired by the department of Veterinary Science. They decided to test the formalin fixed PML tissue to determine whether it would be satisfactory for EM study. (Formalin fixation is not the ideal way to prepare tissue for electron microscopy.) Zu Rhein selected smaller PML lesions rather than large confluent ones for study. When they viewed the first ultrathin section on the EM screen, they saw that it was packed with virus!

---

[3] Byron Waksman, personal communication, 2003.
[4] Elliott Mancall, personal communication, 2004.

What Zu Rhein saw on the EM screen looked very familiar. She had been active in teaching neuropathology in the veterinary school as well as the medical school. Recently she had read about canine oral papilloma in the thesis of a veterinary pathology student. The "intranuclear crystalloid aggregates of virions" in the human PML lesions resembled those found in the dog papillomas [7].

In September 1964 she traveled to New York with the Epon blocks from her PML brains. On arriving at Montefiore Hospital for her sabbatical, she showed Dr. Harry Zimmerman the first EM prints. He was impressed. Since he was president of the Association for Research in Nervous and Mental Disease (ARNMD) he was able to quickly add her as a speaker at the organization's upcoming annual meeting. In December, she presented her material at the symposium on "Infections of the Nervous System." In her lecture Zu Rhein pointed out not only that the virions looked like papova virus but that the particles in her material were about the same size as polyoma virus in the papova virus group. On the expert panel at her talk was one of the world's great virologists, Dr. Albert Sabin.

Zu Rhein's suggestion that PML was caused by polyoma virus aroused emotional responses. Sabin was highly critical. By Zu Rhein's recollection, he referred to her work as "deplorable" and rejected the idea that one could identify a virus by morphologic evidence [2]. After the session, however, Dr. Richard Johnson, a neurovirologist at the Cleveland Metropolitan General Hospital, praised her work and congratulated her with a hug. Later, Johnson recalled, Sabin had disdainfully commented to him, "She thinks there are warts in the brain" [2]. (At the time, the human wart virus was the only papova virus known to cause disease in human beings.) In the published version of the proceedings Sabin's discussion is more polite [8].

Zu Rhein and Chou published their findings in 1965 [9]. Silverman's independent confirmatory electron microscopic observations were published in the same year [10]. Later in 1965, Zu Rhein attended the meeting of the American Association of Neuropathologists. She listened to Harvey Shein's lecture about polyoma virus induced cytopathic change in human cell culture. His findings in fetal spongioblasts and astrocytes reminded Zu Rhein of the cytopathology of PML [7].

Three years later (1968), Zu Rhein had her opportunity [7]. She received a call from the VA Hospital in East Orange, New Jersey about a suspected case of PML. She flew to New Jersey for the autopsy, sliced the fresh brain, selected numerous pieces and flew back to Madison, Wisconsin. At midnight she transferred the tissue on ice to Dr. Duard Walker, a microbiologist. For years he tried unsuccessfully to harvest virus from tissue cultures of this material.

Another opportunity came in 1970 [7]. One Sunday, Zu Rhein was in her laboratory, where she received a call from the VA Hospital in Wood, Wisconsin. There a PML patient was about to be autopsied. Forthwith, she and Dr. Walker drove to Wood and sampled the fresh brain of John F. Cunningham. Dr. Billie Padgett in Walker's lab tried a different method to demonstrate virus. She developed a modification of the culture system used by Dr. Shein for polyoma virus. With this method virus was grown from John Cunningham's brain on March 24, 1971. In honor of the brain donor the agent was named the JC virus. Eventually, using her special method, Dr. Padgett also cultured JC virus from the East Orange brain [11].

20.1 Final Comments

By clinical analysis alone, a neurologist recognized that the "first" PML patient was suffering from a unique disease. It was an immunologist not a pathologist who first noticed the intranuclear inclusions in PML. After the pathologists accepted his observation, they were hesitant to comment on the significance of the inclusions. No doubt this hesitancy stemmed from the pathology of PML being so unlike that of the known viral encephalitides. When the use of a newer technology, electron microscopy, provided visual evidence of the viral particles in the PML lesions, some virologists were skeptical. They were so accustomed to nonmorphologic methods that some felt a visceral antipathy to the images of Zu Rhein and Chou. Resistance also came from their fixed idea that the only human disease caused by polyoma virus was the cutaneous wart. When usual virologic methods failed to yield virus, a modified method succeeded. Many investigators from the fields of neurology, neuropathology, immunology, and virology participated in developing knowledge of a mysterious disease. Tenacity and hard work were essential to success. By studying the PML story one can gain many insights into the challenges one faces in advancing neurology or any other field of medicine.

References

1. R. Laureno. *Raymond Adams: A Life of Mind and Muscle*. New York, Oxford University Press, 2009.

2. K. Khalili, G. L. Stoner. *Human Polyomaviruses*. John Wiley & Sons, Inc., New York, 2001.

3. K. E. Astrom, E. L. Mancall, E. P. Richardson. Progressive multifocal leuko-encephalopathy; a hitherto unrecognized complication of chronic lymphatic leukaemia and Hodgkin's disease. *Brain* 1958; **81**: 93–111.

4. J. W. Henson, D. N. Louis. Edward Peirson Richardson Jr. (1918–1998) and the discovery of PML. *J Neurovirol* 1999; **5**: 325–326.

5. J. B. Cavanagh, D. Greenbaum, A. H. Marshall et al. Cerebral demyelination associated with disorders of the reticuloendothelial system. *Lancet* 1959; **2**: 524–529.

6. E. P. Richardson. Progressive multifocal leukoencephalopathy. *N Engl J Med* 1961; **265**: 815–823.

7. G. M. Zu Rhein. Reflections on my family history, my youth, and my professional career. Autobiography. *J Neuropathol Exp Neurol* 2012; **71**: 1149–1162.

8. Association for Research in Nervous and Mental Disease, H. M. Zimmerman, ed. *Infections of the Nervous System: Proceedings of the Association. December 4–5,1964, New York, NY*. Baltimore, Williams and Wilkins Company, 1968.

9. G. M. Zu Rhein, S. M. Chou. Particles resembling papova viruses in human cerebral demyelinating disease. *Science* 1965; **148**: 1477–1479.

10. L. Silverman, L. J. Rubinstein. Electron microscopic observations on a case of progressive multifocal leukoencephalopathy. *Acta Neuropathol* 1965; **5**: 215–224.

11. B. L. Padgett, D. L. Walker, G. M. Zu Rhein et al. Cultivation of papova-like virus from human brain with progressive multifocal leucoencephalopathy. *Lancet* 1971; **1**: 1257–1260.

Index

abscess, *95*
  secondary, 93–95
acute toxic exposure,
    neurologic effects on, 82
acute transneuronal change
    (diaschisis), 61
Adams, Raymond, 46
Adams, Raymond D., 20, 41, 97
agnosia, 11
  Sigmund Freud, 9
alcohol withdrawal, 26
allergic encephalomyelitis, 97
Alzheimer's disease, 25, 33
American Association of
    Neuropathologists, 99
amnesia, 2
  anterograde, 1
  caused by a unilateral
      lesion, 7
  causes of, 7
  due to bilateral lesions, 7
  memory tests and, 6–7
amnesic syndrome, 1, *3*, *4*, 7
  anatomy and memory
      relationship to, 5
  inferomedial temporal lobe
      bilateral resection of
      the, 1–2
  multiple territories, 4–5
  terminologies used with, 7
amoebae, 85–86
amygdala-anterior
    hippocampal
    hemorrhage, *5*
amyotrophic lateral
    sclerosis, 17
anatomy
  amnesic syndrome and, 5
  olfactory system, 87
anesthesia
  distal, 15
  social and legal aspects of,
      69–71
anterograde amnesia, 1
anterograde atrophy, 59
anterograde transneuronal
    atrophy, *60*
antiepileptic medicine, 41
aphasias, 2, 9, 12

Armand Trousseau and, 9
apraxia, 10
  classifications of, 10
  Hugo Liepmann and, 9
Association for Research in
    Nervous and Mental
    Disease (ARNMD), 99
asterixis, 41–43
  causes of, *41*, *42*
Astrom, Karl-Erik, 97
ataxia, 18, 80
  Friedreich, 55–56
  gait, 75
atrophic fibers in
    denervation, *49*
atrophy, anterograde, 59
auditory perseveration
    (palinacousis), 32

bacteremia, 89
basal forebrain, 4
basal forebrain damage, *4*
basal ganglia disease, 75
Bender, Morris, 17
bifrontal disease, grasp reflex
    and, *36*
bifrontal lesions, grasp reflex
    and, *37*
bilateral hippocampal
    infarction, *2*
bitemporal atrophy, MRI, *3*
brain
  brain death, 69,
  degenerative disease of
      the, 25
  forebrain disease, 33, 39
brain diseases, 15, 22, 41, 72, 73
  degenerative, 2, 31
  grasp reflex and, 33
  liver cure and, 73
  liver disease and, 72, 74
brain/spinal cord lesion, 59
Briquet syndrome, 22

canine oral papilloma, 99
carbon monoxide
    poisoning, 66
cardiovascular medications,
    hallucinogenic, 26

central nervous system
    disease, 30
central nervous system lesions
    transneuronal distant effects
    of, 61
central pathway, the, 55–57
cerebral artery distribution
    infarction, *11*
cerebral degeneration, 25
cerebral hemorrhage, 93, 94
cerebral infarction, *95*
cerebrovascular disorders, 89
Charles Bonnet Syndrome, 29
Cleveland Metropolitan
    General Hospital, 78
Cobb, Stanley, 52
contralateral focal lesion, grasp
    reflex and, *35*
conversion, 22, 23
  reactions, 23
copper neurotoxicity, 72
Creutzfeldt Jakob disease,
    progressive dementia
    and, 19

degenerative brain diseases, 2
dementia, 10, 69
  hallucinations and, 25
depression, 19, 22, 91
  diagnosis of, 21
  malingerers and, 20
deprivation phenomena,
    hallucinations and, 30
Dimethylmercury, 82
disordered vestibular system,
    hallucinations and, 30
dopaminergic drugs,
    hallucinations and, 26
dorsiflexion, 41

electric shock, 21
electroencephalographic and
    video recording, 16
electromyographic
    recording, 16
electrophysiologic study, 16
emotion
  intense, 19
  patients overwhelmed by, 19

THE EINSTEINIAN REVOLUTION

The Einsteinian Revolution

THE HISTORICAL ROOTS
OF HIS BREAKTHROUGHS

HANOCH GUTFREUND
& JÜRGEN RENN

PRINCETON UNIVERSITY PRESS
PRINCETON & OXFORD

Published by Princeton University Press
41 William Street, Princeton, New Jersey 08540
99 Banbury Road, Oxford OX2 6JX

press.princeton.edu

All Rights Reserved

ISBN 9780691168760
ISBN (e-book) 9780691256498

Library of Congress Control Number: 2023940551

British Library Cataloging-in-Publication Data is available

Editorial: Eric Crahan and Whitney Rauenhorst
Production Editorial: Terri O'Prey
Jacket Design: Chris Ferrante
Production: Danielle Amatucci
Publicity: Matthew Taylor and Kate Farquhar-Thomson
Copyeditor: Susan Matheson

This book has been composed in Arno

Printed on acid-free paper. ∞

Printed in the United States of America

10 9 8 7 6 5 4 3 2

CONTENTS

Introduction

THIS BOOK is based on a monograph written by one of the authors (J. R.), published in German in 2006: *Auf den Schultern von Riesen und Zwergen—Einsteins Unvollendete Revolution* (On the shoulders of the great and small—Einstein's unfinished revolution). It explores the history of Einstein's transformation of our concepts of space, time, matter, gravitation, and radiation. This revolution can be traced back to his pioneering papers of 1905, in which he began to question the classical understanding of these concepts, shaking the very foundations of classical physics. His ideas challenged the assumption that light is a wave, gave striking proof for the existence of atoms, led to a new understanding of space and time (which came to be known as the "special theory of relativity"), and identified mass as a form of energy. Attempts to fit Isaac Newton's well-established law of gravity into the framework of the special theory of relativity did not succeed, at least not without ignoring basic principles of mechanics. Although this problem did not lead to urgent empirical challenges, it led Einstein in 1907 to question the special theory's concepts of space and time, and inspired him to continue the revolution with his 1915 general theory of relativity.

What we call here the "Einsteinian Revolution," emerging from his work in the early twentieth century, was merely the beginning of a major transformation of the knowledge system of classical physics.[1] This process spanned much of the century and eventually saw the establishment of quantum physics and general relativity as the two major conceptual frameworks that represent the two unreconciled pillars of modern physics. Shortly after formulating the general theory of relativity, Einstein, dissatisfied with this conceptual dichotomy, embarked on a search for a unified understanding of physics, an endeavor he pursued until the end of his life.

The main goal of this book is to dispel the popular myth that Albert Einstein, the unconventional scientific genius, instigated an overwhelming scientific revolution through pure thought alone. This myth tends to blind us to the historical conflicts that Einstein was involved with, as well as to the conditions shaping the transformation of knowledge systems connected with his work. In trying to understand the origin of the innovation that is the hallmark of Einstein's contributions, it is tempting to seek out personality traits that relate to his individual creativity. However, any attempt to understand the birth of modern physics as the outcome of individual accounts of discovery will encounter paradoxes. Consequently, an understanding can only be reached by carefully reviewing the long-term history of the evolution of knowledge. This book thus focuses on Einstein's enduring contributions to science in the context of the evolution of knowledge.

The plan to produce an English version of this book prompted us to rethink its structure and the presentation of its core messages. During this process, we found that a much more extensive revision was necessary to incorporate the many insights we had gained throughout the course of our collaboration. Numerous books on various aspects of Einstein's life and science have been published since the German version appeared, including four we coauthored. Our aim with this book is to highlight more clearly and concisely the historical origins and the unique features of the Einsteinian revolution. We also intend to make this book more accessible to a broader community of readers through its style and presentation.

We suggest that satisfactory answers to the historical questions raised by Einstein's breakthroughs of 1905 and 1915 require a new approach to the puzzling issue of scientific revolutions. The concept of scientific revolution entered the historiography of science and popular culture through the influential book *The Structure of Scientific Revolutions,* published in 1962 by the physicist and historian of science Thomas Kuhn. Although no longer popular in historical accounts, it still offers—at least with regard to the development of physics between the seventeenth and twentieth centuries—a decent overview of the alternating periods of continuous growth (referred to as "normal" phases) and profound conceptual transformation (referred to as "revolutionary" phases). The latter are interpreted as resulting in "paradigm shifts."[2] A paradigm is characterized by a general agreement within the scientific community on basic practices of problem-solving related to a specific system of knowledge. Kuhn's notion of a scientific revolution implies the rather disruptive replacement of an existing paradigm with a new one, leaving it unclear exactly how such transitions occur.

We argue that a thorough analysis of the scientific breakthroughs in which Einstein was involved will lead to a revision of the Kuhnian premise that a scientific revolution signifies an entirely new beginning in which previously accepted ideas and practices are discarded and eventually wholly overcome. In reality, what we call here "the Einsteinian revolution" is much more complex, extends over generations, and is thus much more interesting. We demonstrate that it did not result from a paradigm shift amounting to a fundamental break, caused by a crisis of "normal science," but was part of a long-term process of knowledge transformation. In this transformation, an accumulation of incremental changes eventually led to the emergence of new concepts, similar to the creation of a new species in biological evolution. Thus, when describing the nature of the Einsteinian revolution, we prefer an evolutionary perspective, replacing the notion of a "paradigm shift" with what we call a "transformation of a system of knowledge."

This process of transforming or restructuring existing knowledge can be described as a "Copernicus process,"[3] an analogy that uses the arguably most famous example in the history of science

of the restructuring of an existing system of knowledge. Copernicus created a new astronomical system by shifting a formerly peripheral celestial body, the sun, to the center. Rather than starting with a tabula rasa, he essentially adapted the complex
mechanism of planetary astronomy inherited from Greek and
Arabic astronomy.

Such a transformation of knowledge does not discard the knowledge that came before, but repurposes it in a process of reflection
that changes the architecture of knowledge while leaving many
building blocks intact. Furthermore, the so-called Copernican
revolution, understood as the upheaval of an entire scientific
worldview, spanned more than a century, extending from the mid-
sixteenth century to the age of Newton. This revolution involved
numerous scientists, including Galileo and Kepler, whose ingenuity contributed to many fields of knowledge within astronomy and
physics. Structural changes in systems of knowledge, popularly
known as scientific revolutions, often resemble this long and comprehensive Copernican revolution, encompassing several phases
and requiring a massive communal effort.

We describe the Einsteinian revolution as an analogous transformation of the system of knowledge of classical physics. In this
context, we highlight the notion of "borderline problems" and
their fundamental role in this process. In the nineteenth century,
physics was composed of three core areas—mechanics, electrodynamics, and thermodynamics—each with their own characteristic structures of knowledge and methods of investigation.
However, tensions had been building since the mid-nineteenth
century as these three areas of physics slowly began to shift their
relative positions. With regard to their conceptual foundations,
electrodynamics and thermodynamics were moving further and
further away from mechanics, the primary continent of physics.
Electrodynamics and thermodynamics also encroached upon
each other's boundaries, with specific borderline problems raising
the risk of conflict not only with mechanics but also with one another. These were the systems of knowledge embodied by the

organization of physics at the beginning of the twentieth century when Einstein became a scientist. It took him less than twenty years to accomplish this decisive first phase of the transformation of classical physics. During this time, he established the premises that both the quantum theory and the general theory of relativity would later be based on. Through the subsequent effort of many scientists over several decades, comprehensive knowledge systems would eventually emerge from the initial seeds. Einstein's starting point was precisely the problems at the borders between the three major continents of physics.

This book is composed of six main sections, each divided into topical sections. Section I is devoted to the multidimensional character of this "Einsteinian revolution." We present a timeline of his scientific achievements, which we return to in greater detail in the following sections. The brief account of his intellectual trajectory is interwoven with biographical events that are relevant to the development of his scientific work. Einstein's personal biography does not explain everything, as some of his biographers want us to believe. But it does provide us with some clues about his unique perspective that enabled him to become a scientific pioneer. We also discuss Einstein's interaction with society at large and the interplay between his life as a scientist and his public and political activities. We do so in relation to the question of how the intellectual developments integral to the emergence of modern physics from classical physics were rooted in larger societal changes, particularly those that led to the rise of the chemical and electrotechnical industries in the so-called Second Industrial Revolution.

In section II, we place the Einsteinian revolution in a larger historical and philosophical framework of the evolution of knowledge. We emphasize the role of mental models in the historical reconstruction of thinking processes. In this context, we describe Einstein's own epistemological credo and his mode of thinking. Referring to the title of the original version of this book, we show that Einstein stood not only on the shoulders of giants, such as Galileo and Newton, but also on the vast body of shared scientific, technical, and practical knowledge accumulated over generations. To provide another example of a Copernicus process, we briefly refer to Galileo's preclassical mechanics: an intermediate stage between Aristotelian and Newtonian mechanics. Comparing some of the features of Galileo's theory of motion and its role as a scaffold for building classical mechanics with Einstein's conceptual innovations is enlightening.[4] To conclude this section, we discuss some of the other widely discussed approaches to the problem of scientific change.

Section III describes the world of physics at the time when Einstein had completed his years as a student at the Polytechnic in Zurich. We describe the rise of the mechanical worldview, rooted in Newtonian mechanics, and its demise after the emergence of the novel concept of fields and of the classical Maxwell-Lorentz theory of electrodynamics based on the concept of an all-pervading ether as a carrier of these fields. The third domain of physics was thermodynamics, which Einstein regarded as the ideal physical theory because it was independent of detailed assumptions on the constitution of matter or radiation and thus extremely helpful in guiding his search for new ideas and principles.

At the end of the nineteenth century, the physics community was puzzled by three problems at the borderlines between these three domains of physics: the problem of black-body radiation (a conflict between thermodynamics and electrodynamics and central to future quantum physics); the riddle of fluctuation phenomena, such as Brownian motion (a borderline problem between mechanics and thermodynamics and central to statistical physics); and the failure to detect the motion of the earth through the ether (a borderline problem between mechanics and electrodynamics that eventually gave rise to relativity theory). We discuss these in detail and demonstrate how the problems specifically, and borderline problems more generally, triggered changes in the structure of knowledge that are characteristic of transformations of knowledge.

Section IV is devoted to Einstein's miraculous year, 1905, when he was working at the patent office in Bern. We argue that only by

recognizing his breakthroughs as steps within an extended Copernicus process does it become possible to understand how the scientific research of a young patent office employee could have such
far-reaching consequences. His success is rooted in a transformation
of the knowledge of classical physics accumulated over generations.
He achieved the breakthroughs of his miraculous year by reinterpreting the solutions to the borderline problems that the masters of
classical physics had provided. We emphasize both the role of Einstein's interest in atomistic notions that connect diverse areas of
physics and his search for observable fluctuation phenomena during the years 1902 to 1905. This search led him to deviate radically
from nineteenth-century traditions of optics and electrodynamics
and to the groundbreaking papers of 1905. Although, at first glance,
the papers of Einstein's miraculous year seem to deal with separate
domains, we demonstrate that they are actually closely related and
represent a unified vision of physics, which, however, could not be
accomplished as originally envisaged.

Section V describes Einstein's convoluted road from the special
to the general theory of relativity. This is a well-documented chapter
in the history of science and has been described by many authors,
including in our book wholly devoted to this topic: *The Road to Relativity*. Here, we briefly describe this process, emphasizing the main
obstacles, dilemmas, and insights that will support its characterization in the final section as a transformation of a system of knowledge.
With the establishment of special relativity as a new framework for
dealing with space and time, a new borderline problem emerged between this new kinematics (laws of motion) and the classical theory
of gravitation. How could Newton's law of gravitation—conceiving
gravity as an instantaneous attraction between masses—be adapted
to this new framework that prohibited the instantaneous propagation of such physical effects? We discuss Einstein's struggle with this
problem over several years and show how he finally arrived at a new
relativistic theory of gravitation after having first constructed an intermediate theory that served as a scaffolding for formulating the
field equations of general relativity in 1915.

Although this was a decisive step, it did not mark the end of this Einsteinian revolution. We follow the further development of general relativity over the course of roughly fifteen years after its completion. We refer to this period as the formative years of general relativity.[5] During this period, Einstein, together with a small community of colleagues, explored the basic consequences of the field equations. We focus mainly on the tension between the heuristics that guided Einstein on his road to the general theory of relativity and the actual implications of the framework created in 1915.

Finally, in section VI we take a further look at the Einsteinian revolution as a transformation of the system of knowledge, this time presenting it as a chapter in the long history of physics. Within this context, we discuss the unique features of the Einsteinian revolution that made it so perplexing to observers, both then and now, including to Einstein himself. General relativity was not motivated primarily by new empirical results but instead was guided by ultimately elusive heuristics and based on the knowledge of classical physics, and yet it gave rise to nonclassical insights incompatible with the framework that Einstein's research was originally based on. Another characteristic feature of general relativity is its long evolution from its genesis to its gradual shift to the periphery during its "low-water mark" period,[6] and its eventual rise to a second pillar of modern physics, next to quantum physics, in the critical period of its renaissance in the mid-1950s. The theory was then finally understood by a growing scientific community as a generally applicable physical framework in its own right, which finally led to the "golden years" of the 1960s when this theoretical framework was connected with new astrophysical discoveries, becoming the foundation of relativistic astrophysics and cosmology.

We conclude this section, and the book, with a comprehensive summary, recapitulating the central points of the previous sections, thus ending the reader's journey through a convoluted and exciting road of discovery.

We indicated above that numerous books on various aspects of Einstein's scientific achievements, on their consequences, and on his personal life have been published since the publication of the original German version of this book. Many of them are mentioned in the footnotes or references lists. Nevertheless, we would like to list several of those books, which were written with a broader historical perspective and hence fit into the evolutionary narrative of science history. This listing may be helpful to readers who wish to explore the topics discussed by us in greater detail. In particular, the recently published book by one of us (J. R.), *The Evolution of Knowledge: Rethinking Science for the Anthropocene*, reframes the history of science and technology within a much broader history of knowledge. It discusses the structural changes and modes of transformation of knowledge throughout history and across scientific disciplines and human practices.

Among the books on Einstein's scientific achievements, we mention only a few. *The Cambridge Companion to Einstein*, edited by Michel Janssen and Christoph Lehner, brings together fourteen essays by leading historians and philosophers of science introducing the reader to the scientific work of Albert Einstein; Jed Buchwald's *Einstein Was Right*, a compendium of essays on the prediction and confirmation of gravitational waves; Daniel Kennefick's books *Traveling at the Speed of Thought* and *No Shadow of Doubt* on gravitational waves and on the confirmation of the general theory of relativity; Jean Eisenstaedt's *The Curious History of Relativity* on how black holes saved the theory of general relativity; Roberto Lalli's book on *Building the General Relativity and Gravitation Community During the Cold War*, and the work of the Max Planck Institute for the History of Science group on the renaissance of general relativity in the 1950s and 1960s; the recently published book by Michel Janssen and one of us (J. R.) on *How Einstein Found His Field Equations*. For books on Einstein's public and political activities, we mention the book by David Rowe and Robert Schulmann, *Einstein on Politics*, and Ze'ev

Rosenkranz's book *Einstein Before Israel* and his two books on Einstein's travel diaries: *The Far East, Palestine, and Spain, 1922– 1923* and *South America, 1925*.

Finally, we acknowledge the many sources of influence and support in the publication of this book. This book is shaped directly and indirectly by many years of collaboration with scholars at the Max Planck Institute for the History of Science. The German text of the original publication from which this book is derived was translated with great care into English by Dieter Brill and amended by Donald Salisbury, both of who also made many helpful suggestions. Our thanks also go to the incomparable and unrivaled Laurent Taudin who drew the accompanying illustrations. A friendly word of thanks is due also to the Albert Einstein Archives at the Hebrew University of Jerusalem, in particular Chaya Becker, and to the Collected Papers of Albert Einstein (the Einstein Papers Project) at the California Institute of Technology in Pasadena under the direction of Diana Buchwald for permission to cite passages from Einstein's work and correspondence and more generally for providing Einstein scholarship with it most valuable resource. Thanks also to Jascha Schmitz and Abigail McFarlane for their assistance with the editorial work. We are indebted to our editor at Princeton University Press, Eric Crahan, for his unfailing support. Finally, we acknowledge with appreciation and gratitude the invaluable and professional editorial management of Lindy Divarci.

THE EINSTEINIAN REVOLUTION

I

The Einstein Phenomenon

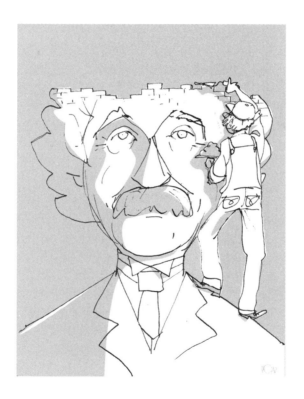

Preview

At the beginning of the twentieth century, Albert Einstein was twenty-one years old, recently graduated from the Polytechnic, the Federal Institute of Technology (now ETH) in Zurich, and desperately searching for a position that would allow him to provide

1

for the family he intended to create with his fellow student Mileva Marić. About twenty years later, in 1921, after profoundly changing the understanding of the physical world as it was then seen by the scientific community, he won the Nobel Prize in Physics. At the end of the century, he was chosen by *TIME* magazine as "Person of the Century," followed by Mahatma Gandhi and Franklin Roosevelt.

The first phase of the Einsteinian revolution began in 1905, the so-called miraculous year, when Einstein was still employed by the patent office in Bern, Switzerland. Thus, the critical papers he produced during that year were conceived and written outside the realm of the centers of learning where the questions he addressed were extensively debated and researched by the prominent players in the contemporary arena of physics. In these papers, Einstein profoundly modified the classical concepts of space, time, matter, and radiation. This raises questions: How could Einstein, as an outsider, cause such a revolution in physics? And, following on from the first question, what is a scientific revolution? Numerous Einstein biographies have attempted to answer the former. Thomas Kuhn and many historians and philosophers of sciences have attempted to answer the latter. This book is neither a biography nor another philosophical analysis of a scientific revolution. It is not even a scientific biography. The biographical discussion in this first section treats both personal and scientific aspects and is intended, for the case of Einstein's upheaval of physics, to lay the groundwork for answering both of these questions in subsequent sections.

This requires going beyond the scope of his personal scientific biography, by placing this upheaval in the broader context of the history of science and the evolution of knowledge. We also critically look at Kuhn's description of the nature of scientific revolutions, with his notion of change of paradigm[1] having become a popular way of interpreting such upheavals. We instead present the Einsteinian revolution as a transformation of the knowledge system of classical physics that spanned several decades. Systems of knowledge are understood here as comprehensive unities of theories, concepts, and practices, including the instrumentation and the knowledge required to utilize them. They are socially transmitted via education, shared practices, textbooks, and the material culture included in such instrumentation.

That we are dealing with a more complex, protracted process than is suggested by the notion of a "paradigm shift" is suggested by the dual nature of Einstein's "relativity revolution," exemplified by the revolution of space and time that began in 1905 with his formulation of the special theory of relativity, which shortly after was seen to be incomplete. Attempts to fit Newton's well-established law of gravity into the framework of this theory did not succeed, at least not without abandoning basic principles of mechanics. Although this problem did not lead to urgent empirical questions, it brought Einstein to question the special theory's concepts of space and time and inspired him to continue the transformation of knowledge with his 1915 general theory of relativity.

While Einstein was working, beginning in 1907, on the implications of relativity for the understanding of gravity, his papers on the constitution of matter and radiation advanced his career and eventually led to his call to Berlin in 1913. There was hope that he would make decisive advances toward a theory of matter that would connect both physics and chemistry, but Einstein concentrated primarily on the problem of finding a new theory of gravity. He pursued this quest despite the resistance of his established colleagues and, initially, with few prospects for success. Eventually, however, in 1919, his prediction of the bending of light due to gravitation was spectacularly confirmed during a solar eclipse expedition. Thus, the myth of Einstein as a solitary genius was born.

Einstein was committed to the search for a comprehensive scientific worldview, a quest that first emerged in the context of his early readings of popular scientific literature and philosophical textbooks. It evolved during his further scientific odyssey and later formed the framework of his *Autobiographical Notes*. Einstein's scientific achievements were developed in loose conjunction with his views on epistemology and the philosophy of science. These views also guided him on his road to general relativity and in his later quest for a unified field theory. His commitment to these views, however, made him a dissident of the emerging and widely accepted quantum worldview.

The extent to which Einstein's achievements constituted revolutionary breakthroughs, or rather represented a continuation of the work of his predecessors, was an issue that he was aware of himself. When considering Einstein's contribution to the evolution of physics as a transformation of the knowledge systems of classical physics, we must enter a dialogue with his own epistemological reflections. Indeed, understanding his breakthroughs from the perspective of a historical epistemology, as is proposed here, owes much to his own thinking about conceptual transformations in science. We return to this dialogue throughout the book.

a. Childhood and Youth

In the following discussion, we concentrate on the intellectual landscape of physics that the breakthroughs of 1905 and 1915 emerged from, as well as the dynamics of Einstein's interaction with this landscape. These dynamics do, of course, involve his early personal development, which affected the way that he later appropriated the shared knowledge of contemporary physics. For this reason, we briefly review his youth and family background.

Einstein's introduction to science was already favored by his birth in Ulm, Germany, in 1879, into an assimilated Jewish family whose livelihood was in the field of electrical technology. In 1880, the Einstein family moved from Ulm to Munich, where Einstein's father, Hermann, together with his brother, the engineer Jakob Einstein, founded a firm producing generators, and arc and incandescent lamps, as well as telephone systems.

When Albert was about ten years old and enrolled in the Luitpold-Gynasium in Munich, his parents invited a young, orthodox Jewish medical student from Lithuania, Max Talmud, to their home to teach young Albert about the principles of Judaism. Talmud surpassed their expectations, and to their dismay, young Albert demanded that they observe the rules of the Sabbath and respect kosher in the home. However, this period was short-lived and later referred to by Einstein as a "religious paradise of youth."[2] Still, Talmud had a lasting impact on Einstein's life. He gave young Albert a geometry book and, in later recollections, Einstein would refer to the encounter with this book as the impetus that led to him to become a scientist. The possibility to prove surprising statements with certainty, such as the claim that the three altitudes in a triangle intersect at one point, seemed miraculous to him. The sense of wonder generated by the possibility of reaching unexpected truths through pure thought alone remained with him throughout his life.

Talmud also recommended that Albert read the popular books on natural science by Aaron Bernstein, a Jewish author, reformer, and scientist from Danzig, Poland, who earned a reputation as a popularizer of science. He had been a supporter of the failed 1848 democratic uprising and since then had hoped to promote the ideals of progress and democracy through the popularization of science. His books offered readers a fascinating and encyclopedic overview of contemporary natural science. Reading Bernstein's books provided Einstein with a remarkably broad knowledge that also familiarized him with the international spirit of science, including some of its philosophical and political implications. Through these books, the young Albert learned how concepts such as "atoms" or "ether" could help to uncover mysterious and surprising relations between different areas of knowledge that were otherwise separated by specialization into various scientific disciplines. Furthermore, several of the conceptual tools used by Bernstein and other authors to establish connections between different areas of physics and chemistry made an impression on Einstein and arguably influenced his understanding of the readings and lectures he would later encounter as a student.

Behind the numerous ideas and speculations that Einstein developed as a student and discussed with his friends was a fascination with the notion that one can discover unity in natural phenomena by using mental models and thought experiments. This fascination also had its roots in his earlier reading of popular scientific books. At the age of sixty-seven, Einstein still remembered this formative educational experience:

> When I was a fairly precocious young man I became thoroughly impressed with the futility of the hopes and strivings that chase most men restlessly through life. . . . As the first way out there was religion, which is implanted into every child by way of the traditional education-machine. Thus, I came—though the child of entirely irreligious (Jewish) parents—to a deep religiousness, which, however, reached an abrupt end at the age of twelve. Through the reading of popular scientific books I soon reached the conviction that much in the stories of the Bible could not be true. The consequence was a positively fanatic [orgy of] free-thinking coupled with the impression that youth is intentionally being deceived by the state through lies; it was a crushing impression. Mistrust of every kind of authority grew out of this experience, a skeptical attitude toward the convictions that were alive in any specific social environment—an attitude that has never again left me, even though, later on, it has been tempered by a better insight into the causal connections.[3]

A "fanatic [orgy of] free thinking" and a "mistrust of every kind of authority" remained with him throughout his scientific journey, in his political activities and philosophical thinking. Einstein's introduction to the natural sciences of his time through the reading of Bernstein's books inspired his hope of achieving a conceptual unity of their numerous specialized branches. As a result of having such reading material as a starting point, Einstein developed a different view of physics than many of his established physicist colleagues, who sometimes lacked the vision of the overarching connections between the special topics they were investigating.

These readings shaped young Einstein; science became his orientation in life and a replacement for religion. For him, science held the promise that with its aid one could rise above the void of earthly hopes and ambitions. The popular books by Bernstein, in particular, portrayed science as a human enterprise, not only to be revered but also one in which one could participate. In contrast to contemporary compartmentalized academia, Bernstein drew no sharp boundaries between the sciences or between science and life.

Advancements in electrotechnology during this time led to a rapid increase in electric lighting in urban areas. The Einstein family's involvement in this increasing electrification provided the young Albert with rich intellectual stimuli and challenges. In 1885, the enterprise expanded, employing up to two hundred people, until competition with large firms in the increasingly specialized electrical industry prompted the Einsteins to move their business activities to Pavia in Northern Italy in 1894, following the loss of a major municipal contract for the electric lighting of central Munich. Albert had to stay in Munich to continue his studies at the Luitpold-Gymnasium, one of the most progressive high schools in Germany in mathematics and science instruction at the time. Contrary to popular misconceptions, he achieved excellent grades not only in mathematics and the sciences but also in the humanities. But the program was too authoritarian for his taste and, at the end of the year, Albert suspended his formal schooling to join the family in Italy. With his father's assistance, he succeeded in renouncing his German citizenship, with the consequence that he was no longer subject to compulsory military service.

After only two years, the firm established in Pavia had to be sold in 1896, and a new firm was founded in Milan, which was also liquidated after two years. Following this, the Einsteins embarked on a new direction, installing power plants for electric lighting in small towns close to rivers, which were used as a power source. This venture turned out to be moderately successful and created the expectation that young Albert might join the activities of his father. Despite his father's attempt to persuade him to join the family business, he was deterred by his extensive exposure to the uncertainties of the business world, with its harsh competition and threat of financial uncertainty. Several documents from this time demonstrate that the young adolescent had other plans for his life. In a school essay on his future plans, dated 1896 and written in French, he stressed that he preferred the independence of a scientific profession, mentioning his inclination for abstract and mathematical thinking.[4] This, however, was not the only reason for paving his own path. At an early age, he already felt estranged from the bourgeois concerns of his family. In letters to friends, he mocked their philistine attitude and extolled the benefits of solitary living, akin to that of the philosopher Arthur Schopenhauer.

The young Einstein was aware of the central topics of physics even before his formal academic studies. Inspired by the family business, he developed his own scientific ideas on electricity and magnetism. They centered around the physical meaning of the mysterious ether, considered an elastic substance that fills all of space and acts as a carrier of electromagnetic phenomena and light. At the age of sixteen, he wrote an essay, "On the Investigation of the State of the Ether in a Magnetic Field." This essay may be considered his first scientific paper, which he sent to his beloved uncle Caesar Koch. In an accompanying letter, he admitted that the text was "rather naïve and imperfect, as might be expected from such a young fellow like myself."[5] Still, the content of the letter demonstrates a distinct imagination and curiosity. In this first scientific work, he investigated the alteration of the ether caused by the magnetic field around an electric current. Such an alteration was thought to affect the velocity of propagating electromagnetic waves within it. These were the first indications of the problems at the borderline between mechanics and electrodynamics that would still intrigue him in 1905, forming the point of departure for the special theory of relativity.

At the same time, another problem occupied his mind. In one of his most well-known thought experiments, he posed the question: What does a light beam look like to somebody moving alongside it at the speed of light? This raises the question of the velocity of a light beam measured by an observer moving at a certain velocity in relation to it. Einstein would answer this question ten years later in the context of the special theory of relativity.

In Italy, Einstein devoted himself to studying for the entrance examination for the Polytechnic, the Federal Institute of Technology in Zurich, later the Eidgenössische Technische Hochschule (ETH). He was permitted to take this test even though, at sixteen, he was two years younger than the required admission age. His first attempt resulted in failure. He passed mathematics and physics but was unsuccessful in modern languages, zoology, and botany. To improve his chances of admission, Einstein followed the suggestion of the director of the Polytechnic and enrolled in a Swiss secondary school in Aarau, a town outside of Zurich. After completing his studies there with impressive marks, he passed the entrance exams in the summer of 1886, becoming one of the youngest students ever admitted to the Polytechnic at age sixteen and a half.

b. The Student Years

As a student of physics at the Polytechnic from 1896 to 1900, Einstein first had to hone his knowledge of the physics of the time before he could shape his already abundant ideas into substantial scientific contributions. This period of learning did not proceed without conflicts and disappointments; he hated rote learning and the mindless memorization of facts. He learned a great deal through independent study and reading. The main mission of the Polytechnic was to train engineers. In Einstein's year, there were only five students on the science track. Among them was Marcel Grossmann, a student of mathematics who became Einstein's close friend.[6] For the lecture contents, Einstein often relied on Grossmann's notes. Also among the science students was Mileva Marić, who came from Serbia and began her studies of mathematics at the Polytechnic in 1896 as the only woman in her class. The friendship between Albert and Mileva soon evolved into a love story, with the prospect of becoming a work-and-life partnership, although Einstein's parents disapproved. Their marriage in 1903 ended in a bitter divorce in 1919.

As a student, Einstein continued to explore his wide-ranging interests. This is now well documented by the love letters he and Mileva exchanged.[7] These letters are an invaluable historical resource, providing insight into Einstein's intellectual development during this time. They reveal a whole range of previously unknown scientific interests, among them his participation in experiments concerning X-rays, which had recently been discovered, as well as his passion for research on metals. Additionally, Einstein's early correspondence indicates that he was an eager reader of contemporary textbook literature and contributions to professional journals. From these letters, we also learn about his self-assuredness in criticizing the work of renowned scientists. This is one manifestation of the mistrust of authority that he acquired in his earlier years from reading the books of Bernstein.

Einstein's student years were shaped by a certain ambiguity in his relation to mathematics. In his autobiographical recollections, the accomplished scientist, who meanwhile had since come to recognize the powers of mathematics, reflects on his student years, wondering what he may have missed and why he chose physics rather than mathematics as the primary focus of his life. Mathematics appeared to him to consist of a diversity of domains of detailed specialization, and any one of them could consume a lifetime. Only after years of research did he realize the fundamental role of mathematics in gaining physical insights, citing his struggle to develop a general theory of relativity and his search for the field equation in particular.[8] In 1912, he wrote to Arnold Sommerfeld that he had gained great respect for mathematics, "whose more subtle parts, I considered until now, in my ignorance, as pure luxury!"[9]

In contrast, in physics he learned early on to sense which pieces of the extensive and seemingly disparate collection of experimental data to disregard and which would lead to fundamental insights. Einstein's assistant in the 1940s, Ernst Straus, recalls that Einstein often told him about his student-years dilemma between mathematics and physics. As a student, he thought he would never be able to decipher which of the many beautiful questions in mathematics were pertinent and which were peripheral. In physics he could see which were the most central questions.[10] The problems he chose to work on at the beginning of his career confirm the older Einstein's recollection of young Einstein's dilemmas and choices.

A short time after completing his studies, Einstein submitted a doctoral dissertation to Alfred Kleiner, professor of physics at the University of Zurich. He submitted it to the university because, at that time, the Polytechnic was not yet authorized to grant doctoral degrees. The thesis no longer exists, but we know that it dealt with molecular forces in gases. Einstein wrote to Mileva that Kleiner would not dare reject the thesis. Kleiner did not reject it, but after reading it, he suggested that Einstein should withdraw it voluntarily. Apparently, Kleiner did not like Einstein's criticism of the work of leading physicists, including Ludwig Boltzmann. Einstein reluctantly withdrew it.

Following his failure to secure a position at the Polytechnic in 1900, Einstein briefly worked as a teacher in a secondary school outside of Zurich. In 1902, he left this position and moved to Bern, applying for a position at the Swiss patent office there. For the first time in the history of the patent office, the announcement of a vacant position specified that applicants must have a university education with a background in physics. Einstein began his work at the patent office in June 1902 as a "Technical Expert Class III." It was his friend Grossmann who helped him find and secure this position when he was desperately in need of a job. This position enabled the intensive and difficult scientific work that preceded his breakthrough in 1905.

c. Einstein in Bern— The Miraculous Year and Beyond

The correspondence with Mileva also provides a glimpse into a youthful Bohemian world where Einstein's rebellious spirit was formed, and where his resistance to the authority of the physics community found support and encouragement. This attitude was formed during his student years and continued to develop during his years in Bern. He was surrounded by friends with whom he could discuss fundamental questions of science without having to respect disciplinary boundaries or the authority of established paradigms. In this community of rebels, which had much in common with the community of Bohemian artists of the same period, scientific questions became questions about life itself. Einstein met his close friend, Maurice Solovine, a young student of philosophy, when Solovine responded to Einstein's advertisement in the *Newspaper of the City of Bern*, offering private lessons in mathematics and physics to students and pupils. However, instead of conducting lessons on physics, they spent their time together exchanging ideas about the open problems of physics. Their first encounter evolved into a lifelong friendship. They decided to read books by prominent authors together and discuss them. They were soon joined by the mathematician Conrad Habicht in this endeavor. The meetings usually took place in Einstein's apartment and lasted until late into the evening and sometimes into the early hours of the morning. They called these meetings "Akademie Olympia" (Olympia Academy). Solovine reported that Marić attended the meetings, listened attentively, but never took part in the discussions. The "Akademie" did not last long, as Habicht left Bern in 1904 and Solovine in 1905. Einstein often cited this group's gatherings as an episode that contributed to his scientific work in years to come. Throughout his life, he would prefer this academy to the official ones.

The favorite readings at the social meetings of the Olympia Academy were works that critically reviewed conceptual and methodological questions of contemporary science. These included books by philosopher-scientists Ernst Mach and Henri Poincaré, as well as philosophers, such as Baruch de Spinoza and David Hume, but also writers like Miguel de Cervantes and Charles Dickens. As such, this academy and its circles were by no means an immature college clique but a serious collective of thinkers.

In addition to Solovine, Habicht, and Mileva, another friend— Michele Besso—was also one of Einstein's most important influences. They met as students in Zurich, where Besso studied mechanical engineering. They later became colleagues at the patent office and continued their intensive discussions on the foundations of physics. A supportive and challenging discussion partner, Besso came to Bern just at the right time for Einstein. They talked on their way to and from work, and whenever they found the time. In Einstein's 1905 paper on relativity, Besso was the only person to be acknowledged because, as Einstein later recalled, the decisive idea came to him during a conversation with Besso. We return to this in detail in section IVf.

In the years 1902 to 1904, Einstein published three papers on statistical mechanics. He derived the laws of thermodynamics from the statistical behavior of the components of matter (atoms, molecules). This was a continuation of the pioneering work by Boltzmann and a parallel to the work of Josiah Willard Gibbs. We discuss these papers and the new elements they introduce in detail in section IVa. Here, we only wish to emphasize that Einstein's work was based on the conviction that atoms and molecules exist and were part of his self-induced mission to demonstrate their reality, which was not yet accepted by many prominent physicists and even chemists at the time. Einstein's work on statistical mechanics was a milestone on his road to revising the foundations of classical physics. In 1905, it provided the theoretical tools for understanding black-body radiation, for demonstrating the existence of atoms, and for transiting to modern statistical and quantum physics. His other historic work from the same year was what later came to be called the special theory of relativity, which revised the Maxwell-Lorentz theory of the electrodynamics of moving bodies. It introduced a new understanding of the concepts of space and time and established the equivalence between mass and energy expressed in the well-known scientific equation, known even beyond the world of physics, $E = mc^2$. This combination of five characters has become a cultural symbol associated with Einstein's name. It appears on numerous commercial products, and it seems that virtually every country in the world has issued a postage stamp featuring this equation.

One refers to the year 1905 as Einstein's miraculous year because of his outstanding revolutionary achievements. But, the circumstances of these achievements are also miraculous. Einstein was only twenty-six years old and was not working at an academic institution but at the patent office as a clerk. Consequently, everything he did was essentially done in his free time and on his own. In addition to his scientific research, he devoted time to another activity, apparently to increase his income. He published reports in the *Annalen der Physik* on articles that appeared in scientific journals outside of Germany, particularly in France and Italy. In 1905, he published twenty-one such reports.

Einstein worked at the patent office from 1902 until 1909. These seven years were extremely productive and creative. In 1905, in addition to the famous papers, he also completed his doctoral dissertation, which served as the precursor to his paper on Brownian motion. Because of his dissertation, he was promoted to "Technical Expert Class II" with an increase in salary of 4500 francs a year. In 1908, the University of Bern appointed him *Privatdozent* of theoretical physics. This position is roughly the equivalent of an American adjunct professor. Finally, in 1909, he secured his first full-time faculty appointment as *Extraordinariat* (essentially the position of an associate professor) of theoretical physics at the University of Zurich. In the same year, he was awarded an honorary degree by the University of Geneva. In September of that year, he was invited to a conference of German-speaking scientists in Salzburg, where he first met Max Planck. Wolfgang Pauli referred to Einstein's talk at that conference as one of the cornerstones of modern physics. Two years later, in 1911, he was appointed full professor (*Ordinarius*) at Charles University in Prague. In the same year, he was invited to participate in the first Solvay conference. These conferences brought together the leaders of the European physics community to discuss the problems raised by the emerging quantum physics. The first Solvay conference hosted twenty renowned participants, including Planck, Marie Curie, Poincaré, and Lord Rutherford. Einstein, at the age of thirty-two, was the youngest participant. His involvement at this conference marked his transition from patent office clerk in Bern to scholar at the forefront of physics.

One may wonder what would have happened if Einstein had worked at a university as an assistant to an experienced and known professor. Maybe he would have had to get involved in an ongoing research program and adapt to the dominant academic environment. We can safely conclude that the fate that brought him to the patent office at the beginning of his scientific career benefitted him and the world of science.

d. A Tale of Three Cities— The General Theory of Relativity

The special theory of relativity increased a tension that already existed between electrodynamics and Newton's theory of gravity. Electrodynamics is concerned with effects that propagate in space with a very high but finite velocity. Newton's law of gravity, however, does not seem to be directly reconcilable with the demand that gravitational effects should also propagate in space with a definite speed, demand that had become a fundamental requirement on any physical interaction as a consequence of special relativity.

Like a few of the other contemporary physicists, Einstein concentrated on the solution to this "remaining problem" of conflict between classical mechanics and special relativity. One of the basic principles of mechanics challenged by Einstein's attempt to incorporate gravitation into his special theory of relativity was Galileo's principle. This principle states that all bodies fall at the same rate regardless of their mass or their constitution. For Einstein, it was inconceivable that such a fundamental principle be abandoned, as initially seemed to be required by an adaptation of Newton's law to special relativity. He, therefore, decided to maintain Galileo's principle and sought a generalization of his original relativity theory that would allow for this. Einstein began his work on the problem

of gravitation in 1907. He soon arrived at the "equivalence principle," which states that the effects of a homogenous gravitational
field are equivalent to the inertial effects in a linearly accelerated
frame of reference. The formulation of this principle allowed him
to reach several surprising insights very quickly, such as his prediction that the direction of light propagation and its frequency are
affected by the action of gravity. This was a formative step on Einstein's journey to the general theory of relativity. However, it took
eight more years until it was complete in November 1915.

Section V of this book is a detailed analysis of Einstein's convoluted road to reach this goal. Here we present a short account of this
process to set the stage for a discussion, in the following section, of
Einstein's pathway to general relativity in detail. This short account
mirrors the overview in our book *The Road to Relativity*, which describes Einstein's odyssey as a tale of three cities—Prague, Zurich,
and Berlin—each representing a phase of this process, using the
breakthrough of 1907, when he was still in Bern, as a starting point.

A short time after his appointment as an adjunct professor at
the University of Zurich, Einstein was offered an even more prestigious position as a full professor at the German-speaking part of
Charles University in Prague. Despite appeals from University of
Zurich students to university leaders to make every effort to keep
Einstein in Zurich, he moved to Prague in April 1911. There he
wrote eleven papers, six devoted to relativity. In the first paper, he
discussed the bending of light and the gravitational redshift, which
he had already discovered in 1907 but now discussed as observable
effects. In the Prague papers, he focused on developing a consistent
theory of the gravitational field based on the equivalence principle. Just like in Newton's theory, and unlike in the final theory of
general relativity, the gravitational potential was still represented
by a single scalar function. Nevertheless, some basic features of the
final theory were already formed then. Among them was the understanding that the source of the gravitational potential is not
only the mass of physical bodies but also the equivalent mass of
the energy of the gravitational field itself.

In 1911, Grossmann was appointed dean of the mathematics-physics department of the Polytechnic. One of his first initiatives as dean was to ask Einstein if he would consider returning to Zurich to join the Polytechnic. Einstein agreed, declining an earlier offer from Utrecht and an opportunity to go to Leiden, where he would have been close to the Dutch physicist Hendrik Antoon Lorentz. Whatever reasons he had for choosing Zurich, it was the right decision at the time. By the time he left Prague and arrived in Zurich, he realized that the gravitational potential has to be represented by a mathematical object, a tensor, composed of ten functions of space and time. He also realized that this implied a non-Euclidean structure of space and time, or rather of the four-dimensional entity, spacetime. All this required sophisticated mathematical methods, which Einstein was unfamiliar with at the time.

Shortly after returning to Zurich in August 1912, Einstein began an intensive and fruitful collaboration with Grossmann. This collaboration is documented in Einstein's famous "Zurich Notebook," which allows us to "look over his shoulder" as he struggles with the challenge of reconciling physical insights and mathematical methods.[11] As we see in more detail later, this research notebook from 1912/1913 gives us insights not only into a single scientist's intellectual world but also into the mechanism behind the transformation of a system of knowledge. The notebook constitutes a most important document in the history of science and is of great importance for our understanding of the origins of the general theory of relativity.

The Zurich Notebook essentially contains the blueprint for the final, generally covariant theory but, as later described in section V, Einstein abandoned this theory because he had not yet reached a full physical understanding of its mathematical implications. Instead, with Grossmann, he published the "Outline of a Generalized Theory of Relativity and of a Theory of Gravitation," which has since been termed the *Entwurf* theory (*Entwurf* means outline in German). Although this theory did not meet Einstein's initial requirement regarding its mathematical features, he convinced himself that this was the best that could be done and was satisfied with it until the summer of 1915.

In 1913, shortly after Planck was elected secretary of the Royal Prussian Academy of Sciences, he launched a campaign to elect Einstein to the academy and bring him to Berlin. In July 1913, he went to Zurich with the influential Berlin physical chemist Walther Nernst, to present a three-part proposal to Einstein. They offered him: membership in the academy with generous financial support, directorship of the Kaiser Wilhelm Institute of Physics without administrative duties, and a professorship at the University of Berlin without teaching obligations. Einstein accepted and moved to Berlin. Shortly after he arrived, World War I broke out. Confronted with the realities of the war, he stepped down from the ivory tower of science to become a political opponent of Germany's involvement in the war. In Berlin, Einstein encountered the phenomenon of anti-Semitism and became increasingly aware of his Jewish identity. At that time, his relationship with Mileva deteriorated to the point of separation, and she and the children returned to Zurich. In the midst of all this, Einstein ardently pursued his scientific work. He continued to work on the *Entwurf* theory and suggested new arguments for its validity. In 1914, he summarized this theory in a review article, "The Formal Foundation of the General Theory of Relativity."[12] It took him less than a year to regret it. His doubts about the *Entwurf* theory began to form in the summer of 1915. He eventually abandoned it and, in a spurt of creativity and hard work, completed the general theory of relativity in November of that year.

Einstein joined Planck, Nernst, and many others in Berlin, the world capital of physics at the time. Even during the hardships of the war years, the city maintained an inspiring atmosphere and working culture in the physics community. Gerald J. Holton, a pioneer of Einstein scholarship in the historical and philosophical context, addressed the question:

How much did these facts contributed to Einstein's unique ability and daring to develop, between 1915 and late 1917, his General Relativity Theory in Berlin? Could he have done so if he had accepted a grand offer from a city in another country?[13]

Holton's clear answer was:

No other man than Einstein could have produced General Relativity, and in no other city than in Berlin, with its critical mass of close colleagues at the Academy and the University– Max Planck, Walther Nernst, Max von Laue, Fritz Haber, among many.[14]

On closer inspection, however, these prestigious colleagues were less interested and offered less support to Einstein's struggle with general relativity than his Zurich friends and colleagues, Grossmann and Besso. It was not until 1919, when a British solar eclipse expedition, under Sir Arthur Eddington's direction, observed the deflection of light rays in the sun's gravitational field as predicted by general relativity, that Einstein's theory was widely accepted, and he became world-famous. The confirmation of a theory created by a Jewish German holding a Swiss passport by an English expedition so shortly after the end of World War I turned out to be an international media event, confirming the universal character of the scientific enterprise.

e. The Emergence of a Quantum Worldview

Around the end of the nineteenth century, one of the prominent problems on the agenda of classical physics was a borderline problem between thermodynamics and electrodynamics, which concerned the thermal equilibrium of electromagnetic radiation in a cavity enclosed by reflecting walls. The distribution of the energy of this radiation over the different frequencies, namely, the spectrum of the radiation, had been measured with ever greater accuracy because of the technical relevance of this problem for modern industry. This spectrum depends only on the temperature of the cavity and not on the shape and composition of its walls. The phenomenon itself is known as "black-body radiation." A black body is the mental model of an ideal source of thermal radiation that is assumed to absorb all incident electromagnetic radiation. This concept, coined by Gustav Kirchhoff, became the basis of theoretical and experimental studies of electromagnetic radiation in thermal equilibrium. Until the very end of the nineteenth century, all attempts to formulate a theory that could adequately explain the shape of the energy distribution failed.

In 1900, following five years of work on this problem, Planck derived a formula, which describes, with great accuracy, the observed frequency distribution of black-body radiation. His path to this result was anything but straight, and it led him to explore the limits of the conceptual system of classical physics, introducing the notion of a discrete energy quantum. Confronted with Planck's result, Einstein knew he needed to go beyond those limits. For Planck, on the other hand, the notion of an energy quantum was a merely mathematical device that, at most, explained how energy was absorbed or emitted when electromagnetic radiation interacted with matter. He was reluctant to accept the revolutionary consequences of his own discovery and the quantized nature of radiation. Thus, he unwillingly became the pioneer of the quantum revolution. In contrast, in his light quantum paper of 1905, Einstein was the first to realize that not only was Planck's formula a break with classical theories of radiation but also that the introduction of quanta cannot be restricted to just one branch of physics.

Einstein's first contribution to broadening the quantum hypothesis began in 1907 when he extended his quantum ideas to the study of the thermal behavior of solids. He could derive a formula for the specific heat that was in better agreement with experiments than classical explanations. "This quantum question is so extraordinarily important and difficult that everybody should take the trouble to work on it," Einstein wrote to a colleague in 1909.[15] Yet initially its study attracted only a few outsiders. Slowly, interested scientists began networking; their exchanges and cooperation led to a gradual understanding of the true dimensions of the problems being faced.

Einstein's result happened to match a line of investigation pursued by Nernst, who had formulated a heat theorem that was later elevated to the third law of thermodynamics. Nernst was so impressed with the parallels between Einstein's work and his own that he used his experimental results as an excuse to visit Einstein in Zurich. He thus became one of the most prominent supporters of Einstein and was the driving force behind his invitation to the Solvay conference and his call to Berlin. Nernst and his colleague Haber expected a significant contribution from Einstein in connecting the conceptual breakthroughs of theoretical physics with the experimental research on physics and chemistry that was increasingly being pursued, with the invitation to bring both disciplines closer together. This would align with the clear relationship, particularly in Germany, between the chemical industry and advances in physical chemistry. In this industry, there was significant interest in attaining a deeper theoretical understanding of chemical processes. Of particular importance were the insights that could be derived from the emerging atomic and molecular understanding of these processes as well as from that of their thermodynamic properties. Thus, Einstein was called to Berlin to modernize chemistry, but he devoted most of his time to solving the ancient riddle of gravity. Yet he did not turn away completely from the conceptual changes within physics that were connected with the emerging quantum theory, and that were inspired by his work on the quantum nature of radiation and matter between 1905 and 1912.

The spectral analysis of chemical compounds, especially the multitude of spectral line patterns seen in a flame sample, could be interpreted as clues to an extremely complex internal structure of atoms and molecules. Such a structure, however, could not be reconciled with knowledge derived from classical physics. In 1913, Niels Bohr constructed an atomic model based on the astronomical model of a planetary system. In order to explain the spectral line patterns, Bohr's model, later elaborated by Sommerfeld and his school, assumes that electrons circle in discrete orbits. An atom's emission and absorption of light are associated with a transition of electrons between such fixed orbits. This combination of classical and quantum building blocks resulted in a kind of semi-classical atomic theory that later became the springboard for the full quantum theory.

For a long time, Einstein searched in vain for a theory of light that could be considered a fusion of wave and particle theories. In 1916, in two groundbreaking papers, he developed a model of the interactions between atoms and radiation, providing additional insight into the particle properties of light quanta. He showed that light particles must possess a direction and an impulse, similar to particles of matter. He further introduced the idea of stimulated emission of light quanta, which he referred to as a "brilliant idea" in a postcard to Besso.[16] Forty years later, this brilliant idea inspired the invention of lasers. Although Einstein received the 1921 Nobel Prize in Physics for his law of the photoelectric effect, the light quantum hypothesis, which forms the basis of this law, was still met with widespread skepticism in 1922. It was Compton's experiment in 1923 that led to the breakthrough that quelled these doubts. The experiment showed that X-rays collide with electrons in accordance with the classical model of particle collision and in blatant contradiction to the idea of light as a wave. His results were the first that convinced a majority of physicists of the justification of the light quantum hypothesis.

In his doctoral dissertation in 1924, Louis de Broglie showed that applying wave properties to particles is also plausible. Using his idea of matter waves, he could explain key components of Bohr's atomic model. Einstein was elated by this idea. It was fortuitously timed, as the need for new foundations of quantum physics was becoming ever more apparent. Analyzing the interaction of light and matter (in which Einstein's ideas from 1916 play an important role) paved the way for establishing these new foundations. The basis of a new conceptual beginning emerged from re-interpreting formulas that describe the scattering (dispersion) of light on atoms. Based on this, in 1925 Werner Heisenberg published an authoritative paper effectively founding quantum mechanics as we know it. His formalism could be extended to a calculus of matrices and interpreted as a quantum translation of the dynamical equations of analytical mechanics, as was soon realized by Born and Pascual Jordan. He showed that this theory, rather than simply using numbers, involved infinitely large tables of numbers, called matrices. One of the most well-known implications of the new quantum mechanics is Heisenberg's uncertainty principle. It states that two complementary physical parameters, like the position and the momentum of a particle, cannot be measured simultaneously with any degree of accuracy.

Following Einstein's thoughts about the dualism of waves and particles, Erwin Schrödinger took a different route to complete the quantum theory. In 1926, he expanded de Broglie's idea of matter waves by introducing a wave equation for electrons, where its solutions were states of the Bohr-Sommerfeld atom. Soon afterward, Schrödinger found proof that his formalism was essentially equivalent to Heisenberg's. In Schrödinger's formulation of quantum mechanics, the state of a system (e.g., a particle) is characterized by a "wave function," which is a function of parameters like the position (q) and momentum (p) of a particle and time. According to a rule formulated by Born, the wave function can be interpreted as predicting the probability of finding a definite value of the parameter q (or p) at a given time. This probability can also be found empirically by reproducing the same state many times and averaging the results of many measurements of that parameter. Let us look at two ways to interpret the result of a single measurement of, say, q. One possibility is that the value measured is the value of that parameter before the measurement. In that case, the wave function is not a complete description of the system because it only tells us what we know from many measurements.

The other possibility is that the measured value, implied by the wave function, is produced by the measurement itself, namely, that no objective value of that parameter, independent of measurement, exists. In that case, the wave function describes the system completely.

The difference between these two possibilities was at the core of the grand debate between Einstein and Bohr in the 1920s, particularly at the Solvay conference in 1927. Bohr interpreted Heisenberg's uncertainty principle as an expression of the limited applicability of our concepts to the microworld. He argued that there are complementary pairs of physical qualities of a particle, which cannot be measured simultaneously with an arbitrary degree of accuracy. Einstein reacted by conceiving thought experiments aimed at proving the opposite. Bohr rebutted his arguments by pointing out that measuring instruments are also subject to the uncertainty principle. Einstein did not accept the idea that there is no objective reality independent of observation. He would not abandon the causal nature of classical mechanics or the field theories of electromagnetism and gravitation and would not accept the probabilistic character of quantum theory. He presented one argument after another and invented a succession of thought experiments to challenge the theory. Bohr disputed every argument, but Einstein remained unconvinced. At a later stage, instead of claiming that the theory was wrong, he argued that it was incomplete and would be replaced by a comprehensive causal theory in the future.

The essence of this argument is represented in the, now famous, "Einstein-Podolsky-Rosen Paper," published in 1935.[17] This paper has become known under the label "EPR paradox." The authors argued that the wave function cannot provide a complete description of physical reality. Einstein used the existence of "entangled states" to support his conviction that quantum theory was incomplete. In such states, the properties of different particles depend on one another. Consequently, Einstein concluded that measurements of one particle's location (or velocity) should allow one to infer the values for the other particle, remotely separated from the first one, without actually disturbing it. Thus, he argued that the second particle must have both a definite velocity and a definite position. However, that would mean that quantum mechanics is incomplete since, according to its rules, only one of the two values can be determined exactly. Contrary to Einstein's argument, experiments performed in the 1980s showed that quantum mechanics is *not* incomplete. These achievements were honored by the Nobel Prize in Physics in 2022.

For most physicists, the quantum theory was a final theory and, therefore, a cornerstone of every future comprehensive theory of the physical world. Einstein's opinion was the direct opposite:

It is my opinion that the contemporary quantum theory represents an optimal formulation of the relationships, given certain fixed basic concepts, which by and large have been taken from classical mechanics. I believe, however, that this theory offers no useful point of departure for future development.[18]

He believed that a future fundamental theory of all of physics would be based on the extension of the general theory of relativity. He believed that the general theory of relativity was an intermediate step towards a unified field theory, which would include gravitation and electromagnetism in the same framework and provide a substitute for the probabilistic character of quantum mechanics as the ultimate theory of matter. Einstein devoted the last twenty years of his life to an unsuccessful search for such a theory.

Einstein was an architect of the quantum worldview and made historic contributions to the early stages of its evolution. When the quantum revolution reached its first conclusion in the mid-1920s with the formulation of quantum mechanics and became an all-encompassing fundamental revision of the classical ideas of matter and radiation, Einstein did not join the general consensus. He was a dissident until the end of his life. In his essay "Physics and Reality" (1936), Einstein highlights the success of quantum mechanics and thus indicates the magnitude of the challenge to replace it with another theory:

> Probably never before has a theory been evolved which has given a key to the interpretation and calculation of such a heterogeneous group of phenomena of experience as has quantum theory. In spite of this, however, I believe that the theory is apt to beguile us into error in our search for a uniform basis for physics, because in my belief, it is an *incomplete* representation of real things. . . . The incompleteness of the representation leads necessarily to the statistical nature (incompleteness) of the laws.[19]

f. The Einstein Myth and His Iconic Status

Albert Einstein has left his mark not only on the physics of the twentieth century but also on the public image of science and scientists. The photographs from the second half of his life, in particular, evoke an image of a friendly nonconformist. He was an eccentric who defied authority and convention, to the extent that he did not wear socks and refused to groom his hair. The famous picture of Einstein sticking out his tongue represents a certain unworldliness, a protest against the well-bred majority, but also a shrewd and witty handling of the mass media. The origin of Einstein's myth is not only in the joy of discovery but in a certain detachment from the fragility of the human condition. It is a bemusement akin to that granted only to the gods in the Greek theater of antiquity. But, apart from his outward appearance, how unconventional was the real Einstein? And what role did his nonconformity play in the scientific revolution that he supposedly induced?

Since the beginning of the twenty-first century, the real conflicts, both societal and scientific, that were the source of Einstein's estrangement have largely been forgotten. There is little mention of them in the occasional reports about his discoveries or his love life that find their way into today's headlines. Also, as he has entered the pantheon of cultural history, Einstein has himself become a member of the establishment, as evidenced by the many honors bestowed in his memory. His popularity, even in today's Germany, the country from which he was forced to emigrate, represents a level of normalcy that until recently was unthinkable. The memory of Einstein's tense relationship with Germany and the Germans has begun to fade, giving way to the all-pervading Einstein myth.

One of the unique traits of the Einstein phenomenon is that his work has left its mark on the cultural history of the twentieth century in areas far beyond his expertise. His deep influence is evident in many areas, from philosophy to psychology, and even in art. For example, Jean Piaget, child psychologist and founder of genetic epistemology, referred to a suggestion from Einstein in his analysis of the development of spatial and temporal thinking in children.

The spectacular success of his theory of relativity, in conjunction with his anti-militarist position during the World War I, distinguished Einstein as a symbol of pacifism in the Weimar Republic. This laid the roots for his role as the world's conscience and sage, taking a position on all pressing issues, from German reparations to the condition of Jews from eastern countries living in Germany. Later, after World War II, Einstein continued in this role, engaging in the arms control effort and supporting world government. In 1952 he was even offered the presidency of Israel.

Today, more than sixty-five years after his death, public interest in his life and science continues unabated. Centennials of the milestones of his creativity have been celebrated worldwide through public events, international conferences, workshops, television programs, and a spate of new books. His image decorates so many commercial products and is one of the most recognizable faces on the planet.

Progress in science and new cosmological observations remind us time and again that Einstein was right and also underline the unending nature of the quest for knowledge. When new discoveries related to Einstein's work occur, such as the recent detection of gravitational waves, people around the globe, irrespective of their understanding (or indeed because of their lack of understanding) regarding the discovery, are fascinated by the appeal of science and the iconic image of its most discernible figure—Albert Einstein.

The presence of Einstein in modern culture is all-encompassing—in art and literature, movies and television programs, and also in digital media. In 2008, Don Howard, a prominent scholar of Einstein's science and philosophy, began his generally favorable review of a biography of Einstein by Walter Isaacson with the question, "Still, there are too many books on Einstein. Shall we call for a moratorium?"[20] This question seems not to have been taken seriously. Searching online for books about Einstein published after 2008, we find more than eighty English titles related to his life and specific domains of his activities (this number excludes the numerous children's books, comic books, and books for professional physicists). This increase in publications about Einstein attests to his enduring legacy and presence in the public mind, while also contributing to it. Thus, we can expect this to continue for many years.

Can all this simply be the consequence of his unquestionably groundbreaking research results? Apparently not. So, what is so special about Einstein? His iconic status is certainly also due to specific historical circumstances, in particular, the role of the emerging mass media at the beginning of the twentieth century. Einstein became one of the first media stars of science at a time when the world was hungry for such celebrities. This public image endured throughout his lifetime. It evolved and expanded in many directions and continues even today. Einstein himself contributed to this image in many ways. He was constantly in the public eye. In numerous articles, interviews, correspondence with peers, and public addresses, he expressed his views on various public, political, and moral issues, such as nationality and nationalism, war and peace, and human liberty and dignity, relentlessly denouncing all forms of discrimination.

Einstein's views and activities outside of physics were not simply accessories to a life devoted to science; they were evidently driven by the same inner urge as his quest for scientific knowledge. These two aspects of Einstein's commitments and activities reflect, in his own personality, the fundamental tensions of science in the modern world. This is probably the most profound reason why Einstein is still very much alive today and will continue to be so in the foreseeable future: science is becoming increasingly relevant to all aspects of modern societies, but science also raises questions about the capability of humankind to understand the natural world and its role in it, and how to utilize this understanding to shape its own fate. Einstein endures as the pioneer who squarely confronted this human condition, not just as a brilliant scientist but also as a thoughtful philosopher and a caring humanist, aware of both his individual and our collective limits.

Taking a predominately biographical perspective, one might reasonably assume that Einstein's unconventional stance, above all, created the conditions for his scientific revolution and its subsequent impact on culture in general. Indeed, his status as an outsider in physics appears to have made his extraordinary achievements possible. It is undoubtedly important to consider the biographical circumstances that made the Einsteinian revolution possible, which we have already done to some extent in this section and will continue to do so in sections IV and V. But focusing exclusively on a personal biographical perspective brings with it the risk of propagating the Einstein myth. Ultimately, this myth ascribes to his personality or to his personal situation a simplified version of what actually was the outcome of a complex process. Indeed, one of the factors at play was his unique genius. However, one must also take into account the cultural environment in which he lived and worked and recognize that his breakthroughs were a part of the long-term intellectual development of science. The latter requires taking a more extensive historical perspective than is typically assumed in biographical accounts that instead pay great attention to every minute detail of Einstein's life. Taking an extensive historical perspective demands a discussion of the standing of the Einsteinian revolution in the history of physics and the evolution of knowledge.

II

Ideas on Progress and
Revolutions in Science

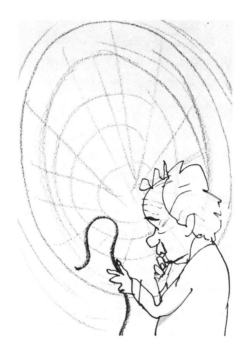

Preview

Einstein's scientific achievements have radically changed our understanding of the physical world. They have been, and continue
to be, the source of ongoing discoveries and of the expansion of
different systems of knowledge. Moreover, their technological

consequences have, in many respects, changed our daily lives. The origins and sources of Einstein's work have typically been described in numerous books and articles within the context of his personal and scientific background and placed within the wider context of the state of physics at the end of the nineteenth century. In this book, we intend to place the Einsteinian revolution in a broader historical and philosophical framework. Both his scientific work and his philosophical reflections provide an important case study for better understanding the evolution of knowledge, without claiming that this evolution follows a universal pattern, as was suggested by Kuhn and others. Moreover, a close analysis of Einstein's upheaval of physics will help us describe some characteristic features of the evolution of knowledge in terms that make use of the rich traditions found in philosophical and historical epistemology.

Philosophers and historians of science have addressed questions such as: How do systems of knowledge evolve? What triggers change? What is the nature of scientific revolutions and how do they affect the structure of knowledge? Considering the role of mental models has proven useful when addressing these questions. With the help of mental models, we can identify, explore, and account for some relevant properties and processes of our complex environment through simple thought experiments akin to those used by Einstein. Assimilating new objects and processes into a mental model constantly changes it by enriching its reservoir of experience. The result is a gradual adaptation of mental models to fit different contexts and to enable their occasional integration. In science, this process is often accompanied by epistemological considerations. Einstein was guided by such epistemological and philosophical considerations in formulating new theories, in transforming existing bodies of knowledge, and in his endless quest for a unified theoretical framework. Hence, understanding Einstein's life in science requires paying attention to the mental models he used, as well as looking closely at his epistemological credo and mode of thinking.

Humankind's knowledge is embodied in instruments and symbol systems that help to transmit this knowledge from generation to generation. These external representations can endure over long periods of time. Novelty in science can emerge because of the possibility of using traditional instruments and symbols in new ways. The expansion of systems of knowledge may set the conditions for their transformation through a "Copernicus process."[1] Such a transformation *shifts* the conceptual focus of a system of knowledge, analogous to the shift of the so-called Copernican revolution, which made a previously marginal celestial body (the sun orbiting the earth, according to the Ptolemaic system) the center of a new cosmic edifice. In a Copernicus process, the knowledge that has been passed down is not rejected but *reordered* and *reinterpreted*. Progress in science is thus achieved by the combined action of *cumulative transmission* and *changes in its architecture* that are induced by reflecting on the accumulated knowledge. In this book, we will comprehend Einstein's scientific breakthroughs in this manner. In contrast, Thomas Kuhn famously rejected the notion of gradual progress when, in 1962, he introduced the notion of a disruptive paradigm shift, which ultimately leads to a new worldview that is "incommensurable" with the previous one.

We argue instead that such transformations take place more gradually and that disruptive change is often the result, not the presupposition, of the transformation of systems of knowledge. A striking example is the transformation from the preclassical mechanics of Galileo and his contemporaries to the classical mechanics of the Newtonian era. While preclassical mechanics was still deeply rooted in the Aristotelian system of knowledge, its greatest discoveries contained the seeds of the radically different system of knowledge of classical mechanics. In this context, we ask whether such a "Copernicus process" can also explain Einstein's revolutionary achievements as the culmination of a longer transformation process of classical physics. Despite the revolutionary outcome of Einstein's work, several circumstances support the view that the origins of statistical mechanics, special relativity, the light quantum hypothesis, and the atomistic interpretation of Brownian motion are rooted in a similar development. In other words, these revolutionary achievements can be understood essentially as reinterpretations of the "outermost" results at the boundaries of classical physics. Within this context, Einstein no longer appears as an isolated pioneer of the twentieth century but rather as a scientist who helped to overcome these boundaries by exploring the limits of classical physics and by building new foundations in the process. We conclude this section with a summary of the most widely discussed approaches to the problem of scientific change.

a. The History of the Philosophy of Progress

The most commonly acknowledged feature of science by most scientists and the general public is its "cumulative" nature. As Isaac Newton asserted, following Bernard of Chartres, "If I have seen further, it is by standing on the shoulders of giants."[2] In other words, in science, each step builds on the previous one; therefore, in retrospect, the long-term development of science resembles steady growth. It is progress in the literal sense, interrupted temporarily, at most, by external disturbances such as wars or revolutions. Scientific progress is similarly self-evident in traditional studies of the history of science.

The survival of modern technological society seems to depend primarily on progress in science. Considered in this light, any doubts about progress in science are apparently merely a matter of esoteric academic debate. Scientific progress seems to be an unstoppable forward-striding golem whose pace establishes, for good or evil, the rhythm of modern industrial and technological societies. In short, there are good reasons to believe that science progresses, as evident in its perceived role in modern society and in the self-image of practicing scientists. However, reconciling this with the phenomenon of scientific revolutions is another matter. (We use "scientific revolutions" here in the sense of major conceptual changes—changes that Kuhn attempted to explain with his notion of "paradigm shifts.") Many historical accounts avoid rather than address this issue, occasionally burying any discussion of it in a wealth of factual details. Philosophers have been more forthcoming in trying to explain the special character of scientific knowledge but sometimes at the expense of historical facts. Nevertheless, before addressing the issue, let us briefly review the historical roots of the scientists' self-image as being part of a history of progress.

There is a widespread understanding of scientific progress that individual scientific insights not only build upon each other but also consistently increase the scope of a scientific worldview. This ultimately is supposed to lead to a comprehensive view of nature and could potentially be expressed in a universal formula or a unified "theory of everything." However, many scientists doubt that such a universal theory will ever be formulated. Or they suspect that such a theory would be in continual need of improvement.

Closely related to the notion of progress in science and its cumulative character is the relationship between our thinking and the external world; in other words, how do we know anything about the world? One much discussed answer to this question comes from the ancient Greek philosopher Plato. Through his famous cave allegory, he described the relation between the external world and the world of ideas. He likened the external world to a cave that portrays sensory impressions we receive from the world as mere shadows. People who experience nothing but these shadows throughout their lives will inevitably mistake them for real things. But once freed from the confines of the cave, they will realize that they previously saw nothing but a faint reflection of true reality. Accordingly, only through philosophical reflection or scientific investigation can we overcome the inadequacies of our senses and finally recognize the world of ideas as true reality.

An opposing point of view was formulated in the eighteenth century by David Hume, who assumed that all our knowledge ultimately comes from our experience in the form of sensory impressions. But we cannot deduce ideas or concepts from such experiences alone. Essential concepts, such as the causal relations between events, cannot be deduced from sensory experiences. According to Hume, one can, at most, form a certain belief or expectation that nature is uniform or regular.

The German philosopher Immanuel Kant accepted Hume's viewpoint that concepts such as space, time, or causality cannot come from experience alone but asserts that the mind inevitably functions in terms of them. From the seemingly indisputable validity of the fundamental statements of mathematics and natural sciences, Kant inferred that the origin of such statements is not to be found in sensory experience. If this was not the case, what would allow us to be so certain of the transitive law—if distance A is larger than distance B, and distance B is larger than distance C, then A must be larger than C? Kant, unlike Plato, located the literal "extra"-sensory origin of this certainty not in an objective world of ideas but in the innate human cognitive capacity itself. Therefore, such conclusions are, in a certain sense, preprogrammed into our awareness. They are valid a priori—prior to all experience—and thus can never be refuted by our awareness.

According to Kant, what we observe through our experience is not pure sensory impressions but rather phenomena which are a composition of sensory stimuli and our mental categories. What then is the relationship between these phenomena and the external world? In Kant's view, the external world is ultimately unknowable. All that we can know are the phenomena. He supposed that these phenomena do, in some sense, come from something outside, the so-called "things in themselves." But we can say nothing about the things in themselves because anything we say refers only to the concepts and categories available in our minds.

In light of this, Kant believed he could explain the basic stability of scientific progress as well, since all experience that has yet to be acquired must, by its very nature, conform to the structure of our inherent faculty of knowledge. It was therefore only natural that Kant also attempted to describe the outline of this architecture, which he called the *Metaphysical Foundations of Natural Science*

(1786).[3] According to him, this outline would provide an orientation for all future developments of scientific research but would itself remain essentially unaffected by these developments. Kant was convinced that this outline could be derived from the laws of reason, whose validity must be presumed prior to all experience. In other words, he envisioned a kind of thought machine, for which our experiences constitute nothing more than raw empirical data. With the help of immutable mechanisms, these experiences are then processed into the rational insights of natural science. Among the unchangeable components of this thought mechanism, Kant included a fixed a priori understanding of space and time.

In the following, we discuss Einstein's epistemological thinking. Here, we only wish to point out that he categorically rejected the position that certain concepts and assertions are part of our a priori knowledge, independent of experience. Without explicitly mentioning Kant, he wrote:

> I am convinced that the philosophers have had a harmful effect upon the progress of scientific thinking in removing certain fundamental concepts from the domain of empiricism, where they are under our control, to the intangible heights of the *a priori*. . . . This is particularly true of our concepts of time and space, which physicists have been obliged by the facts to bring down from the Olympus of the *a priori*.[4]

Indeed, the elementary concepts of space and time were changed fundamentally through the scientific breakthroughs associated with Einstein.

But long before these breakthroughs, the rapid pace of scientific progress had made clear that its robust character could hardly be explained by the seemingly universal mode of operation of Kant's thought mechanisms. The inadequacy of Kant's original approach led others to attempt to identify and describe stable features of science that are not so directly related to its contents as in Kant's scheme, such as a general scientific method. Many such efforts have been made since the beginning of the early modern era. One such attempt is associated with a philosophical movement called "logical empiricism," originating in the so-called Vienna Circle after World War I. Strongly influenced by philosophers such as Ernst Mach, Moritz Schlick, and Ludwig Wittgenstein, the proponents of this movement attempted to reduce all scientific questions to statements dealing with direct experience and to clarify their relations by means of logic. The source of these empirical statements, which concurrently represented the model of the rational acquisition of knowledge, was increasingly sought after in physics.

In practice, however, it has turned out to be difficult to validate any of these philosophical images of science with what historians of science have taught us about the actual development of science. On closer inspection, for instance, identifying purely empirical statements independent of a theoretical framework is hardly possible. The philosophy of science's predicament regarding the search for universal rules that govern its progress came to a head with the publication of Kuhn's work. He convincingly argued that the very criteria of scientific success were themselves features of historically specific paradigms and hence subject to change.

This insight did indeed turn out to have a liberating effect, at least for the history of science, which, now more than ever before, began to take the *cultural contexts* of scientific progress into account. But this extension toward a cultural history of science has long since also contributed to discrediting science itself. And once the genie of skepticism had been released, getting it back into the bottle was challenging. Historian of science Gerald Holton, in *Science and Anti-Science* (1993), explains that every case study in the history of science that takes a closer look at a personality or discovery, with a view to its cultural, technological, and social contexts, implicitly fosters doubt not only in traditional myths but also in the authority of science itself, which still appears to rely on these myths.[5] The closer the focus, the more the purely coincidental and the "all too human"[6] come to light and, consequently, the more difficult it is to separate science from its contexts. Unintentionally, the cultural history of science thus often reinforces a widespread popular tendency. Personal contexts, in particular, bring larger-than-life heroes of science history, such as Einstein, a little bit closer to our small, familiar world of ordinary men and women. What is more relevant for our work is that as science appears to be more contextually interwoven into specific historical situations, comparing different episodes in the history of science has become harder.

In the last few decades, however, studies in the framework of a cultural history of science have provided us with a more realistic picture of the evolution of science than the heroic tales from the last century. Even if such studies have occasionally overestimated the importance of local conditions in structuring scientific content, they have dismissed the outdated ideas that most traditional studies in the history of science were implicitly based on. They opened the door to a new understanding of the production of scientific knowledge, including its social and material contexts.

b. How Did Einstein Think?

To lay the groundwork for the description of both the Einsteinian revolution, which marked the transition from classical to modern physics (discussed in sections IV and V), and its standing and unique nature in the evolution of physics (discussed in the final section of this book), we now describe Einstein's mode of thinking and his epistemological views. We closely follow our discussion of this issue in *Einstein on Einstein* and *The Formative Years of Relativity*.[7]

In numerous accounts of his scientific endeavors, Einstein stressed the importance of epistemological and philosophical considerations for his scientific work. These considerations guided him in his student years and throughout his life. For him:

> The reciprocal relationship of epistemology and science is of noteworthy kind. They are dependent on each other. Epistemology

without contact with science becomes an empty scheme. Science without epistemology is—in so far as it is thinkable at all—primitive and muddled.[8]

As a student and young scientist, Einstein was fascinated by Hume and the possibility of revising established scientific concepts in light of new empirical knowledge. In his *Autobiographical Notes*, he credited Hume for having realized that essential concepts, such as the causal relation between events, are matters of convention.[9]

Einstein's early readings of philosophers such as Hume or philosopher-scientists such as Mach and Henri Poincaré had made him aware of the delicate relation between fundamental concepts such as space, time, and experience. Hume's empiricism, Mach's positivism, and Poincaré's conventionalism were essential to the creation of special relativity because they encouraged Einstein to explore new notions of space and time. His philosophical awareness was, however, much broader than mere background knowledge, and this enabled him to address concrete physical problems with a greater epistemological sensibility than his contemporaries. The very development of his theories of relativity made it necessary for Einstein to engage himself in philosophical thinking in order to resolve foundational ambiguities of the emerging theory of general relativity.

Much later, at about the same time as he was writing the *Autobiographical Notes*, Einstein addressed the relation between knowledge and sensory experience in an essay devoted to the epistemology of Bertrand Russell. In this essay, he also posed the question: "What precisely is the relation between our knowledge and the raw material furnished by sense-impressions?" What he specifically had in mind was: "What knowledge is pure thought able to supply independently of sense perception?"[10] Although concepts and hypotheses derive their meaning from their connection with sensory experiences, that connection is, according to Einstein, "purely intuitive, not itself of logical nature." Only "the relations between the concepts and propositions among themselves are of a logical nature . . . according to firmly laid down rules."[11] Einstein expresses this idea even more strongly in his remarks on Russell's theory of knowledge:

> As a matter of fact I am convinced that even much more is to be asserted: the concepts which arise in our thought and in our linguistic expressions are all—when viewed logically—the free creations of thought which cannot inductively be gained from sense-experiences.[12]

The "logically unbridgeable" gap between certain concepts and sensory experiences is not easily noticed because they are so intimately combined in our everyday thinking.

Akin to philosophers of conventionalism, such as Pierre Duhem and Poincaré, Einstein emphasized the freedom to choose concepts but stressed, even more so than these philosophers, the creative character of this freedom in productive thinking: "All our thinking is of this nature of a free play with concepts."[13] This insight is the basis of Einstein's own epistemological credo:

> All concepts, even those closest to experience, are from the point of view of logic freely chosen posits, just as is the concept of causality, which was the point of departure for this inquiry in the first place.[14]

This notion is expressed more succinctly in an unpublished note, which Einstein intended to include in a forthcoming edition of the *Autobiographical Notes*:

> Everything that is conceptual is constructive and cannot be logically derived directly from experience. Thus, we have complete freedom in choosing the fundamental concepts on which we base our representation of the world. It all depends on how well suited our construction is for bringing order into the chaos of our world experience.[15]

In a similar vein, Einstein discussed forming concepts from sensory impressions and the emergence of a "real world" from such

concepts and relations between them in his fundamental essay
"Physics and Reality":

The connection of the elementary concepts of everyday thinking with complexes of sense experiences can only be compre-
hended intuitively and it is unadaptable to scientifically logical
fixation. The totality of these connections—none of which is
expressible in conceptual terms—is the only thing which dif-
ferentiates the great building which is science from a logical but
empty scheme of concepts.[16]

Turning to the more psychological aspects of the question,
"What precisely is thinking?," Einstein stressed that thinking begins with the formation and manipulation of concepts generated
by the mental ordering of images and memories produced by sensory impressions that appear repeatedly in different contexts. He
found it natural that "thinking goes on for the most part without
the use of signs (words) and beyond that to a considerable degree
unconsciously."[17] Verbalization of the thought process is a secondary stage and is needed only to make thinking communicable.

Einstein summarized, in similar terms, his introspective psychological account of the nature of thinking in a letter to the
French mathematician Jacques Hadamard, who at the time was
conducting a psychological survey of mathematicians to explore
their mental processes. In this letter, Einstein responded to a series
of questions posed to him by Hadamard:

The words or the language, as they are written or spoken, do
not seem to play any rôle in my mechanism of thought. The
psychical entities which seem to serve as elements in thought
are certain signs and more or less clear images which can be
"voluntarily" reproduced and combined. There is, of course, a
certain connection between those elements and relevant logical
concepts. It is also clear that the desire to arrive finally at logically connected concepts is the emotional basis of this rather
vague play with the above-mentioned elements. But taken from

a psychological viewpoint, this combinatory play seems to be the essential feature in productive thought—before there is any connection with logical construction in words or other kind of signs which can be communicated to others.[18]

A dimension often neglected when recounting the remarkable story of the interaction between physics and reflections on physics in the early twentieth century is that of psychological investigations of the cognitive and creative processes in science. Such investigations were central to the work of Max Wertheimer, one of the founders of Gestalt psychology, who was in close contact with Einstein since at least 1916. Einstein sympathized with the views of Wertheimer on the holistic character of conceptual constructions and also of the processes by which they change. Like Wertheimer, Einstein was interested in the "productive" character of thinking. His epistemological credo thus took the empirical roots of knowledge for granted but stressed the creativity of human thinking and its psychological depths beneath the level of conscious awareness.

In 1916, Wertheimer interviewed Einstein to find out more about the creative process that led to the establishment of special relativity and the first steps toward general relativity. This process is described in Wertheimer's *Productive Thinking* as a drama in ten acts, from the sixteen-year-old Einstein's thought experiment about an observer riding on a beam of light to Einstein's version of Newton's rotating bucket experiment that led to general relativity (see section Va). Regarding Einstein's thought process that led to the general theory of relativity, Wertheimer writes:

Every step had to be taken against a very strong gestalt—the traditional structure of physics, which fitted an enormous number of facts, apparently so flawless, so clear that any local change was bound to meet with the resistance of the whole strong and well-articulated structure. This was probably the reason why it took so long a time—seven years—until the crucial advance was made.[19]

He summarizes his analysis of Einstein's thinking by saying:

> Scrutiny of Einstein's thought always showed that when a step
> was taken this happened because it was required. Quite gener-
> ally, if one knows how Einstein thought, one knows that any
> blind and fortuitous procedure was foreign to his mind.[20]

Einstein's epistemological views changed over the years. In the
formative years of relativity (a period discussed in section V), Einstein increasingly distanced himself from the kind of radical empiricism and positivism of Hume and Mach that had previously
fascinated him. In a lecture honoring the sixtieth birthday of Max
Planck, titled "Motives for Research" (*Motive des Forschens*), Einstein asserts: "The supreme task of the physicist is to arrive at those
universal elementary laws from which the cosmos can be built up
by pure deduction."[21] The emphasis here is on "pure deduction."
Einstein would not have made such a statement in the earlier phase
of his scientific development. It marks a departure from Hume's
and Mach's empiricism. An even sharper departure from that doctrine is expressed in Einstein's recollection of the lesson he learned
on his road to the general theory of relativity, a lesson that was,
however, tainted by his contemporary search for a unified field
theory following a purely mathematical strategy[22]:

> I have learned something else from the theory of gravitation:
> no collection of empirical facts however comprehensive can
> ever lead to the setting up of such complicated equations. . . .
> [They] can be found only through the discovery of a logically
> simple mathematical condition that determines the equations
> completely or almost completely. Once one has obtained those
> sufficiently strong formal conditions, one requires only little
> knowledge of facts for the construction of the theory.[23]

The departure from strict empiricism is marked, as Einstein
emphasized, by recognizing the role of free thinking as a constitu-
tive element of science. This conviction resonates with the con-
ventionalist position that philosopher-scientists, such as Poincaré

and, in particular, Duhem, had taken. But it would hardly do justice to portray Einstein as a philosopher-scientist, trying to fit him into one of the numerous categories that historians of philosophy have used for classifying an epistemological position. Einstein, obviously referring to himself, explains that a physicist is different from a philosopher. The physicist cannot rigidly adhere to a particular epistemological position. On different occasions, he may sound like a realist, an idealist, a positivist, and even a Platonist. This may sound to a systematic epistemologist like "epistemological opportunism." However, the historian and philosopher of science Don Howard remarked on this statement: "But when viewed in its proper historical setting, it emerges as an original synthesis of a profound and coherent philosophy of science that is of continuing relevance today, the unifying thread of which is, from early to late, the assimilation of Duhem's holistic version of conventionalism."[24]

c. The Role of Mental Models

Which concepts can a historian use to describe the thought processes leading to Einstein's scientific breakthroughs? Following the lead of his own reflections in sympathy with the insights of Gestalt psychology and its emphasis on the holistic character of cognitive structures, we make use of the concepts of cognitive science which stands in its tradition. Cognitive science has some promising tools to offer to the history of knowledge, such as the concept of a "mental model." Mental models represent a particular form of cognitive structure that is especially suited for drawing conclusions and tracing changes that are based on incomplete information. Additionally, this concept is also suitable for understanding how scientific knowledge is dependent on common experience and subject to correction. With the help of these models, we can replace common anachronistic accounts of verification and falsification in the history of science with a more appropriate view of the development and transformation of knowledge. The resulting image is neither one of linear cumulative development nor of disruptive change. Mental models can be adapted to new experiences without abandoning the underlying cognitive framework. With them, we can understand changes in conclusions as resulting from changes in an experiential context. Mental models connect present and past experiences by embedding new experiences into a cognitive structure formed through past experiences. And finally, mental models form a connecting link between different forms of knowledge—from practical to theoretical. With them, we can understand the implicit reasoning processes inherent in the activities of the practitioners who use them.

The elaborate edifices of scientific theories typically encompass numerous mental models that help to make them applicable to more concrete forms of knowledge, such as the understanding of a "body," of "movement," or of a "living being," which are not necessarily defined within a theory but rather constitute prior knowledge presupposed by it. Mental models are typically content-specific and not universally valid. They allow for the theoretical description and explanation of specific frameworks of reasoning and their changes through history. Mental models bridge various levels of knowledge and represent the same object in various forms, ranging from the technical knowledge of artisans up to the theories of scientists.

How do mental models help us to explain changes in systems of knowledge? The assimilation of different objects and processes into a mental model constantly changes the model itself by enriching its scope of experience. The result is gradual adaptation and modification, and occasional integration of different models applied to the same object or situation. The application of mental models may also itself become the object of reasoning that produces new knowledge in a process of reflection.

Studies in cognitive science have shown that even in early childhood the realization that objects can be moved by applying force to them leads to the inverse conclusion that every perceived movement must have been caused by a mover exerting a force upon it.

In other words, the experience of forces as causes of motion is converted into an interpretation of perceived motions as being caused by force exerted by a mover. At the same time, it is expected that (under otherwise equal conditions) a greater force must cause a stronger motion. This set of expectations may be viewed as a typical example of the formation of a mental model, which in this case is called the motion-implies-force model. The experiences represented by this model are so general that we may assume that the motion-implied-force model is probably acquired by people in every culture over the course of their ontogenetic development.

Einstein refers to a childhood experience in his *Autobiographical Notes* (and on several other occasions throughout his life) when he was four or five years old and he received a compass from his father. The motion of the magnetic needle did not meet little Albert's expectations, which were shaped by the idea that motions are either caused by touch or force, or are part of the natural constitution of the world, like the falling of heavy objects. Little Albert was evidently using the mental model of motion-implies-force. The deviation of an experience from intuitive physics represents a conflict with a fixed world of concepts. It left Albert with a sense of "wonder." Looking back at this experience, Einstein perceived clashes between experiences and conceptual frameworks or preconceived mental models as a driving force behind our thinking.

Another childhood episode that inspired a sense of wonder occurred when Albert received a little book on Euclidean geometry. This led to his realization that certain unexpected assertions could be proved with certainty, such as the intersection of the three altitudes of a triangle meeting at one point. Only later did he realize that this particular wonder—based on the impression that certain knowledge of the objects we experience can be obtained through pure thought alone and thereby supporting a Platonic or Kantian epistemology—actually rested on problematic assumptions.

Nevertheless, the wonder of being able to gain surprising insights by thinking alone stayed with Einstein. He was indeed the master of thought experiments, which played a crucial role in several of his scientific discoveries. Thought experiments are, however, not premised on the existence of a priori knowledge but rather work with mental constructions, enabling one to explore the consequences of existing knowledge and to reflect on them from a new perspective, which may lead to novel insights—even without actually carrying them out as real experiments.

In light of Einstein's emphasis on the nature of conceptual constructions as free creations of the human mind, their success in helping us orient ourselves in the world must itself come as a surprise, or rather, as a wonder. This larger sense of wonder, related to the comprehensibility of the world, is thus at the core of his epistemological conviction:

> The very fact that the totality of our sense experiences is such that by means of thinking (operations with concepts, and the creation and use of definite functional relations between them, and the coordination of sense experiences to these concepts) it can be put in order, this fact is one which leaves us in awe, but which we shall never understand. One may say "the eternal mystery of the world is its comprehensibility."[25]

In the following sections, we present a number of mental models, demonstrating their role in changing specific structures of knowledge and highlighting their features in conjunction with what we have already covered.

d. Restructuring Systems of Knowledge—
A Copernicus Process

In the following, we argue that we can understand conceptual transformations as a restructuring of existing systems of knowledge, preserving much of the underlying empirical knowledge but revising its cognitive architecture, for example, the nature and order of the mental models constituting their architecture. Using an analogy with biological evolution, we may expect that a gradual knowledge evolution could also lead, in the long run, to the emergence of new knowledge structures, just as in biology new species may emerge from long-ranging processes of gradual changes. This possibility rests on an inner variability of the system. In biology, this variability is assured by the occurrence of genetic mutations, through which individuals are produced with new characteristics. In the case of a system of knowledge, the variability derives from the exploration of inherent potentials embodied in its material and symbolic means. This exploration is typically a social process within a scientific community that produces a constant inner differentiation of the system of knowledge.

The growing internal complexity, in turn, increases the possibility of generating new results, with a concomitant broadening of the scope of the system of knowledge. The new results can either be experimental outcomes or theoretical conclusions. In biology, new species arise when events create conditions that enable a divergence of a descendant generation (progeny), especially through the spatial separation of populations. Similarly, the emergence of new systems of knowledge requires that certain conditions be fulfilled.

In biology, such events are often imposed externally on diverging populations. For example, a decreasing water level might cause one lake to divide into several smaller lakes, therefore preventing the exchange of genes between the separated populations of one species of fish. In the dynamics of knowledge development, the decisive engine of divergence often lies within the system itself but may also be triggered by external challenges, such as different areas of application of a knowledge system. In fact, the exploration of a system of knowledge by a community of practitioners focusing on a new set of problems typically leads to inner tensions, ambiguities, and even contradictions that trigger a restructuration of the system of knowledge. The starting point for such restructuring can often be traced to challenging objects or borderline problems of the existing theories. The process may lead previously incidental elements in an increasingly complex and unstable system to become the cornerstones of a new edifice of scientific knowledge. The resulting structure is largely new but consists, for the most part, of the building blocks that were already at hand. The historian of science Michel Janssen supplements the biological analogy with an architectural metaphor of arches built upon scaffolding, a metaphor that is also used in evolutionary theory to explain the path-dependency of certain developments. In the first phase, one often sees the construction of a "scaffolding" that uses the existing materials, namely, the elements of the existing knowledge system to cope with a challenging problem. This "scaffolding" may eventually serve to guide and support the development of a radically novel knowledge system, which he calls "the arch." This process is more than just "normal science"—it constitutes a highly creative effort that may take considerable time and typically involves an entire scientific community.[26]

The reflection giving rise to such a restructuring is called here a "Copernicus process," in analogy to what is probably the most famous example in the history of science for this kind of restructuring of an existing system of knowledge; it ultimately established a new worldview but in a process involving many actors and stretching over centuries. Let us take a closer look at one of the episodes in this longer range process, the preclassical mechanics of Galileo and his contemporaries.

e. An Example of a Copernicus Process— The Galilean Revolution

Galileo is generally known for his contributions to observational astronomy and his defense of the Copernican view of the planetary system. They were related to the engagement of Galileo and his contemporaries in the transformation of the Aristotelian conception of motion. We will return to this example more than once.

The core of the Aristotelian theory of motion is the intuitive mental motion-implies-force model, stating that there is no motion without a mover in contact with the moving body. The failure of this model to identify a mover led to the exclusion of two types of motion from the motion-implies-force model: first, the motion of celestial bodies, and second, the motion of heavy objects falling to the center of the earth as well as the ascending motion of light objects in the opposite direction. Aristotle referred to these motions as "natural" motions, which do not require an external cause, as opposed to "violent" motions, which are the subject of his theory of causation of motion by force.

The phenomenon of flying projectiles challenged the motion-implies-force model. When a projectile is thrown into the air it continues to move without being driven by a detectible cause. What is the force in direct contact with the flying object that maintains its motion after it leaves the thrower's hand? One traditional, but rather implausible, answer to this question suggested by the motion-implies-force model involves the medium (air) surrounding the flying object. The initial motive force of the throwing hand moves the surrounding medium, which then acts as the motive force in contact with the object.

An alternative theory, based on an extension of the motion-implies-force model, became a starting point for a more plausible explanation of inertial phenomena that were otherwise difficult to integrate into the Aristotelian paradigm. This extension, which served as a kind of scaffolding for the later conception of the inertial principle, was achieved by modifying the concept of force. The force that causes a motion could be conceived as an entity that is transferred from the mover to the moving object. This transferred force was typically designated as an "impressed force" (*vis impressa*) or as an "impetus." Impetus is the cause of continued motion. It allows motion in a vacuum and is not necessarily self-dissipating.

Aristotelian physics persisted over centuries. It formed the basic knowledge taught at Medieval European universities, and any attempt to create an equally general theory of nature had to build upon this body of knowledge, even if its goal was to revise the Aristotelian system. This explains why Galileo and his contemporaries combined an anti-Aristotelian attitude with an adherence to basic Aristotelian assumptions, a characteristic feature of the pre-classical mechanics of the early modern period.[27]

To demonstrate the departure from Aristotelian physics and entry into the realm of classical mechanics, we consider the pivotal case of projectile motion. To understand how this motion functions according to classical mechanics, we need two principles that are in direct contradiction to Aristotelian natural philosophy, the principle of inertia and the principle of superposition of motions. With these assumptions, the laws of projectile motion easily follow: According to the principle of inertia, a projected body moves uniformly in the direction of its projection. Simultaneously, it falls downward in accelerated motion as determined by the law of free fall. The two motions superpose to form the projectile's parabolic trajectory.

Let us next consider the special case of a horizontally shot projectile. Galileo's conceptual framework was Aristotelian in the sense that he still distinguished between the "natural" motion of free fall and the "violent" motion of propagation in any other direction. The violent motion requires a cause, communicated to the object through the projecting agent. But in the special case of a horizontal shot, Galileo found it plausible to assume that this communicated force, the impetus, is preserved, as he saw this in analogy to the uniform motion of a body along a horizontal plane which, for him, constituted an intermediate case between violent and natural motion in which the impetus is conserved. For the case of a horizontal shot, he could thus infer that, if the trajectory of the projectile resembles a parabola, the vertical motion must follow the law of fall, with spaces traversed being proportional to the square of the time elapsed. Galileo can be said to have "discovered" parabolic projectile motion through experiments where he rolled balls on inclined surfaces, which he conducted with Guidobaldo del Monte in 1592. Turning this argument around, he could derive the parabolic shape of the trajectory from the law of free fall and the assumption that motion along the horizontal is uniform.

This treatment of projectile motion exhibits such a close and direct connection to the principles of classical physics that it is hard to avoid the conclusion that Galileo must also have had these principles at his disposal. Such a conclusion thus naturally leads to the claim that Galileo is the founder of classical mechanics. But a closer historical examination of Galileo's work shows that, for the generic case (that is, the case of oblique projection), he failed to provide proof for the parabolic shape of a projectile's trajectory, just as he did not succeed in finding a consistent derivation of his law of free fall despite many years of effort. The reason was that his thinking was still deeply rooted in the knowledge system of Aristotelian dynamics, which stipulates that there cannot be a force-free motion, for example a uniform motion along the direction of an oblique shot, an assumption used in classical mechanics to derive the parabolic shape of an oblique trajectory.

It was left to Galileo's distinguished but lesser-known disciples to formulate the concepts of classical mechanics that are not explicitly found in Galileo's work. Nevertheless, the classical principles of inertia and the superposition of motions can be easily "read into" Galileo's texts. Indeed, before Galileo had finished his last work, the *Discorsi*, his pupil Bonaventura Cavalieri published in 1632 the first derivation of the trajectory of an obliquely thrown projectile. Cavalieri's derivation uses the principles of inertia and superposition comparable to that of modern accounts. But does this mean that Cavalieri was the true creator of classical mechanics? Was he the youthful revolutionary who dared ponder that which had not crossed the mind of the obstinate Galileo? This is the interpretation proposed at the end of the nineteenth century by one of the first interpreters of Galileo's manuscripts, Raffaello Caverni.

But this interpretation is not very convincing in view of the fact that Cavalieri's derivation is not part of a systematic treatise on motion but is mentioned in passing in a book about concave mirrors. He does not emphasize the use of the principles of inertia and superposition. On the contrary, Galileo accused Cavalieri of stealing from him through his premature publication, thereby taking credit for his forty years of work. In his defense, Cavalieri claimed to have stated what was already generally known as Galileo's achievement. Indeed, Cavalieri is not the only disciple of Galileo who made derivations of the parabolic trajectory using the new concepts. But what seems natural in the works of almost all Galileo's disciples cannot be found in the works of their master, whose thinking was still rooted in Aristotelian concepts, although he succeeded in exploring their limits.

Another student of Galileo, Evangelista Torricelli, clearly states in the introduction to his book on the motion of heavy bodies (which contains the basic principles of classical mechanics) how little Galileo's disciples identified themselves as revolutionaries:

> We will consider here the science of the movement of heavy bodies and projectiles, with which many have dealt, but which, as far as we are aware, has been derived in a geometric way only by Galileo. We admit that, as he reaped this field with a seemingly large scythe, there can be little left for us but to gather the chaff by following in the wake of this diligent reaper, heedless of whether he has discarded the chaff or it has simply been thrown away; if however we are not even able to find this then we can at least pick the cornflowers and violets that grow on the paths; perhaps with these flowers we may even be able to form a not too contemptible wreath.[28]

Thus, in the transition from preclassical to classical mechanics, the "errors" of preclassical mechanics did not need "correcting"; rather, the results of preclassical mechanics could simply be reinterpreted by the next generation, who were then essential in forming a newly constructed system of knowledge, the system of classical mechanics. This is an exemplary case of a Copernicus process where previously marginal elements such as the assumption of a "conserved motion," assumed a central role in the new system.

The later sections of this book will show that, similar to Galileo's disciples, Einstein took the problematic assumptions of the theories of his predecessors as the point of departure for a new system of knowledge. So, in a sense, the new system inherited the old one but was transformed via a Copernicus process. With the introduction of new concepts of space, time, gravitation, matter, and radiation, the new system could not be reconciled with the former. We will use the Copernicus process initiated by Einstein to flesh out the ideas on the theory of historical development that have been illustrated above. We will show that by using such a framework, progress not only loses its paradoxical character but is itself a manifestation of human creativity. Upon reflection, the source of scientific innovation and the conditions for dealing responsibly with the possibilities of science ultimately prove to be of the same nature, while not being always aligned with each other.

f. The Einsteinian Revolution and Changing Worldviews

For anyone who wants to understand the course of science history not just as a sequence of contingent events or as the outcome of the creativity of a genius, Einstein's contributions to the emergence of the two fundamental theories of modern physics, relativity and quantum theory, raise a number of puzzling questions. Clearly, some of the causes for these developments are associated with processes beyond intellectual history, for example, industrialization or national ambitions. Other causes bear the mark of Einstein's personal perspective on science, such as his quest for a unified worldview. These causes also involve the influence of his immediate environment, such as that of his circle of bohemian friends. But taking a step back from Einstein's biography and its immediate context, one cannot avoid the impression that one is witnessing a larger-scale process with its own dynamics, a process that is not just about societal developments or personal fortunes but about the development of knowledge as a dimension of science that cannot be reduced to that of its actors, its institutions, and their contexts.

This brings us to the phenomenon of the existence of both long periods of stability and periods of profound changes in the worldview of science. Examples of such profound changes in physics are the revolutions associated with the names of Copernicus, Newton, Faraday, and Maxwell. In the Copernican revolution, the earth lost its central place in the universe and took on the role of one among several planets orbiting the sun. In the Newtonian revolution, the terrestrial and the cosmic realm became subject to the same universal laws of motion, whereas before, in the Aristotelian cosmos, these distinct realms were each subject to its own laws. Newton introduced an absolute physical space with no preferred locations and directions, and asserted that events anywhere could be tracked relative to a clock measuring absolute time. According to the Aristotelian worldview, heavy objects tend to move toward their natural home, the center of the earth, whereas the Newtonian worldview sees them moving subject to a gravitational force. That force arises from action at a distance, that is, without any intervening material contact. In the revolution associated with Michael Faraday and James Clerk Maxwell, absolute space becomes occupied by an all-pervading ether that carries all physical interactions with finite speed. These interactions were conceived as being due to fields, which in turn were initially understood as distortions of the ether.

The revolutions associated with Einstein's name can, broadly speaking, be described similarly. Absolute space and time were subsumed by the special theory of relativity and replaced by concepts of space and time that are dependent on the relative state of motion of an observer. Moreover, space and time were merged into the single new concept of spacetime, taking the place of Newton's absolute space and time, to set the stage for physical interactions. In the general relativity revolution, an independently existing spacetime *stage* was abandoned, and spacetime now became a *field* that participated in physical processes itself. In the quantum revolution, radiation ceased to be conceived as a wave phenomenon within a universal ether and acquired properties of both fields and particles. Similarly, matter acquired a dual nature: under certain circumstances it exhibits particle-like behavior, and under others it behaves like a wave. Statistical laws were no longer a manifestation of our ignorance of the details of physical processes but a reflection of a fundamental indeterminacy in the laws of nature.

This short review of scientific revolutions in physics stands in stark contrast to the previously described cumulative view of the history of science, with its underlying assumption that steady and

gradual scientific progress is an enduring characteristic of knowledge development in science. This contrast stimulated the famous
1962 study on the structure of scientific revolutions by Thomas
Kuhn. He saw the history of science not as a continuous accumulation of knowledge but as characterized by deep disruptions and
radical upheavals of comprehensive worldviews, whereby one prevailing "paradigm" succeeds another. Kuhn conceived a paradigm
as a consensus shared by scientists that follows from common practices of problem-solving, a common understanding of theories, the
knowledge they comprise, and relevant research objectives. When
this consensus is taken for granted in scientists' day-to-day work,
they are said to be conducting "normal science." When unexpected
results come to light, anomalies that cannot be made to fit into prevailing theories propel the paradigm into a crisis. After a phase of
fundamental scientific controversy known as "extraordinary science," a new paradigm is established. For Kuhn, the replacement of
classical physics with modern physics represented just such a paradigm shift.

With scientific revolutions recognized as also being dependent
on cultural, social, and psychological factors, their structures became comparable to those of political and cultural revolutions.
Thus, the history of science became a legitimate part of a comprehensive cultural history. But, in contrast to politics or art, completely dismissing the idea of progress in science is difficult. Kuhn
and his successors could not provide a satisfactory answer to the
question of how such paradigm shifts can be reconciled with this
intuition of a progressive accumulation of knowledge in science.
Nor could they convincingly explain the origin of a new paradigm.
According to Kuhn, the new paradigm does not build on its
predecessor but entirely replaces it.

Does a perspective exist that permits us to reconcile cumulative
and gradual progress in science with the possibility of scientific
revolutions? Evidently, such revolutions overturn truly fundamental categories of our understanding of the world, yet the cognitive
process of science does not have to restart after each revolution.

The scientific revolutions associated with Einstein's name offer excellent examples of this paradox. In spite of their profound implications for our understanding of the world, the centuries of preparatory work on which today's scientific worldview is based were not simply discarded in the aftermath of the Einsteinian revolutions. Rather, the discoveries of Copernicus, Galileo, Newton, and Maxwell are simultaneously refuted and confirmed in this revolution. How is this possible? How can the feasibility of progress be reconciled with the fact that scientific revolutions happen? In the following sections of this book, we try to answer some of these questions by reconstructing Einstein's breakthroughs in physics as transformations of knowledge.

g. Other Historiographic Perspectives on Progress in Science

This book is devoted to the presentation and historiographic analysis of the Einsteinian revolution. In this context and for the purpose of comparison, we also mention the Copernican and Galilean revolutions. Other developments that have been traditionally labeled a "revolution" are: the chemical revolution, the Darwinian revolution, and the geological revolution. More recently, there is: the molecular biology revolution and the artificial intelligence revolution.

The historiography of science has often attempted to describe such scientific turning points by searching for common characteristics of their origins, evolution, and consequences. In the twentieth century, epistemological and historiographic reflections on science developed into different perspectives on how science evolves.[29] Early in the twentieth century, such reflections were shaped by a closer interplay between science and philosophy, as promoted by philosophers of the Vienna Circle, such as Moritz Schlick, who interacted with prominent scientists like Einstein. But by the mid-1930s some of these philosophers retreated to a formal analysis of language or rather abstract discussions of "the" scientific methodology, which resulted in a deep rift between a historical and philosophical epistemology of science.

We have already mentioned several times the bold attempt by Kuhn to place the different phases in the evolution of science into the scheme of "shifting paradigms." He described the history of science as a series of long periods of normality during which scientists are guided by a generally accepted view—a "paradigm." Occasionally, the normal evolution of science is interrupted by times of crisis, when new observations in a certain area of science are incompatible with the existing paradigm. Under such circumstances, the area of science enters a time of "revolutionary science" when a new paradigm may be created.

Kuhn's analysis of the structure of scientific revolutions concentrated exclusively on a community of academic experts, disregarding broader epistemic communities and contexts, and was shaped by the ideological controversies of the Cold War, in particular by the opposition to Marxist views that emphasized such contexts. Such views were articulated, for example, by Boris Hessen, director of the Physics Institute at Moscow University, who presented a scholarly study on the "Social and Economic Roots of Newton's Principia" in 1931. Another study of the relation between science and the economic and technological conditions was presented in 1935 by the Marxist economist Henryk Grossmann.[30] Hessen and Grossmann independently developed a view of science as one kind of labor within the system of social production. One of their main messages was that material conditions and social factors—including the experience of practitioners, such as artisans or technicians—as well as ideologies, beliefs, and political and philosophical worldviews can affect the evolution of science. Their thesis about the enabling role of technology for gaining scientific knowledge, which differs from widely spread prejudices against Marxism as implying a determinist relation between science and economic conditions, had virtually no influence on the history of science before the 1970s. In contrast, Kuhn's perspective implied that economic structures, technological developments, and practical conditions are largely irrelevant to the history of science. By his account, discoveries are almost isolated, mystical achievements of individuals that occur while the majority of the scientific community continues to practice normal science.

A different model of the evolution of scientific knowledge is associated with the name of the Polish bacteriologist, physician, and historian of science Ludwik Fleck. In 1933, he sent a manuscript to Schlick titled "The Analysis of a Scientific Fact: Outline of Comparative Epistemology." Fleck hoped that Schlick could help him publish this work, which offered a new perspective on science as a collective enterprise, arguing that the historical development of all knowledge is a socially conditioned collective enterprise. To describe the collective enterprise, Fleck introduced notions such as "thought collective" and "thought style."[31] A thought collective is a community of individuals who mutually exchange ideas or maintain intellectual interaction. Members of a specific collective speak about things that would not cross their minds if they were alone or would not talk about if they were in another collective. Thus, a thought style characteristic for that group emerges. A certain collective mood that causes the members of that group to act in a certain way also emerges. For Fleck, thinking is a collective activity. It results either in an idea that is accepted by those who take part in this social activity or in a worldview that is only clear to the members of the collective. What we think and how we perceive depends on the thought collective to which we belong.

For Fleck, the history of scientific knowledge is related in fundamental ways to social mechanisms like education and tradition. In the letter to Schlick, he criticized traditional epistemology and, in particular, the emphasis of the Vienna Circle on the primacy of sensations in the acquisition of scientific knowledge:

I could never shake the impression that epistemology examines not knowledge as it actually occurs, but its own imagined ideal of knowledge, which lacks all its real properties. . . . The statement that all knowledge originates in sensations is misleading,

because the plurality of all human knowledge stems quite simply from textbooks . . . Finally, the historical development of
knowledge shows some remarkably common aspects as well,
such as for instance the particular stylistic closeness of the respective systems of knowledge, which demands an epistemological investigation. These prompted me to treat a scientific
fact from my area of expertise epistemologically.[32]

The "scientific fact" analyzed in Fleck's book was a major medical
problem of the time—venereal disease. He demonstrated his ideas
by showing how a community of medical practitioners together
came to an understanding of syphilis based on earlier, traditional
notions of causation, which then led to the development of the
Wassermann test used to detect the disease.

Another view of progress in science is based on the notion of
"dialogue" as an alternative to the emphasis on the notion of "paradigm." This is the essence of Mara Beller's analysis of the quantum
revolution.[33] Beller argues that the notion of a paradigm has dog-
matic ideological roots and totalitarian implications. She is particularly critical of the notion of incommensurability implied by
the tensions between old and new paradigms. Kuhn (as well as
philosopher of science Paul Feyerabend) suggested that scientific
theories (concepts, paradigms, worldviews) separated by a scientific revolution are incommensurate. He used the term *incommensurability* to describe the miscommunication between pre- and
postrevolutionary scientific traditions, claiming, for example, that
the Newtonian paradigm is incommensurable with its Cartesian
and Aristotelian predecessors in physics and that Antoine-
Laurent Lavoisier's paradigm is incommensurable with that of
Joseph Priestley's in chemistry. These competing paradigms supposedly use fundamentally different concepts and methods to
address different problems, limiting communication across the
revolutionary divide.

Beller points out that Kuhn himself, in his analysis of the Copernican revolution, which was published five years before his *The*

Structure of Scientific Revolutions, demonstrated that a scientific revolution does not have to be a complete Gestalt switch of concepts, meanings, and practices. She argues that

> historians of science find it increasingly difficult to build their narratives in Kuhnian terms. . . . Rather than dogmatic commitment to a rigid set of ideas, scientific creation—be it during the Copernican, chemical, or quantum revolution—is often characterized by the ingenious mingling and selective appropriation of ideas from different "paradigms."[34]

Beller also strongly disagrees with Kuhn's assertion that rigid adherence to paradigms produces more originality and creativity in human endeavors. In contrast to his structure of incommensurable paradigms and commitments to paradigms, Beller adopts a dialogical approach, which

> perceives communications between friends and foes alike as the precondition of all scientific creativity. Unlike the concept of a paradigm, which by its nature excludes the "other," the dialogical approach celebrates the existence of other minds as indispensable for scientific advance.[35]

This is the basis of Beller's "dialogism"—a dialogical philosophy and historiography.

Here, we have mentioned one view of the evolution of science inspired by Marx's historical materialism, and we briefly described three others, based on the notions of "shifting paradigms," "thought collective," and "dialogue," mentioning only the main proponents of these perspectives. Our historiographic analysis of the Einsteinian revolution is based on the idea of a "transformation of knowledge," a process that occurred on the background of the Second Industrial Revolution, opening up new material conditions for knowledge generation in the sense of the Hessen-Grossmann thesis, within a broad dialogue among friends, colleagues, and peers, just as Beller describes it—from the Olympia Academy, to the collaboration with Einstein's friends Michele Besso and Marcel Grossmann, and the extensive correspondence and exchange with scientists and philosophers. Thus, this transformation of knowledge was in part also the result of a collective thought process in the sense of Fleck. Therefore, our analysis includes insights from these other views on scientific revolutions and proposes an answer to some of the challenges raised by the original Kuhnian scheme. It also includes Michel Janssen's architectural metaphor, mentioned earlier, which claims that new theories are built like arches on scaffolds provided by the elaboration of old theories.

Let us conclude this discussion with Einstein's own view on his grand achievements. During his visit to Italy in 1921, in his lectures on the theory of relativity at the universities of Padua and Bologna, Einstein addressed the central point of the ongoing debate on the nature of the theory of relativity by emphasizing the benefits of an evolutionary view of scientific progress. He asserted that the theory of relativity was not a revolution but the result of a slow and constrained evolution. He argued that: "No fairer destiny could be allotted to any physical theory, than that it should of itself point out the way to the introduction of a more comprehensive theory, in which it lives on as a limiting case."[36]

III

The Continents of Classical Physics and the Problems at Their Borders

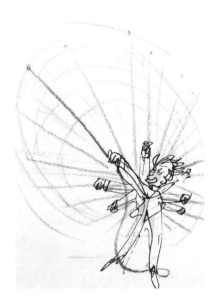

Preview

By the nineteenth century, physics had developed into a discipline with a strong conceptual basis and institutional framework. Teaching and research as well as numerous technical applications formed its backbone, along with a rich system of publication. The starting point of this development was classical mechanics, as established in the seventeenth and eighteenth centuries with basic concepts like space, time, force, and motion, which seemingly provided a generally valid framework for all physics and formed the foundation for a mechanistic worldview. In the mid-nineteenth century, however, new areas with independent conceptual foundations emerged in the form of the theories of thermal and electromagnetic phenomena giving rise to three "continents" that constituted the world of classical physics—mechanics, electrodynamics, and thermodynamics. Indeed, in the second half of the nineteenth century, tensions had been building while these three continents, slowly but surely like tectonic plates, were shifting their relative positions.

Electrodynamic and thermodynamic phenomena could be related to mechanical concepts in terms of mental models that explain those nonmechanical processes with the help of hidden mechanisms. The most prominent mental models were atomism and the all-pervading ether. The latter was thought to be a mechanical medium that was required to support electromagnetic phenomena. Most notably, the ether was regarded as the carrier of light waves, in analogy to air carrying sound waves.

But friction at the borders, where these continents were starting to overlap, produced tremors. Borderline problems arose between mechanics and electrodynamics, between thermodynamics and electrodynamics, and between mechanics and thermodynamics. We discuss these problems in detail and their consequences for the underlying hidden mechanisms. Einstein's monumental success was in demonstrating the possibility of finding solutions to the borderline problems of classical physics that did justice to the available empirical knowledge. Each of these solutions taken by itself appeared to be both a triumph of classical physics and a contribution to its demise, as will be shown in the next section. Together they eventually led to the relativity, quantum, and atomic revolutions.

Keeping the history of nineteenth-century science in mind is essential for understanding the roots of scientific revolutions that led to the rise of modern physics. The state of physics described in this section represents the intellectual arena that the young Albert Einstein took his first steps in as a creative scientist.

a. Classical Mechanics as a Comprehensive Worldview

Mechanics is one of the most ancient fields of physical knowledge. The first theories of mechanics go back to Greek antiquity. In the scientific revolution of the early modern period, mechanics played a pivotal role, culminating in Isaac Newton's famous *Principia* of 1687. But it was the year 1666 that was recognized as Newton's miraculous year, thanks to a poem by the British poet John Dryden, "Annus Mirabilis." The poem describes the year's unprecedented events: the victory of the British fleet over the Dutch fleet and the Great Fire of London, which was considered a miracle because it destroyed the city and gave the king an opportunity to rebuild it in a more modern style.

During that year, twenty-four-year-old Isaac Newton realized that the force that makes an apple fall from a tree is the same force that keeps the moon in its orbit around the earth, thus bringing together the laws of terrestrial and planetary motions in a single framework. He also invented differential and integral calculus, which enabled him to derive the motion of planets in the solar system and to explain the laws deduced from astronomical observations by the astronomer Johannes Kepler. In the same year, he also explored the spectral nature of light, which led to his theory of colors. A "miraculous year" indeed, no less impressive than Einstein's in 1905.

In Newtonian mechanics, the "motion-implies-force" model of preclassical mechanics is replaced by the "acceleration-implies-force" model. This model implies a separation of motions of physical bodies into two classes: motions that demand a causal explanation by a "force" and the so-called inertial motions that are dominated by the principle of inertia and do not require a cause. Inertial motions include all straight, uniform motions of bodies, as well as the state of rest, whereas all accelerated motions must be viewed as being caused by forces. Since a given motion can appear accelerated as well as uniform depending on the point of reference, this separation is unique only relative to a certain frame of description, say a laboratory that is localized at a certain place at a certain time, and thereby represents a "frame of reference." In Newtonian mechanics, "absolute space" serves as such a frame, as does any frame that moves with uniform, straight-line motion relative to absolute space. The concept of an "inertial system" was introduced in the late nineteenth century to designate such frames of reference that move uniformly along straight lines relative to absolute space. The assertion that the laws of Newtonian mechanics should be valid when formulated in any of these inertial systems is called the "principle of Galilean relativity."

If a body is accelerated with respect to an inertial system, it must be subject to a force that one or possibly several other bodies exert on it. The magnitude of the acceleration depends on the magnitude of the force as well as the resistance with which the body opposes the force. In classical mechanics, this resistance is an internal characteristic of the body, called "inertial mass." In addition, bodies possess another kind of mass in Newtonian mechanics, the "gravitational mass." The latter, unlike the former, does not measure the resistance against the action of a force but represents the origin and source of a force itself, the gravitational force. According to Newton's law of gravity, this force is proportional to the product of the gravitational masses of two bodies that attract each other, and is inversely proportional to the square of their distance. Although the two kinds of masses in Newtonian mechanics have conceptually very different functions, they are equal to each other. This remarkable coincidence has implications for free-fall motion due to gravity; namely, all bodies fall with the same acceleration, irrespective of their mass.

Newton created the basis for what became an all-encompassing mechanical worldview, elaborated in the eighteenth and nineteenth centuries, which applied to areas far beyond mechanics proper. As a student, Einstein was fascinated by this extension into other areas: "What made the greatest impression upon the student, however, was not so much the technical development of mechanics or the solution of complicated problems as the achievements of mechanics in areas that apparently had nothing to do with mechanics."[1] As examples of the impressive range of mechanics, he adduces the theory of sound, hydrodynamics, the theory of light, the kinetic theory of heat, and, in particular, the capability to deduce the basic laws of thermodynamics from a statistical theory of classical mechanics. The most widely known example of an extension of mechanics beyond its immediate domain of applicability is indeed the explanation of heat by atomic motion. This development will be discussed below in section IIIc.

Newton's concept of absolute space was criticized by Ernst Mach. Newton inferred the existence of absolute space from his well-known thought experiment of two buckets filled with water, where one of the buckets is rotating and the other is not. The water surface is curved only in the rotating bucket. One cannot say this effect is due to a relative motion between the two buckets. The curved water surface clearly distinguishes between the two. According to Newton, the existence of absolute space can be inferred from its effect on the rotating water. Mach objected to this interpretation, claiming that it was in fact possible to consider the effect as being due to a relative motion between bodies. He claimed that if one takes into account the existence of distant stars, then one does not have to assert that the water surface is curved due to rotation with respect to absolute space but can explain it as being due to rotation with respect to these distant stars.

Mach criticized the metaphysical character of the concept of absolute space and argued that the concept of motion, or even of inertial mass, cannot be applied to a single body in "absolute space," as claimed by Newton. Instead, he suggested that all classical mechanics should be rewritten in terms of relative motions of bodies, and that the concepts "inertial mass" and "inertial system" should be redefined in this fashion. Mach conjectured that

"inertial forces," the apparent forces acting on bodies in accelerated frames of reference, such as centrifugal forces, which cause
the curvature of the water level in a rotating bucket, are due to the
interaction with distant masses in the universe.

Einstein was deeply influenced by reading Mach. He accepted
Mach's criticism of Newtonian mechanics and rejected the notion
of absolute space as an entity that could act but could not be acted
upon. We discuss this point in detail in section V in the context of
Einstein adopting Mach's position on his road to general relativity.
It took him many years, until around 1930, to realize that this epistemological position is ultimately untenable.

We elaborate on Einstein's critique of mechanics in section V.
Here, in summary, we can say that, aside from clashes with empirical evidence, classical mechanics harbored a number of internal
tensions. One tension was the contrast between an action at a distance, the characteristic feature of Newton's law of gravitation, and
the field concept introduced by magnetism. A second tension was
between gravity conceived as a property of space, suggested by its
universal character and in particular by the equivalence of gravitational and inertial mass, and its explanation as a force in Newton's
theory. The first tension was sharpened through the rise of special
relativity and both tensions were resolved through the introduction of the general theory of relativity.

b. Electrodynamics and the Ether Concept

In the mid-nineteenth century, Michael Faraday, a self-educated,
creative British experimentalist, showed that electrical and magnetic phenomena were closely related. James Clerk Maxwell unified these experimental findings in the four fundamental equations
of electromagnetism that carry his name. According to Lorentz's
electron theory, discussed below, these equations introduced the
concept of electric and magnetic fields as new physical entities that
exist everywhere in space. These fields are generated by electrically
charged particles that determine their behavior. They are continuous

functions of the coordinates of space and time. Einstein referred to the "electric field theory of Faraday and Maxwell" as "probably the most profound transformation of the foundations of physics since Newton's time."[2] It eventually replaced discrete material particles with continuous fields as the fundamental physical entities, thus introducing a new physical worldview that was, however, only fully unfolded in the later work of Heinrich Hertz and Hendrik Lorentz, as we discuss below. Einstein mentions Faraday and Maxwell in his *Autobiographical Notes*, comparing their newly emerging worldview with the old worldview of Galileo and Newton. While Faraday and Galileo, guided by intuition, achieved basic insights and performed some fundamental experiments, Maxwell and Newton developed comprehensive theories, including an exact mathematical formulation. In the *Notes*, Einstein recalls the deep impression that Maxwell's theory made on him:

> The most fascinating subject at the time that I was a student was Maxwell's theory. What made this theory appear revolutionary was the transition from action at a distance to fields as the fundamental variables.[3]

Maxwell's equations relate the spatial rates of change of electric and magnetic fields to their temporal change and the electrically charged particles. Such relations between rates of change of physical quantities are represented by the mathematical language of "partial differential equations." It turned out that changing electric fields produce changing magnetic fields, and vice versa. The result is a propagating electromagnetic wave, moving at a speed of ca. 300 million meters a second. The confirmation of the prediction of electromagnetic radiation by Hertz was an important triumph of Maxwell's theory. A corollary to that prediction was the realization that light is such an electromagnetic wave. This conclusion led to the incorporation of optics into the theory of electromagnetism, thus concluding one of the most prominent unification schemes in the history of physics. It combined the seemingly different phenomenological domains of electricity, magnetism, and optics into one theoretical framework.

Faraday, Maxwell, and other scientists of that time postulated that all space is filled with a medium called "ether." They supposed that this medium could support internal stresses, which would represent the electric and magnetic fields. Thus, this medium transports physical effects from place to place, representing a shift away from the action-at-a-distance feature of Newton's law of gravity. Such an ether must resemble an incompressible solid medium but be permeable enough to not disturb motion, such as that of the planets. In other words, as Einstein formulated it, the ether must lead a "ghostly existence alongside the rest of matter."[4] As we have pointed out above, the concept of the ether was shaped according to the familiar mental model of a medium that carries waves, analogous to air as the medium for the propagation of sound waves. The velocity of light appears explicitly in Maxwell's equations. Thus, these equations are different in different inertial systems. The ether could provide a state of rest and thus form an embodiment of Newton's absolute space.

An invisible mechanism anchored in intuitive and practical knowledge typically has more properties than only those properties needed to explain physical processes. Even if, for example, the electrodynamic ether is assumed not to be directly accessible through ordinary mechanical experience, it must nonetheless be understood as a mechanical medium. However, constructing a mechanical model of this ether that fulfilled the necessary requirements turned out to be extremely difficult: this model had to allow for the richness of electromagnetic and optical phenomena contained in Maxwell's theory, but it also had to be compatible with physical knowledge from other areas. To explain the properties of light alone, the ether needed to be an elastic medium that nevertheless could not offer appreciable resistance to the motion of giant physical masses like the earth and the sun. Moreover, from the assumed nature of the ether as a mechanical medium, the ether must either be at rest or in motion with respect to the macroscopically observable bodies embedded in it. The question of which of these two alternatives applies turned out to have significant ramifications for the treatment of the borderline problems of the electrodynamics and optics of moving bodies. The suggestion, based on experimental observations—such as the stellar aberration and the Fizeau experiment, measuring the speed of light in flowing water—was that ether is indeed at rest. Consequently, experimentally detecting the motion of the earth with respect to the ether should be possible. But attempts to actually measure an "ether wind" failed. The best-known experiment of this was performed in 1887 by Albert Michelson and Edward Morley, and was designed to measure the difference between the speed of light propagating in the direction of the earth's rotation and the speed in the perpendicular direction. No such expected difference was found. As we shall see later, this did not at first lead to scientists abandoning the underlying mental model but rather to assuming specific effects of the ether on the dimensions of material bodies moving in this hypothetical medium.

The extension of Maxwell's theory to include optical phenomena caused significant difficulties. To describe optical properties of matter and phenomena such as metallic conductivity, the field was also assumed to exist within matter. Empty space (ether) and the interior of a material body were treated equally. Matter as a carrier of the field could have velocity; the same also applies to ether. Thus, the theory of electromagnetism inherited all the problems that had been the subject of discussion in the context of optics since the beginning of the century.

These difficulties were removed by Lorentz, albeit at the cost of further complicating the theory. In his modified theory of electromagnetism, ether is stationary and its behavior is determined entirely by the laws of electrodynamics. To describe the electromagnetic behavior of ordinary matter, Lorentz, in addition to the ether, introduced atomism as another invisible mechanism into his theory. According to his electron theory, matter consists of elementary particles that are electrically charged. Properties of matter—like conductivity and optical refraction—are determined by the behavior of these particles.

According to Lorentz's theory, charges interact only through the ether by generating fields and by being subject to forces exerted by those fields. Their motion is determined by the Newtonian equations of motion. Thus, Lorentz succeeded in integrating the laws of electrodynamics and of Newtonian mechanics. There is, however, one fundamental difference: the force between the particles is propagated by the field and does not act at a distance.

But a theory based on a stationary ether had to address a number of serious problems. The motion of a body in an ether at rest ought to have observable consequences. Since the ether model implies that the speed of light must always be the same relative to the stationary ether, irrespective of the state of motion of the body that radiates the light, the violation of the relativity principle seems to be an unavoidable consequence of the model. For instance, if the speed of light is measured in two laboratories that move with respect to each other, then the two measurements cannot yield the same result because at least one of the laboratories must necessarily be in motion with respect to the ether. But if this is the case, then the ether model cannot be reconciled with the principle of relativity of classical mechanics, which states the same physical laws must hold in two laboratories, each representing an inertial system that is moving in a fixed direction and at constant speed with respect to the other. So, at this point, the explanation of optical effects by an ether model encountered a paradox. On the one hand, an essentially stationary ether was required by the observations of aberrations and experiments of the kind conducted by Fizeau; on the other hand, the motion through this ether did not have the physical effects that it ought to have according to the ether model. This paradox constitutes the borderline problem of Einstein's paper "On the Electrodynamics of Moving Bodies."[5]

c. Thermodynamics, the Kinetic Theory of Heat, and Atomism

The emergence and development of thermodynamics, the third subdiscipline of classical physics, was, to a large extent, connected to the needs of the industrial revolution. Of particular significance was the introduction of the steam engine and the practical need to improve its efficiency. The related science was concerned with heat phenomena, although no consensus on the fundamental nature of heat could be reached for a long time. But this was irrelevant as far as the formulation of the fundamental laws of thermodynamics was concerned. The first law was a statement concerning the interchangeability of heat and mechanical energy under the right circumstances. James Prescott Joule measured the heat generated by a paddle wheel turned by a weight falling from a certain distance. The heat produced was found to be proportional to the mechanical energy released in the process. Conversely, heat engines transform heat into mechanical energy.

The second law of thermodynamics precisely defined the circumstances under which such conversion could take place. There were several seemingly different but equivalent formulations of this law. One of these asserted that operating an engine cyclically such that heat was entirely transformed into useful mechanical output was never possible. In other words, no heat engine can perform with 100 percent efficiency; there will always be wasted energy. Now, in addition to familiar characteristics like temperature, pressure, and energy, another property was assigned to a physical system, dubbed its "entropy" by Rudolf Clausius. The second law could also be reframed to assert that the total entropy of an isolated physical system could not decrease under any circumstances. Among the three main subdisciplines of physics at the time, thermodynamics probably enjoyed the most sophisticated and abstract mathematical formulation, again in the form of partial differential equations.

The development of thermodynamics as an independent physical subdiscipline was related to the development of the idea that heat can be conceived as an irregular motion of the microscopic constituents of matter. The so-called kinetic theory of heat was the first example of the use of statistics in a physical theory. The laws of thermodynamics relate different aspects of the large-scale regular behavior at the macroscopic level that emerges from average properties of the complicated irregular motion at the atomic level. The explanation of heat by atomic motion, as elaborated in the nineteenth century, was a striking example of the extension of mechanics beyond its immediate domain of applicability. It formed a bridge between two of the three continents of the physics of the time. It used atomism as an invisible mechanism for the understanding of the macro-scopic phenomenology of thermodynamics.

Atomism, the theory that matter consists of tiny, indivisible units, was used with increasing frequency during the nineteenth century to explain phenomena in many different areas of physics and chemistry, although at first there was no substantial empirical basis for these explanations in the sense of direct evidence for the existence of atoms. Late nineteenth-century atomism differed from that of antiquity or early modern times in that it was a flexible conceptual tool rather than a basis for universal theories of nature. Prominent examples include the kinetic theory of gases, as de-veloped by Maxwell and Boltzmann, and the Lorentzian atomistic version of Maxwellian electrodynamics, the so-called electron theory. Atomistic models were also used in inorganic and organic chemistry and in the ion theory of electrolytic conduction.

The further development of the kinetic theory of heat led to a change in understanding the relation between a whole and its parts. Originally it was plausible to assume that a single atom be-haves no differently from a collection of atoms in any fundamental sense. The first indication that this assumption leads to difficulties within the kinetic theory of gases was the contrast between the slow diffusion of gases and the high speeds of atoms demanded by kinetic theory. Another difficulty emerged in connection with the discussion of borderline problems between mechanics and ther-modynamics due to the contrast between the irreversibility of macroscopic changes and the reversibility of atomic motion. We will come back to these difficulties in more detail in the discussion on Brownian motion.

The kinetic theory of heat gave certain aspects of thermodynam-ics the status of borderline problems between mechanics and thermodynamics. This applies particularly to the irreversibility of heat processes, one of the main differences between thermodynamics and mechanics. If two fluids of different temperatures are mixed, the mixture will assume an intermediate temperature. But according to the second law of thermodynamics, this process is irreversible—the mixture will never separate spontaneously into a colder and a hotter component, at least not unless work is performed. In contradistinction to the processes described by thermodynamics, the laws of mechanics do not change if the direction of time is reversed. This contrast eventually became one of the most important problems in the further development of the kinetic theory of heat. The kinetic theory of heat made the transformation process between mechanical and thermal energy in heat engines plausible and thus supported the new thermodynamics, a fact that made it even more urgent to resolve the conceptual clash between thermodynamics and mechanics. The further development of the kinetic theory eventually led to the creation of modern statistical mechanics. In the following section, we discuss statistical mechanics as a bridge leading from nineteenth-century physics to the foundations of modern physics formulated by Einstein.

In his *Autobiographical Notes*, Einstein emphasizes the role of mechanics as a foundation of the atomic hypothesis and thus of those parts of science related to it, not just the kinetic theory of heat but also chemistry.[6] However, in 1900, little was known about the actual microscopic reality of chemical atoms. It must have been a provocation for the young Einstein that his philosophical hero, Ernst Mach, whose critical assessment of mechanics as a foundation of all physics he so agreed with, denied the existence of atoms. Mach is famously said to have responded to a believer in the existence of atoms: "Have you seen one?"[7] As if provoked by this question, the young Einstein feverishly explored atomistic ideas and, in particular, a demonstration of the actual existence of atoms as a powerful tool to pursue the construction of a scientific worldview. He applied this tool in the most diverse fields of physics, capillarity theory, the theory of solutions, the electron theory of metals, gas theory, and even the theory of light. It was this broad perspective that eventually brought him to recognize more clearly the fissures in the mechanical worldview.

d. Borderline Problems of Classical Physics

The tripartition of classical physics into mechanics, electrodynamics, and thermodynamics did not lead to peaceful coexistence between these three branches and their theoretical foundations. In the late nineteenth century, attempts were undertaken to lay a unified theoretical foundation of physics, building on the different conceptual frameworks of these subdisciplines, which were considered as competing starting points for such a unification. Thus, scientists at the time discussed a mechanistic worldview, an electrodynamical worldview, and another that was bound to the basic concepts of thermodynamics, in particular to the fundamental role of energy for all of science.[8]

In addition, there were numerous unsolved problems concerning the relation between these different branches of knowledge and their inner structure. In fact, in practically every field of investigation, there was a competition between a number of different theoretical approaches. These alternatives differed variously in their deductive organization of knowledge, their modification of aspects of the underlying theoretical framework, their concentration on various specific problems, or their suggestion of different quantitative laws for observable phenomena. A particular role was played by those problems that required the application of two or all three of the fundamental branches of classical physics: the "borderline" problems of classical physics.

One such borderline problem was that of heat radiation in equilibrium, the subject of one of Einstein's revolutionary papers in 1905. The problem emerged at the intersection of the theory of heat and radiation theory, which was part of electrodynamics. As discussed above, here it was found that radiation, enclosed in a cavity at thermal equilibrium, has heat properties independent of all specific features of the cavity, such as the properties of its material. Experiments revealed that, at a given temperature, the intensity of radiation in the cavity is distributed in a universally valid manner over the various frequencies. The universal energy distribution of this radiation was described with great accuracy by the radiation formula proposed by Max Planck in 1900. Planck's radiation formula solved this special problem at the border between electrodynamics and thermodynamics in a form that is still valid today. However, this revealed a foundational crisis: the classical view of a continuum of waves of all possible frequencies could not be reconciled with Planck's radiation formula. Instead, entirely new, nonclassical concepts were necessary to reach a physical interpretation of the energy distribution of radiation in thermal equilibrium as described by this formula.

The problem of Brownian motion, also the subject of a paper by Einstein from his *annus mirabilis*, was a borderline problem between mechanics and thermodynamics. The rapidly fluctuating motion of small particles suspended in a liquid had been known practically since the invention of the microscope. The detailed investigations of the English physician and botanist Robert Brown made clear that this could not be a biological phenomenon. The explanation of this motion by collisions of the suspended particles with the atoms of the liquid was rather obvious if one accepted the atomic theory as developed by Maxwell and Boltzmann. However, the difficulty that follows from this explanation is that the speed of the suspended particles following from this explanation did not seem to correspond to the observations. As it turned out, this problem could only be solved by introducing the nonclassical concept of a stochastic motion without a well-defined speed.

Finally, the problem of the electrodynamics of moving bodies arose in the border region between mechanics and electromagnetism and became the birthplace of relativity theory. Lorentz had made increasingly successful efforts to develop a theory that would do justice to the empirical knowledge of the problems in this border region. However, he did not succeed in bringing the basic assumptions of this theory into agreement with the other subdisciplines of classical physics. As it turned out, to harmonize the basic principles of electrodynamics and mechanics, one must introduce new, nonclassical concepts of space and time.

In other words, all the key conceptual breakthroughs of early twentieth-century physics emerged from borderline problems of classical physics. These problems were generated by the development of physics at the turn of the twentieth century. Every attempt to understand the origin of the 1905 revolution will fall short if this pattern is not taken into account. Only against this backdrop is the uniqueness of the perspective that Einstein brought to these problems—and his reasons for concentrating his efforts on their resolution—distinguishable. There were other ways of addressing these problems that did not call into question the compatibility of concepts from different subfields of classical physics. For example, Planck regarded the problem of heat radiation essentially as a special problem in the theory of heat; Boltzmann regarded fluctuation phenomena, like Brownian motion, as problems in mechanics; and Lorentz regarded the electrodynamics of moving bodies as a concern only for electrodynamics and not for the foundations of mechanics. In the remainder of this section, we discuss these borderline problems in greater detail.

e. Between Thermodynamics and Electromagnetism—Black-body Radiation

A celebrated borderline problem of classical physics was that of heat radiation in equilibrium, briefly described above. Such radiation is known as "black-body radiation." A black body is the mental model of an ideal source of thermal radiation that is assumed to absorb all incident electromagnetic radiation at every wavelength. This concept, coined by Gustav Kirchhoff, became the basis of theoretical, as well as experimental, studies of electromagnetic radiation in thermal equilibrium.

The universal energy distribution of this radiation is asymmetrically bell-shaped. It is skewed towards lower wavelengths with increasing temperature. The wavelength of the maximum of the radiation curve is inversely proportional to temperature. This displacement of the maximum of the black-body radiation curve is called Wien's law. The shape of the curve was described exactly by the radiation formula proposed by Planck in 1900, after five years' work on this problem. The development of an extensive body of experimental research (key contributors were Samuel Langley, Friedrich Paschen, Otto Lummer, and Peter Pringsheim, as well as Ferdinand Kurlbaum and Heinrich Rubens) was crucial to Planck's persistent efforts to derive an empirically adequate law of black-body radiation.

From a modern standpoint, the establishment of Planck's law represents the beginning of quantum theory, but it took several years of effort by Einstein and other colleagues such as Paul Ehrenfest before the incompatibility of Planck's law with classical physics was generally accepted. These efforts were crucial to the "speciation" eventually separating modern from classical physics.

After his dissertation, Planck focused his research program on the second law of thermodynamics and its contrast to the reversibility of mechanical processes. Boltzmann had tried to solve this conflict between mechanics and thermodynamics by giving the second law a statistical meaning, but Planck initially pinned his hopes on electrodynamics. He thought that he had found an irreversible elementary process in the absorption and emission of radiation by an electrical resonator. One can imagine Planck's resonator as a massless spring with a charge attached to one end that can oscillate. Such a resonator is able, for example, to absorb a plane wave and then reemit it as a spherical wave. Planck derived his formula based on the assumption that the absorption and emission of radiation by the walls of the cavity occurs through such resonators. He believed that the properties of the resonators, particularly the phenomenon of radiation damping, ensured their key role in establishing the thermal equilibrium of black-body radiation.

Planck's attempt to use electrodynamics to establish the second law of thermodynamics as a universally valid law is even more remarkable as it initially included a rejection of both atomism and statistical methods—even though these investigations eventually resulted in Planck's radiation law, which implied an atomistic structure of radiation. Planck was initially convinced that, in the conflict between the principles of mechanics on the one hand and thermodynamics on the other, the reversibility of mechanical laws as applied to atomic motion, and therefore atomism itself, would have to be abandoned.

To his disappointment, Planck soon recognized that his research program could not be carried out without statistical assumptions. In 1897, Boltzmann pointed out that the basic equations of electrodynamics are reversible, similar to those of mechanics, and that it was therefore not possible to derive irreversible processes from pure electrodynamics. In his subsequent investigations, Planck gradually introduced the methods of Boltzmann's theory of gases, which he had originally rejected; however, he did so without taking over the atomistic concepts. Instead, he supplemented classical electrodynamics with independent assumptions about the statistical behavior of radiation in thermal equilibrium. For this reason, his original research program had in effect failed, and for him, the search for the thermal radiation law thus took on a central role.

Planck's black-body radiation law was the crowning achievement of his life's work. His formula contains a constant h, which has been named after him and is known to be one of the fundamental constants of nature, eventually becoming a hallmark of quantum theory. Multiplied by the frequency of radiation, it represents the discrete amount of energy exchanged between the heat radiation and the walls of the cavity in an emission or absorption process. With the help of an additional constant in this formula, the Boltzmann constant k, the value of which can be determined from empirical data, one can correctly compute the size of an atom. This was a great achievement, which Planck clearly recognized and which Einstein also acknowledged.

The path to Planck's radiation law was anything but straight. He recalled in his Nobel Prize lecture on 2 June 1920:

When I look back to the time, already twenty years ago, when the concept and magnitude of the physical quantum of action began, for the first time, to unfold from the mass of experimental facts, and again, to the long and ever tortuous path which led, finally, to its disclosure, the whole development seems to me to provide a fresh illustration of the long-since proven saying of Goethe's that man errs as long as he strives.[9]

After repeated revisions, Planck eventually succeeded in deriving the radiation law named after him toward the end of 1900. His derivation uses Boltzmann's formula, which connects entropy with the probability of microscopic arrangements that are compatible with a given thermodynamic state. The entropy is then proportional to the logarithm of this probability. Planck determined the probability of a given energy distribution by applying combinatorial considerations to a set of resonators of different frequencies. The use of Boltzmann-type combinatorial techniques prompted the breakup of the resonator's energy into finite units. In this way, the energy quantum found its way into classical physics. Planck, however, did not consider a quantum structure of radiation itself and did not doubt the classical radiation theory. For him, the quantum of action was associated only with absorption and emission processes. This becomes clear from a letter he wrote in 1907 to Einstein:

Does the absolute vacuum (the free ether) possess any atomistic properties? Judging by your remark that the electromagnetic state in a [finite] portion of space is determined by a *finite* number of quantities, you seem to answer this question in the affirmative, while I would answer it, at least in line with my present view, in the negative. For I do not seek the meaning of the quantum of action (light quantum) in the vacuum but at the sites of absorption and emission, and assume that the processes in the vacuum are described *exactly* by Maxwell's equations.[10]

Like most of his contemporaries, Planck did not try to elucidate the meaning of the quantum of action through new concepts foreign to classical physics but by pushing classical physics into the realm of microphysics, where a new hypothesis may have been required. Only the future would reveal how untenable such an attempt would be, as Einstein later underlined the impossibility of a classical explanation of the equilibrium of heat radiation in his paper on the light quantum hypothesis as well as in his subsequent work on the quantum problem (discussed in section IV).

f. Between Mechanics and Electromagnetism—The Electrodynamics of Moving Bodies

Maxwell's theory held the promise of unifying optical and electromagnetic phenomena into a single theoretical framework. However, by extending the theory of electromagnetism to apply to optical phenomena, it inherited all the problems mentioned earlier that were connected with the supposed motion of the earth through the ether, which, as we have pointed out, had been the subject of discussion in the context of optics since the beginning of the century. Lorentz pursued this integration systematically, beginning with his dissertation in 1875, overcoming most of these problems.

Lorentz's theory is based on the model of a stationary ether. Lorentz assumed that the ether was no longer subject to Newton's laws of motion and that its behavior was determined completely by the laws of electrodynamics. The Lorentzian ether exerts forces on objects contained within it without being subjected to reaction forces itself, as stipulated by Newton's third law according to which action generates an equivalent reaction. To describe the electromagnetic behavior of ordinary matter, which cannot escape the laws of mechanics, Lorentz, in addition to the ether, included atomism in his theory as another invisible mechanism. Matter, according to his assumption, consists of elementary particles that are electrically charged.

Whereas the particles themselves were modeled on the discrete bodies of ordinary mechanical experience and obeyed the laws of mechanics, the charges, according to Lorentz, interact with the ether. The mechanism of this interaction mirrors the interaction between charges and dielectric media in macroscopic electrodynamics. The presence of charges generates a special state of the surrounding ether, corresponding to an electromagnetic "field," which propagates through the ether and can thus influence other charges. According to Lorentz's theory, charges only interact through the ether by generating fields and by being subject to a "ponderomotive" force exerted by the field on electrically charged elementary particles. Lorentz thus succeeded in integrating the laws of electrodynamics and mechanics in his theory by using complicated invisible mechanisms that refer to two entities with totally different characteristics; the cost, however, was a fundamental dualism between fields and matter.

Technically speaking, Lorentz's theory could hardly have been improved. He even succeeding in writing down transformations to derive phenomena in a moving frame of reference from the known laws for a system at rest. Finally, in 1904, Lorentz reached a comprehensive and systematic theory. With his transformations between different inertial frames of reference, he could, in principle, explain all phenomena of the electrodynamics of moving bodies. Henri Poincaré called these transformations "Lorentz transformations," and they were to become a core feature of the later theory of relativity. In its well-developed form, Lorentz's theory already encompassed many of the remarkable phenomena for which the special theory of relativity is known today: the length contraction, as well as the dilation of time for processes observed from different frames of reference, and also the increase of a body's mass with its speed. However, these aspects still had a different meaning in Lorentz's theory.

To explain the absence of any observable effect on the motion of a terrestrial laboratory through the stationary ether, Lorentz had to expand his theory of electrodynamics with additional assumptions about the behavior of bodies moving through the ether. He introduced a new time coordinate for moving systems, "local time," which served as an auxiliary variable depending on local motion with respect to the ether. Additionally, he later introduced the assumption of a length contraction in moving systems to explain the negative result of the Michelson-Morley experiment, which could have detected effects of the motion of the earth through the ether with extremely high accuracy.

This extension of the theory with auxiliary hypotheses loosened the theory's bonds to the conceptual foundations of classical physics. The introduction of special auxiliary quantities for lengths and times in moving systems extended the formalism of Lorentzian electrodynamics through elements whose physical interpretation was problematic from the perspective of classical physics. Yet Lorentz's formulas for the electrodynamics of moving bodies were compatible with all available knowledge and were even in agreement with the principle of relativity of mechanics in practice, which was otherwise incompatible with the foundations of ether-based electrodynamics.

Lorentz associated his transformations between moving systems with an interpretation that differed, however, fundamentally from the interpretation of the later theory of relativity. For him, these transformations served to solve a specific problem of electrodynamics rather than making sure that the principle of relativity could be satisfied. Instead, Lorentz maintained the so-called Galilean transformations of classical physics, which can ensure the validity of the relativity principle only for mechanics. For Lorentz, the transformations he proposed were by no means an alternative to the classical transformations but a supplement. They belonged primarily to electrodynamics and were part of his so-called theorem of corresponding states, in which the previously mentioned auxiliary quantities enabled the prediction of electrodynamic processes in a moving system. According to Lorentz's interpretation, these processes actually abide by quite different laws than the same processes in a frame of reference at rest with respect to the ether. By using his cleverly designed auxiliary quantities, he succeeded in showing that this differently running process leaves no traces in observable phenomena.

To summarize: Lorentz's theory was distinguished by its extraordinary empirical success as well as by the complex construction and argumentation leading to its success. Furthermore, it left many questions that lay beyond its immediate realm of validity unanswered, such as the compatibility of its basic assumptions about the ether with the principles of mechanics. It therefore offered a natural point of departure for a Copernicus process. To what extent can the transition from Lorentz's theory to relativity theory be described as such a Copernicus process? We will discuss this question in more detail in the context of Einstein's criticism of the Maxwell-Lorentz theory. But, in short, the shift of emphasis characteristic of such a process can be described as follows: ether was a central concept of Lorentz's theory, and the new variables for space and time were only auxiliary quantities. As we shall see later, the concept of ether no longer plays a role in relativity theory, whereas the Lorentzian auxiliary variables became the new fundamental concepts of space and time at the center of the new theory. In contrast, the formalism, particularly the Lorentz transformations between relatively moving systems of reference, is left largely untouched by this transformation of the conceptual framework, although it acquires a different interpretation.

g. Between Mechanics and Thermodynamics— The Riddle of Brownian Motion

Brownian motion is the irregular motion of a microscopic particle suspended in a liquid. The first systematic investigation of such motion can be traced back to the botanist Robert Brown, who published his meticulous observations in 1828. He investigated a large number of different particles suspended in a fluid—from plant pollen to fragments of an Egyptian sphinx—and also explored a multitude of possible causes—from currents in the fluid to interaction among the particles to the formation of small air bubbles. In doing so, Brown and his successors succeeded in excluding many potential explanations of the irregular motion of the suspended particles, in particular, the idea that they may be an exclusive property of organic matter and in some way an expression of "life."

Still, Brownian motion did not become a topic of wide interest among physicists, at least not until the mid-nineteenth century. In the meantime, a series of articles appeared about the influence of special circumstances on Brownian motion, for example, the temperature of the liquid, capillarity, convection currents in the fluid, evaporation, light incident on the particle, electric forces, and the role of the environment. Since the mid-nineteenth century, scientists considered the kinetic theory of heat (which meanwhile had become an increasingly useful tool for explaining thermal phenomena on a mechanical basis) as a possible explanation of Brownian motion. The erratic motion of the suspended particles was thought to be caused by collisions with the randomly moving molecules of the host liquid. However, none of these efforts led to a consistent theory of Brownian motion. Those who attempted to establish an explanation of Brownian motion did not realize that it does not have velocity in the classical sense because it is a stochastic process in which the mean-square displacement is proportional to time. An exception was the Polish physicist Marian von Smoluchowski, who developed an adequate theory of Brownian motion at about the same time as Einstein.

From today's perspective these early studies may appear more or less useless, a part of prehistory that one may simply forget. But their collective wisdom proved, in the end, to be crucial in identifying Brownian motion as a special case of heat motion because, first, the experiments, when viewed as a whole, revealed that the phenomenon persistently occurred everywhere. And second, the experiments excluded explanations that were possible a priori and instead relied on specific circumstances under which the phenomenon was produced. Einstein's explanation of Brownian motion was rapidly accepted as proof of the atomic nature of matter; in part this was because for almost a century alternative explanations had been pursued and eventually rejected after thorough testing.

Brownian motion certainly represented a true borderline problem of classical physics in the sense that it was a challenge for classical phenomenological thermodynamics, as well as for its counterpart, the kinetic theory of heat. From the point of view of pure thermodynamics, small particles suspended in a liquid should simply reach thermal equilibrium with the host liquid after a certain amount of time passes and should not continue to move, despite observations to the contrary. From the point of view of kinetic theory, one could indeed consider such a body as a kind of giant atom or molecule that is continually exposed to thermal impulses by the smaller molecules of the host liquid and therefore takes part in their heat motion. From the laws of mechanics, one can then compute the average speed of these "atoms" corresponding to their share of the heat energy. But it turned out to be impossible to relate the calculated speeds of bodies in suspensions to observations of the actual motion of these bodies.

The idea that Brownian motion could be interpreted as a succession of collisions between the suspended particles and the fluid molecules comes as no surprise because kinetic theory emerged as an increasingly useful tool for explaining thermal phenomena on a mechanical basis. Within its frame of reference, multiple factors could explain Brownian motion, such as the fluid's temperature and viscosity, unequal specific heat of particles and fluid, and also particle size and speed. Furthermore, other factors beyond the realm of kinetic theory, for example, electrical interactions, could not yet be ruled out and provided incentive for further investigation. But the potential complexity of the phenomenon was not the only reason why it remained in a kind of "epistemic isolation" and did not become a key theme in the extensive studies on the kinetic theory of heat.

The marginal role of Brownian motion in physics in the nineteenth century is also due to the dominant understanding of kinetic theory. Its actual focus was more concerned with the reconstruction of the laws of phenomenological thermodynamics than the discovery of deviations from these laws, even when these deviations were the statistical fluctuations that necessarily result if the interpretation of heat as a kind of motion is correct. For example, Boltzmann explicitly excluded the possibility that the heat motion of molecules in a gas leads to observable fluctuations. Another likely reason for marginalization was the intrinsic difficulty of applying kinetic theory to Brownian motion. Serious problems arose as soon as quantitative arguments were made. For example, quantitative arguments applied by cytologist Karl von Nägeli and meteorologist Felix Exner led to results that were inconsistent, either with the experiment or with the kinetic theory of heat.

Hence, by the turn of the century, Brownian motion had become a genuine challenge to classical physics, even if the challenge was not universally recognized because the majority of physicists apparently considered this a marginal problem. In summary, after practically all other explanations had been excluded, kinetic theory emerged as a plausible option to explain Brownian motion in principle, but it did not yield a satisfactory quantitative understanding of the phenomenon. This dilemma could be overcome only by its reinterpretation in the course of a Copernicus process, in which the emphasis shifted from the speed of motion of the suspended particles to the fluctuation phenomena that had played only a marginal role in kinetic theory. This decisive shift of focus would be realized by the young Albert Einstein.

h. Borderline Problems in Historical and Cultural Context

Transformations of scientific knowledge do not follow a generic scheme that can be applied to all cultural and historical contexts. They may be triggered by a variety of causes, some of which we refer to as "challenging objects." Challenging objects are phenomena that confront existing theoretical frameworks, which in principle should be applicable to them, with explanatory tasks that cannot be accomplished through the available conceptual means and methods, thus triggering their further development and finally their transformation. One type of a challenging object is what we have already characterized as borderline problems. The unique feature of borderline problems, in general, is that they belong to distinct, sometimes conflicting, systems of knowledge, which they bring together, causing their integration and reorganization. Indeed, when changes happen in highly developed disciplines, the changes are often the result of solutions to problems belonging to more than one domain of knowledge. The role of borderline problems in triggering a change in the structure of previously accumulated knowledge is particularly evident in the transition from classical to modern physics in the early twentieth century. For example, a typical problem of this kind is the previously mentioned problem of heat radiation, which will be discussed in greater detail in section IV. This problem belonged to two different subdisciplines of contemporary physics: the theory of heat and the theory of radiation. These two subdisciplines had independent conceptual foundations that were brought into contact through their application to this specific problem. The exploration of this problem by Planck and Einstein led to conclusions that could not easily be accommodated by one of these domains.

In summary, we claim that it was no coincidence that the scientific revolution generated by Einstein in 1905 emerged from the very borderline problems we have discussed. These borderline problems do not concern isolated questions but rather overlapping zones between the continents of classical physics, where highly developed systems of knowledge collide. The internal conceptual conflicts of classical physics were, in no small measure, brought about by the mental models of ether and atoms, both serving as overarching structures connecting different subdisciplines. Therefore challenges arising at the overlapping zones between the subdisciplines of classical physics necessitated an elaboration and transformation of these conceptual structures. Further discussion of this process in section IV will help us understand why the seemingly specialized papers of the miracle year would eventually lead to the abolition of the ether, to evidence for the existence of atoms, and to the surprising conclusion that light has properties of waves as well as of particles.

The disruptive nature of borderline problems remains inexplicable as long as one entertains the notion that the transition from classical to modern physics occurred in the world of isolated ideas attributed to single individuals. In reality, each borderline problem is the culmination of long traditions of developing systems of knowledge in which many individuals contributed by learning, applying, and researching. Even the bold ideas and philosophical arguments that Einstein used in his contribution to overcome the inner contradictions of classical physics had their roots in such systems of knowledge.

Indeed, the system of knowledge of classical physics comprises not only the familiar, specialized disciplines but also philosophical, popular, and amateur scientific traditions in which lively discussions concerning concepts that had long been part of the established canon of academic science took place. Mach, for instance, questioned basic concepts of Newtonian mechanics, such as absolute space. Poincaré used his popular scientific writings to discuss alternative ways to define the concept of time in physics. But the cultural inheritance of physics at the turn of the twentieth century goes beyond such contemporary analyses of the foundations of physics and also includes the long series of earlier philosophical reflections on nature and science. This inheritance was, however, not canonized but valued very differently by different representatives of the subject, and tended to be eclipsed by increasing specialization.

Paradoxically, the rapid development of specialization into separate disciplines in nineteenth-century science was precisely what revealed that specializing did not necessarily disentangle a problem from a wider context of knowledge. Specialization and the further elaboration of theoretical frameworks and experimental explorations it leads to also brought forth knowledge that belonged to the areas of validity of different subdisciplines and therefore inevitably led to overlaps of different, highly structured bodies of knowledge. These overlaps proved to be a crucial driving force for further developments. When the same natural phenomena is subjected to conceptually distinct perspectives, alternative explanations are likely to proliferate. It was only in seeking clarity on these alternatives that one could appreciate the extent to which the different conceptual systems could be reconciled with each other. Whoever attempted to solve a concrete problem was simultaneously forced to rethink the concepts involved, possibly finding ways to modify or transform them. Any attempt to seek a unified conceptual basis for all physics, as pursued by the young Einstein, had to take seriously the tensions and potential conflicts generated by borderline problems, which typically trigger further elaboration and critical examination of the underlying frameworks. For this reason, the borderline problems of classical physics could become the seeds of their own resolution.

The rapid development of specialization that began in the nineteenth century has continued at an accelerated pace; borderline problems are now a familiar aspect of interdisciplinarity. Today the body of scientific knowledge is structured by a vast and intricate web of disciplines and subdisciplines, characterized by distinct phenomenological domains and modes of research. Research and teaching at universities, however, for the most part is still organized along traditional disciplinary lines. In addition, there are numerous initiatives, within and outside of academia, to establish interdisciplinary research centers focusing on a specific phenomenological domain. A typical example of this is interdisciplinary brain research. In our terminology, the brain thus becomes a borderline problem. However, it is not located on the borderline between only two disciplines but many disciplines.

The understanding of brain function requires input from biology and medicine, physics and statistical mechanics, mathematics and computer science, psychology and linguistics, and more. In fact, all current fundamental problems faced by humankind are of this nature, for example, the transformation of the earth by the global impact of human environmental interventions and their life-threatening consequences, captured by the term *Anthropocene* for this new epoch in earth history.

IV

Classical Physics Put Back on Its Feet—The Miraculous Year

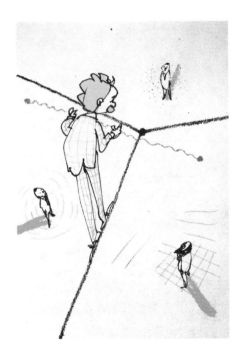

Preview

The exposition of section III showed that even the most outstanding results produced by the masters of classical physics did not yet represent the transition to modern physics. This would not take place until Einstein's miraculous year. Indeed, the solutions to the borderline problems of classical physics found by Max Planck, Hendrik Antoon Lorentz, and Ludwig Boltzmann remained within the conceptual framework of classical physics. Planck's derivation of the radiation law, in particular, did not mark the beginning of quantum theory. Nor can Lorentz's derivation of his transformation equations be conceived of as the first result of relativity theory. These results were, in fact, the culmination of research that had goals other than overcoming classical physics: Planck's primary goal was a deeper understanding of the second law of thermodynamics; Lorentz was striving for a coherent formulation of Maxwell's theory, focusing on the relation between ether and matter; and Boltzmann used kinetic theory to lay a mechanical foundation of thermodynamics.

In contrast, the solutions suggested by Einstein in his revolutionary papers of 1905 dismantled the classical view and sowed the seeds for a completely new one, at least in the case of the special theory of relativity. As already emphasized, *such a breakthrough is conceivable only on the basis of the accumulated knowledge of classical physics gathered over generations.* He reinterpreted the solutions to the borderline problems that the masters of classical physics had developed. From the outset, he considered the borderline problems of classical physics as challenges to the conceptual foundations rather than special problems to be solved within the given classical framework.

For the young Einstein, these challenges initially took the form of speculative counterproposals to classical physics, which he developed with particular attention given to atomistic ideas. His deliberations concerning the atomic structure of matter and radiation became the starting point of his formulation of statistical mechanics, a theory that allowed connections to be made between the general propositions of the science of heat on the one hand and various assumptions about the composition of the microworld on the other. In particular, such connections made the investigation of some of the problematical consequences of a mechanistic worldview possible. Thus, statistical mechanics contributed in a crucial way to the insight that the solutions of the borderline problems were actually incompatible with the foundations of classical physics. By demonstrating this incompatibility with the help of statistical mechanics, for example by showing that Planck's radiation law implied a particle-like structure of radiation under certain conditions, Einstein's speculations eventually achieved the status of revolutionary transformations of classical physics.

Uncovering the mystery of how the scientific research of a young patent office employee could have such far-reaching consequences is only possible by recognizing the structure of the Einsteinian revolution as a Copernicus process involving a reinterpretation of the works of the masters of classical physics. This view is also supported by Einstein's own retrospective account of his road to these revolutionary results in his *Autobiographical Notes*, which has been described as telling "a unique adventure—and a world-shaking one—that took place within the ivory tower of a mind."[1]

As this account confirms, Einstein's papers from 1905 are interrelated in multiple ways. First, they were the result of his pursuit of a wide range of physical interests, from the theory of liquid solutions to electrodynamics. Second, they were also undoubtedly the result of an attempt to confront classical physics with a comprehensive plan that uses atomistic ideas and includes new nonclassical properties to make the connection apparent between previously unconnected areas of knowledge. In this section, we first discuss the role of statistical mechanics as a bridge between classical and modern physics and then turn to the topics of Einstein's 1905 papers: light quanta, the theory of special relativity, and Brownian motion; finally we provide a comprehensive description of Einstein's early work that led to the groundbreaking papers of the miraculous year. The papers of 1905 were the result of a process that transformed the understanding of some of the most significant results of classical physics, which we describe as a Copernicus process. This description fits Einstein's own epistemological credo and his way of thinking, presented in section II.

a. Statistical Mechanics—A Prelude
to the Miraculous Year

Statistical mechanics applies the theory of probability to the study of physical systems composed of a large number of microscopic constituents, specifically, of material particles. It provides a framework for relating the random motion of billions and billions of individual atoms and molecules and their collisions to the thermodynamic properties of macroscopic systems, like temperature, pressure, and entropy. It is also a framework for deriving the basic laws of thermodynamics, on the basis of a set of assumptions about the underlying microscopic processes.

The building blocks of statistical mechanics can be found in the publications of the nineteenth-century pioneers of the kinetic theory of gases, James Clerk Maxwell and Ludwig Boltzmann. Nineteenth-century statistical physics was developed with the aspiration of extending the principles of mechanics to a whole range of thermal phenomena. A solid basis for these hopes was provided by Maxwell's and Boltzmann's work on the kinetic theory of gases. This work was based on the mental model of a gas as a collection of particles that move freely in space and occasionally interact. It was assumed that these interactions would distribute the kinetic energy uniformly over the whole system until a statistical distribution is reached that is characteristic of the state of thermal equilibrium. The kinetic theory of gases can explain many of the properties of macroscopic systems that are covered by "phenomenological" thermodynamics.

In addition, the kinetic theory yields a series of surprising predictions about the microscopic properties of a gas, such as the distribution of their velocities, named after Maxwell and Boltzmann. The distribution of molecules among the different velocities obeys a probability law similar to the well-known Gaussian bell-shaped distribution. It specifies the proportion of the molecules with a particular speed at a given temperature. This distribution is crucial for understanding the fundamental properties of gases conceived as statistical systems. Most notably, it enables the explanation of the transport properties of gases, such as diffusion, on the basis of mechanical and statistical laws.

It was the 1902 book by Josiah Willard Gibbs, *Elementary Principles of Statistical Mechanics* that gave the first general formulation of statistical mechanics as a complete and autonomous theory without limiting it to a specific mechanical system such as a gas. In the same year, and in the two consecutive years, Einstein published three papers on statistical mechanics:[2]

- "Kinetic Theory of the Thermal Equilibrium and of the Second Law of Thermodynamics," 1902;
- "A Theory of the Foundations of Thermodynamics," 1903; and
- "On the General Molecular Theory of Heat," 1904.

These papers originated independently and almost simultaneously with Gibbs's foundational treatise. However, unlike Gibbs, Einstein immediately explored the connections with a wide array of other topics he was pursuing at that time. His interest in the theory of electrons in metals, developed by the German physicist Paul Drude, likely played a role in the emergence of his formulation of statistical mechanics.[3] Einstein was critical of Drude's theory, probably because it lacked an adequate underpinning in statistical physics, which was exactly what Einstein tried to provide with his papers.

Einstein's work on statistical mechanics was guided by his conviction that atoms and molecules really do exist. Although the kinetic theory of gases, based on an atomistic worldview, was remarkably successful by the end of the nineteenth century, many physicists of that time did not accept the reality of atoms. One of the leading critics of the atomistic hypothesis was Mach. For him, the atomistic worldview underlying the kinetic theory of gases was just a speculative hypothesis that helped to explain experimental results. Mach was an empiricist and, for him, any statement not supported by direct observations should not be accepted as part of the description of physical reality. Einstein was strongly influenced by Mach in his formulation of the theory of relativity, the special and the general, but he did not agree with Mach's anti-atomistic views. In the *Autobiographical Notes*, he mentions his belief in atomism as a major incentive for his work on statistical mechanics: "My principal aim in this was to find facts that would guarantee as much as possible the existence of atoms of definite finite size."[4]

The growing significance of atomism at the turn of the century and the conceptual problems that came with it attracted the attention of young Einstein. For him, atomism connected different fields of contemporary science, allowing him to cherish the hope for conceptual unification between different phenomena. He was firmly convinced by Boltzmann's atomistic principles. In a letter to Mileva in September 1900 he wrote:

> The Boltzmann is magnificent. . . . I am firmly convinced that the principles of the theory are right, which means that I am convinced that in the case of gases we are really dealing with discrete mass points of definite finite size.[5]

Another innovative component of Einstein's formulation of statistical mechanics was his view that fluctuations of physical quantities should be taken seriously; he recognized their importance and potential to lead to new results. The thermodynamic properties of a state of a physical system are derived as statistical averages across all the possible microscopic configurations of the positions and velocities of the particles of which the system is composed. Boltzmann and Gibbs argued that fluctuations around these averages are exceedingly small and claimed that they will never be observed in a macroscopic system. Einstein did not accept this conclusion and looked for cases where such fluctuation phenomena, predicted by statistical mechanics, could be observed; otherwise ultimately there would be no need for statistical mechanics other than as a conceptual exercise.

Einstein intensely studied Boltzmann's book *Lectures on Gas Theory* but was not aware of his papers that further elaborated this work. He read the book with his own interests in mind and developed his own interpretation of its results by placing them in a new and broader context. In a letter to Mileva he wrote:

> At present I am again studying Boltzmann's theory of gases. Everything is very nice, but there is too little stress on the comparison with reality.[6]

A few months later, he wrote to his friend Marcel Grossmann (6? September 1901):

> Lately I have been engrossed in Boltzmann's works on the kinetic theory of gases and these last few days I wrote a short paper myself that provides the keystone in the chain of proofs that he had started.[7]

The "short paper" is probably an earlier version of Einstein's first paper of his statistical-mechanics trilogy.

These two quotations indicate that Einstein detected certain shortcomings in Boltzmann's work, although in his later retrospective of the achievements of classical mechanics, he stated more generously that

> it was also of profound interest that the statistical theory of classical mechanics was able to deduce the basic laws of thermodynamics, something in essence already accomplished by Boltzmann.[8]

Einstein is more explicit about the shortcomings of the previous work on the kinetic theory in the opening remarks of his 1902 paper. It begins with the statement that, despite the great achievements of the kinetic theory of heat,

> the science of mechanics . . . has not yet succeeded in deriving the laws of thermal equilibrium and the second law of thermodynamics using only the equations of mechanics and the probability calculus, though Maxwell's and Boltzmann's theories came close to this goal. The purpose of the following considerations is to close this gap.[9]

Einstein mentions Maxwell and Boltzmann but does not mention Gibbs. At the time, Einstein was indeed ignorant of the fact that his paper contained the essential features of statistical mechanics that had been thoroughly discussed by Gibbs a year earlier. The underlying idea developed in Einstein's three papers on statistical mechanics is related to the method of averaging across the fast and random changes of the microscopic state of a system of N particles. Such a state is characterized at each moment in time by the positions and velocities of all the particles. Einstein (and Gibbs) argued that instead of averaging across the temporal changes of this immense set of parameters, one can assume an imaginary "ensemble" of all possible microstates of the system and calculate their average. Such a virtual ensemble denotes a large number of essentially identical copies of one and the same system. All of these copies obey the same dynamics, but they differ in the exact configuration of their atomic constituents: there is a vast number of ways that billions and billions of atoms can zoom about and still make up a gas with the same given volume, pressure, and temperature. The difficult and usually impossible analysis of the time development of a microscopically described system has thus been replaced by the formation of a statistical average across a large number of different copies of the system under consideration. These copies follow the same dynamics but are distributed across all possible initial values that are compatible with the given constraints on the system. Einstein discussed such ensembles of microstates of constant energy and of constant temperature and showed that they gave the same results.

In the first paper, Einstein derived the second law of thermodynamics from the laws of mechanics and the theory of probability. He explored the statistical-mechanical description of temperature and entropy and derived the important equipartition theorem, crucial also to Drude's electron theory, which asserts that the energy of a system in equilibrium is equally distributed among its microscopic degrees of freedom. Einstein concluded that the mechanical aspects of the system do not play a significant role, indicating that the results may be more general. Einstein's second paper essentially frees his statistical mechanics from mechanics,[10] paving the way for applications to several systems beyond mechanics, such as the radiation field, electrons in metals, and others.

Having completed the second paper, Einstein wrote to his friend, Michele Besso:

> After many revisions and corrections, I finally sent off my paper. But now the paper is perfectly clear and simple, so that I am quite satisfied with it. The concepts of temperature and entropy follow from the assumption of the energy principle and the atomistic theory, and so does the second law in its most general form, namely the impossibility of a *perpetuum mobile* of the second kind, if one uses the hypothesis that state distributions of iso[lated] systems never evolve into more improbable ones.[11]

There is significant overlap between Einstein's three papers on statistical mechanics, at least as far as the general method is concerned. However, the third paper contained significant new results. In this paper, he determined the fluctuations in the energy of a system in contact with another system with a very large amount of energy and a constant temperature T. He showed that the average value of the energy fluctuations is related to the constant k, known as the Boltzmann constant, which plays a central role in the molecular theory of heat. It determines the thermodynamic properties of particles of an ideal gas and, specifically, the average energy associated with a single degree of freedom (for example, the kinetic energy of motion of a particle in the x-direction). Einstein found that the Boltzmann constant also appears in the expression of the mean-squared energy fluctuation. The latter is a measure of the thermal stability of the system. This relation provides a new meaning to the constant k.

Einstein then applied this calculation to the energy of the blackbody radiation field enclosed in a cube of side L and showed that if L is equal to the wavelength, λ_m, of the maximum energy component in the energy distribution of the radiation field, then energy fluctuations are of the order of magnitude of the energy itself. This result leads to the surprising conclusion:

> One can see that both the kind of dependence on the temperature and the order of magnitude of λ_m can be correctly determined from the general molecular theory of heat, and considering the broad generality of our assumptions, I believe that this agreement must not be ascribed to chance.[12]

He reported this result to his friend Conrad Habicht:

> I have now found the relationship between the magnitude of the elementary quanta of matter and the wavelengths of radiation in an exceedingly simple way.[13]

The relation between the thermodynamic properties of a gas of material particles and of a radiation field, as established by Einstein's analysis of thermodynamic fluctuations, would play a central role in his conclusion about the quantum nature of electromagnetic radiation.

What enables statistical mechanics to function as a bridge between classical and modern physics? Whereas kinetic theory typically starts with the interaction between the atomistic constituents of a macroscopic system, such as collisions between molecules of a gas, statistical mechanics does not focus on the time development but rather on the concept of "ensemble" averaging mentioned above. It can therefore be applied much more generally than kinetic theory.

There can be little doubt that statistical mechanics, with its important impact on the further development of twentieth-century physics, constitutes an important conceptual innovation in the history of science. That so many of its building blocks can be found in the work of Maxwell and Boltzmann and, consequently, actually predates its creation, suggests that this innovation was largely due to a change of perspective: a reinterpretation of pre-existing results in a new light—in the sense of a Copernicus process. In Einstein's case, this shift in perspective was provided precisely by the multitude of problems that required the application of statistical methods, which did not immediately lie within the range of applicability of kinetic theory.

The wealth of contemporary applications of atomism is hardly reflected in Boltzmann's gas theory, from which Einstein mainly drew his knowledge about the kinetic theory. No wonder that he observed, in his letter to Marić quoted above, that Boltzmann's gas theory contained too little emphasis on comparison with reality. When reading this book, Einstein, with his rich general knowledge about the contemporary applications of atomism, noticed shortcomings that would have easily escaped the attention of less broadly informed readers.

Einstein's formulation of statistical mechanics is a cornerstone of his work prior to the miraculous year. His three papers not only established statistical mechanics independently of Gibbs but also provided the basis for his exploration of heat radiation and also for his analysis of Brownian motion and other fluctuation phenomena as evidence for the existence of atoms.

b. Letter to a Colleague—A Blueprint for Einstein's Copernican Revolution

At the beginning of 1905, after several years of hard work when Einstein wavered between excitement, hope, and despair, the stage was set for a volcanic outbreak of creativity. This decisive breakthrough was announced by Einstein in a letter in mid-May of that year to his friend and companion in the Academia Olympia, Conrad Habicht. Its prescient content makes it a unique letter in the history of the Einsteinian revolution, and it deserves to be quoted almost in full. The letter begins in a mocking tone before concluding with a momentous announcement of the far-reaching insights soon to be published:

Dear Habicht,

Such a solemn air of silence has descended between us that I almost feel as if I am committing a sacrilege when I break it now with some inconsequential babble. But is this not always the fate of the exalted ones of this world?

So, what are you up to, you frozen whale, you smoked, dried, canned piece of soul, or whatever else I would like to hurl at your head, filled as I am with 70% anger and 30% pity! You have only the latter 30% to thank for my not having sent you a can full of minced onions and garlic after you so cravenly did not show up on Easter. But why have you still not sent me your dissertation? Don't you know that I am one of the 1½ fellows who would read it with interest and pleasure, you wretched man? I promise you four papers in return, the first of which I might send you soon, since I will soon get the complimentary reprints. The paper deals with radiation and the energy properties of light and is very revolutionary, as you will see if you send me your work *first*. The second paper is a determination of the true sizes of atoms from the diffusion and the viscosity of dilute solutions of neutral substances. The third proves that, on the assumption of the molecular theory of heat, bodies of the order of magnitude 1/1000 mm, suspended in liquids, must already perform an observable random motion that is produced by thermal motion; in fact, physiologists have observed (unexplained) motions of suspended small, inanimate, bodies, which motions they designate as "Brownian molecular motion." The fourth paper is only a rough draft at this point, and is an electrodynamics of moving bodies which employs a modification of the theory of space and time.[14]

The first paper appeared on 17 March under the heading "On a Heuristic Point of View Concerning the Production and Transformation of Light."[15] It is the only one that Einstein explicitly characterized as "very revolutionary." Here, he introduced his claim that, under certain conditions, light behaves as though it consists of particles with definite energy and color (the light quantum hypothesis). In the nineteenth century, the idea of light as a wave was firmly established through countless experiments and practical applications. No "serious" physicist believed that this theory would ever be called into question. Einstein showed, however, that it was inconsistent with the idea that light can come into thermal equilibrium with matter, thereby attaining the same temperature as the matter with which it is in contact. With the help of his light quantum hypothesis, he was able to explain some previously puzzling phenomena related to the interaction of light and matter.

His next important paper appeared soon after, at the end of April.[16] It was devoted to a new determination of the size of molecules. Although this paper was less "revolutionary" than his other contributions, it finally secured, after the failure of previous attempts, his doctoral degree from the University of Zurich. It was an important precursor to the paper "On the Movement of Small Particles Suspended in Stationary Liquids Required by the Molecular-Kinetic Theory of Heat,"[17] which was completed and submitted eleven days after the completion of Einstein's doctoral thesis.

This was the first time that the law of motion of tiny particles suspended in a liquid was formulated as a law of statistical fluctuations. Einstein showed that the movement can be understood as the elementary process that causes diffusion. This is the same process that is responsible, for instance, for the spread of perfume in the air. He deduced a law for the mean squared displacement of the small particles and found that the size of the atoms could be inferred from the observed displacements. By 1905, physicists were still debating whether or not atoms actually existed or if they were merely a useful theoretical model. Einstein delivered an essential argument for the acceptance of the atomic hypothesis and yet another method for determining the size of atoms. The Brownian motion phenomenon was then still hardly known in detail to Einstein; thus, one can even claim that in this paper he "invented" Brownian motion.[18]

Arguably the most important paper of that year was "On the Electrodynamics of Moving Bodies,"[19] which was submitted in June, only a few weeks after Einstein described it as still unfinished in his letter to Habicht. The title refers to the borderline problem of electromagnetic phenomena associated with moving bodies and moving reference frames, treated earlier by Lorentz and briefly discussed above. Einstein's modifications of the Lorentz theory led, in this paper, to the first formulation of what later came to be known as the special theory of relativity.

But this was not yet the end of the cascade of revolutionary breakthroughs. Einstein drew another important conclusion from his special theory of relativity: mass and energy are equivalent. In another letter that year to Habicht, Einstein refers to the ideas in the paper "Does the Inertia of a Body Depend on its Energy Content?" published in September:

> A consequence of the study on electrodynamics did cross my mind. Namely, the relativity principle, in association with Maxwell's fundamental equations, requires that the mass be a direct measure of the energy contained in a body; light carries mass with it. A noticeable reduction of mass would have to take place in the case of radium. The consideration is amusing and seductive; but for all I know, God Almighty might be laughing at the whole matter and might have been leading me around by the nose.[20]

God had not led Einstein around by the nose. This paper established Einstein's famous relation between mass and energy, later expressed by the formula $E = mc^2$, which brought along with it the potential for further revolutionary changes in physics and technology.

c. The "Invention" of Brownian Motion— The Reality of Atoms

The paper on Brownian motion was not the first of Einstein's 1905 papers. One may argue that it is less revolutionary than the other papers of that year. Nevertheless, we begin our discussion of the Einsteinian revolution with this topic. We are doing so because it is explicitly related to what Einstein defined as the major goal of his studies, namely, to establish "the existence of atoms of definite finite" size. His attempts to achieve this goal, combined with the quest to observe fluctuations around a thermodynamic property of a physical system, such as thermal radiation, motivated by his interest in Planck's groundbreaking work, constituted the driving force for his work leading to the miraculous year. Initially, Einstein thought that the best place to look for such fluctuations was in the case of electromagnetic radiation enclosed in a cavity. However, his search for observable fluctuations eventually led him to a completely different system. He concluded that colloidal particles, large enough to be observed under a microscope, suspended in a liquid, undergo a perpetual random motion due to the thermal motion of the molecules. The latter motion could be described by the molecular-kinetic theory.

In the introductory remarks of his paper on Brownian motion, Einstein writes:

> It is possible that the motions to be discussed here are identical with the so-called "Brownian molecular motion"; however, the data available to me on the latter are so imprecise that I could not form a definite opinion on this matter.[21]

The science historian Martin Klein, referring to this paper, remarked that

> Einstein had *invented* the Brownian motion. To say anything less, to describe this paper in the usual way, that is, as his *explanation* of the Brownian motion, is to undervalue it.[22]

Although Einstein obviously had heard about Brownian motion, he did not have precise empirical data at his disposal, and he derived its properties exclusively from theoretical reasoning. The puzzle regarding the origin of Einstein's article on Brownian motion opens up a number of further questions: How could Einstein predict the unusual properties of a phenomenon purely from theoretical reasoning without empirical data? And how was his investigation of Brownian motion related to the other topics that claimed his attention in 1905? How did Einstein hit upon the problem of Brownian motion, and how could he suggest a solution that apparently escaped his predecessors and most of his contemporaries (with the exception of Marian von Smoluchowski)?

A closer look at Einstein's prior scientific efforts, overshadowed by the famous papers of his miraculous year, provide clues for answering these questions. His perspective on Brownian motion was indeed guided by concepts and methods with which he was familiar from his earlier work. His first two papers, published before the three papers on statistical mechanics, which Einstein later referred to as "my two worthless first papers,"[23] were not so worthless after all. In particular, the second of these papers, with the long title, "On the Thermodynamic Theory of the Difference in Potentials between Metals and Fully Dissociated Solutions of their Salts and on an Electrical Method for Investigating Molecular Forces,"[24] already dealt with several of the topics that would play a key role in his paper on Brownian motion. For example, it dealt with the nature of diffusion and with the application of thermodynamics to the theory of solutions. In 1903, Einstein had already developed an idea of how to calculate the size of ions in a liquid using hydrodynamic arguments and the size of neutral salt molecules using the theory of diffusion. This idea developed into the doctoral thesis "A New Determination of Molecular Dimensions,"[25] which, as mentioned above, he successfully completed in 1905 and submitted to the University of Zurich after earlier failed attempts.

The dissertation suggested a new method for measuring the size of molecules; it showed how to find Avogadro's number (the number of particles, atoms, or molecules in a specific quantity, one mole, of a substance) by investigating the case of large sugar molecules dissolved in a solution. The procedure consisted of writing two equations for two unknowns, from which Avogadro's number and the size of the molecules could be calculated. One equation described the change in viscosity of the solution when sugar molecules are added, whereas the other used a relation between the diffusion coefficient of sugar molecules and the viscosity of the solution. Here the diffusion coefficient determines the speed with which differences in concentration of a dissolved substance equalize. The first equation was derived from rather complex hydrodynamic calculations. The other equation, which relates diffusion and viscosity, proved to also be crucial for the analysis of Brownian motion.

The accumulated effort of Einstein's doctoral thesis and his previous research on the hydrodynamics of solutions, diffusion, and viscosity led to his paper on Brownian motion, "On the Movement of Small Particles Suspended in Stationary Liquids Required by the Molecular-Kinetic Theory of Heat."[26]

In his *Autobiographical Notes*, Einstein recalls the key step that allowed him to make the transition from the treatment of molecules dissolved in a liquid to the treatment of particles suspended in a liquid. He conjectured that such particles contribute to the osmotic pressure in the same way as molecules, of salt or sugar for example, dissolved in the liquid. Osmotic pressure in classical physics is the pressure exerted on a membrane immersed in a fluid, which contains a substance in solution that cannot pass through the membrane from one side to the other. This concept, well understood at the time, was originally introduced solely for the thermodynamics of solutions and was thus applied to dissolved molecules. Naturally, it was used in the derivation of the relation between diffusion and viscosity in Einstein's dissertation. However, its applicability to a collection of suspended particles was not an obvious step.

In his paper, which led to the description of Brownian motion, Einstein again used the viscosity-diffusion equation, this time derived with the methods of his statistical mechanics because only in this way could he justify the application of concepts like osmotic pressure to a collection of suspended particles. He combined the results of his thesis research with those he collected in the study of fluctuations in the context of statistical mechanics. Thus, he had all the connections at hand to build a model of observable fluctuations in a material system, as exemplified by Brownian motion. The result of this combination of previous results and methods was Einstein's derivation of the mean square distance covered by particles in a given time. Experimental measurement of the predicted displacement would provide a new and reliable method for determining the Avogadro number and the actual size of atoms.

Einstein recognized the far-reaching implications of this paper for the conceptual foundations of the two areas of physics brought together by the borderline problem of Brownian motion: thermodynamics and the kinetic theory of heat. From the point of view of phenomenological thermodynamics, he argued, small particles suspended in a liquid should reach thermal equilibrium with the surrounding liquid and should, therefore, no longer exhibit irregular motion. However, from the perspective of kinetic theory, these particles differ from the atoms and molecules of the host liquid merely by their size. Therefore, they should always be subject to collisions with the atomistic constituents of the fluid, and they should themselves participate in this thermal motion. In this way, he used the kinetic theory shrewdly applied to the suspended particles to demonstrate the limits of classical thermodynamics rather than just as its speculative mechanistic underpinning. Einstein emphasized this point in the introduction, concluding that if the predicted behavior of particles suspended in a liquid can be observed,

> then classical thermodynamics can no longer be viewed as strictly valid even for microscopically distinguishable spaces, and an exact determination of the real size of atoms becomes possible. Conversely, if the prediction of this motion were proved wrong, this fact would provide a weighty argument against the molecular-kinetic conception of heat.[27]

In other words, Einstein invented Brownian motion as a border-line problem, revealing the limits of classical physics by sharpening inherent conceptual tensions and turning them into contrasting perspectives. Fortunately, Brownian motion had not only one but many counterparts in physical reality.

While Einstein's paper on Brownian motion influenced a large number of different areas, its main consequence was the acceptance of atomism at the beginning of the twentieth century. This was made clear above all by the pioneering experiments on Brownian motion by Jean Perrin. Perrin started his experiments in 1908 and followed largely the same lines of thought on this subject as Einstein. Most remarkably, Perrin could verify in detail almost all of Einstein's predictions about the statistical behavior of suspended particles. He could, therefore, convert this "invention" of Brownian Motion into striking experimental evidence for the atomic hypothesis. In 1909, Einstein wrote to Perrin that he "would have thought it impossible to investigate Brownian motion with such precision; it is fortunate for this material that you have taken it up."[28] In the *Autobiographical Notes*, Einstein emphasizes the importance of this result to convince the anti-atomists, like Wilhelm Ostwald and Mach, of the reality of atoms. We have already mentioned the anti-atomistic views of Mach. Ostwald was another leading proponent of this opinion. For a time, he was even a prominent supporter of a competing scientific worldview centered on the concept of energy and hence called "energetics." Around the turn of the century, the discussion of energetics led to a great rift between Ostwald and the main proponent of atomism, Boltzmann. Einstein attributed the antipathy of these scholars towards atomic theory to their positivistic philosophical attitude and commented that even scholars of such standing "can be hindered in the interpretation of facts by philosophical prejudices."[29]

Arnold Sommerfeld recalled that the "old fighter against atomistics," Ostwald, once told him "that he had been converted to atomistics by the complete explanation of the Brownian motion."[30] Referring to the work described above, Max Born remarked:

I think that these investigations of Einstein have done more than any other work to convince physicists of the reality of atoms and molecules, of the kinetic theory of heat, and of the fundamental part of probability in the natural laws. Reading these papers one is inclined to believe that at that time the statistical aspect of physics was preponderant in Einstein's mind; yet at the same time he worked on relativity where rigorous causality reigns.[31]

d. Radiation and Matter—The Discovery of Light Quanta (Photons)

Two developments at the beginning of the century drew the attention of the young Einstein to the problem of radiation and became central themes of his intellectual struggles before the miraculous year. One was Planck's derivation of the black-body radiation formula, and the other was Philipp Lenard's experiments on the photoelectric effect. Einstein quickly suspected that Planck's formula, which precisely matched the experimental data, posed a challenge to classical physics, which he defined as a "fundamental crisis." On Lenard's experiments, he wrote to Mileva:

> I just read a marvelous paper by Lenard on the production of cathode rays by ultraviolet light.[32] Under the influence of this beautiful piece of work I am filled with such happiness and joy that you absolutely must share in some of it.[33]

Already in 1901, Einstein expressed doubts about Planck's derivation of his radiation formula. In a letter to Mileva he wrote:

> It's easy to explain what is setting me against Planck's considerations on the nature of radiation. Planck assumes that a completely definite kind of resonators (fixed period and damping) causes the conversion of energy to radiation, an assumption I cannot really warm up to. Maybe his newest theory is more general.[34]

In the *Autobiographical Notes*, Einstein explained his criticism of Planck's work, recalling that both its shortcomings and its implications became clear to him soon after the appearance of Planck's work, but for a time he felt helpless:

> All my attempts, however, to adapt the theoretical foundation of physics to this [new type of] knowledge failed completely. It was as if the ground had been pulled out from under one, with no firm foundation to be seen anywhere, upon which one could have built.[35]

It was his study of the foundations of statistical mechanics in the years 1902 to 1904, which we discussed above, that provided him with the tools to explore Planck's derivation and its consequences. This led to the only paper in the miraculous year that Einstein defined as "revolutionary" (in his letter to Habicht): "On a Heuristic Point of View Concerning the Production and Transformation of Light."[36] The term *heuristic* refers to Einstein's use of the light quantum hypothesis as a speculative assumption to account for Planck's law under certain limiting conditions, without yet providing a full explanation. We return to the term *heuristic* again shortly.

Einstein's paper begins by emphasizing the profound difference between theoretical concepts applied to systems of material particles and Maxwell's theory of electromagnetic processes:

> While we conceive of the state of a body as being completely determined by the positions and velocities of a very large but nevertheless finite number of atoms and electrons, we use continuous spatial functions to determine the electromagnetic state of a space. . . . According to Maxwell's theory, energy is to be considered as a continuous spatial function for all purely electromagnetic phenomena, hence also for light, while according to the current conceptions of physicists the energy of a ponderable body is to be described as a sum extending over the atoms and electrons.[37]

Before formulating his revolutionary proposal, Einstein asserted that "the wave theory of light, which operates with continuous spatial functions . . . will probably never be replaced by another theory."[38] This is because optical observations refer to time averages rather than to instantaneous values. Conversely, observations regarding phenomena of interaction between radiation and matter suggested that the energy of light is discontinuously distributed in space:

> According to the assumption to be contemplated here, when a light ray is spreading from a point, the energy is not distributed continuously over ever-increasing spaces, but consists of a finite number of energy quanta that are localized in points in space, move without dividing, and can be absorbed or generated only as a whole.[39]

Following these introductory remarks, the light quantum paper can be divided into three parts. The first part shows, with the aid of the equipartition theorem of energy, that Maxwell's electrodynamics leads to what later became known as the Rayleigh-Jeans law of the spectral distribution of radiation. It coincided with Planck's formula at low frequencies but implied an unlimited growth of the distribution curve at high frequencies (later called "the ultraviolet catastrophe" by Paul Ehrenfest). This failure of classical electrodynamics to account for the thermal equilibrium of radiation opened up the possibility for a new hypothesis, elaborated in the second part of the paper.

Einstein then derived the entropy of monochromatic radiation in the high-frequency range, corresponding to the range of validity of what was known as Wien's law of spectral distribution, a borderline case of Planck's law. He showed, based on Boltzmann's principle of the relation between entropy and the statistical probability of a thermodynamic state, that the volume dependence of this entropy is represented by the same expression as that of a dilute, ideal gas of particles. He concluded that:

> Monochromatic radiation of low density (within the range of validity of Wien's radiation formula) behaves thermodynamically as if it consisted of mutually independent energy quanta of

magnitude $R\beta v//N$ [v is the radiation frequency, the combination of constants $R\beta/N$ is equivalent to Planck's constant h].[40]

Unlike Planck, Einstein did not use Boltzmann's principle (the relation between the entropy and the number of microstates at a given temperature) to draw conclusions from an assumed probability function to obtain the entropy of the system; such a method would have required that prior assumptions be made about the microscopic state of the system. Instead, Einstein applied the principle in reverse to gain insight into the hidden microscopic structure from the entropy function that is assumed to be known. As previously stated, Wien's law is a good approximation of Planck's law at high frequencies. From the form assumed by the entropy in this range, Einstein could deduce that heat radiation behaves in this frequency range as though it is made up of a collection of independent light particles with energy $E = hv$. Einstein's innovative application of Boltzmann's principle as a heuristic tool was possibly a discovery that he made in connection with his reinterpretation of Wien's law, a reinterpretation that changed a speculative assumption about the corpuscular nature of light (a thought that Einstein had explored for a while without it leading him to definitive results) into a heuristic point of view, helpful to interpret a well-established physical law.

The last part of this paper deals with phenomena of interaction between light and matter that could not be explained by classical physics. Why is there a frequency threshold for the photoionization of a gas? Why is there a frequency threshold for the emission of electrons in the photoelectric effect? Why is the frequency of light emitted in photoluminescence never higher than that of the absorbed light? All these effects can be easily understood if one assumes that each of these processes is composed of events in which a single light quantum is absorbed (or emitted) by an atom.

Finally, in this paper, Einstein used Planck's formula, but he interpreted it differently than Planck. For him, light quanta represented a basic feature of the electromagnetic field. For Planck, the notion of energy quanta was a mathematical device that, at most, explained how energy was absorbed or emitted when electromagnetic radiation interacted with matter. He did not accept that energy quanta represented a physical reality that described the nature of electromagnetic radiation itself. Had he accepted that, he would have had to abandon fundamental assumptions of classical physics. If he had done so, he would have promoted the revolutionary transition from classical to quantum physics, but that was very much against his nature. Planck's formula played exactly that role in this transition, but he left it to others, specifically Einstein, to usher in the revolution.

e. Einstein's Lifelong Contemplation of Light Quanta

Despite the success of the light quantum hypothesis in explaining the interaction between radiation and matter both qualitatively and quantitatively, it was received skeptically by Einstein's contemporaries. Even after Einstein received the Nobel Prize (in 1922 for the year 1921) for his explanation of the photoelectric effect on the basis of the light quantum hypothesis, the American physicist Robert Andrews Millikan characterized Einstein's localized light quanta, in his own Nobel Prize address in 1923, as still lacking confirmation: "But the conception of *localized* light-quanta out of which Einstein got his equation must still be regarded as far from being established."[41]

So how did Einstein have the courage and confidence necessary to publish his paper on light quanta, and why did he not publish it in 1904 when he had already gained essential insights into the nonclassical microstructure of radiation? The concrete answers to these questions are connected with the relation between the microscopic and the macroscopic structure of radiation. This is a relation that did not become clear until Einstein had made significant progress with his work "On the Electrodynamics of Moving Bodies." In 1904, he probably already had arguments questioning the classical theory of radiation and favoring his light quantum hypothesis. All of these arguments turned Einstein's innocent speculations at the dawn of the century on a corpuscular or "emission" theory of radiation, similar to that proposed by Newton in the seventeenth century, into a viable option. As unconventional as it was, such a revitalized corpuscular theory not only aligned with his interdisciplinary atomism but also with the fact that the question "wave or particle" was, at that time, being asked anew— not necessarily for light, but for recently discovered forms of radiation, such as X-rays. Apparently, Einstein had good reason for both his caution in 1904 and his daring in 1905, reasons that were indeed closely connected with his other research. Thus, Einstein eventually published his revolutionary deliberations on the microstructure of radiation as a heuristic point of view.

Einstein discovered a good reason for this move through one of his classical thought experiments. He imagined a reflecting mirror immersed in the radiation field enclosed in a cavity. This mental model allowed him to resume the discussion of Planck's formula of the spectral energy distribution of black-body radiation, which he later published in 1909.[42]

According to Maxwell's classical theory, an electromagnetic wave carries energy and momentum. The change in momentum of an electromagnetic wave caused by reflection from a material surface generates a force on that surface. The radiation field in a cavity can be conceived of as a superposition of wavelets interfering with each other and moving in all directions. Their interaction with a reflecting surface generates a radiation pressure on that surface. In his 1904 statistical mechanics paper, Einstein derived the energy fluctuations of such a radiation field. Using a similar calculation, he could also derive the fluctuations in the radiation pressure caused by the momentum fluctuations.

Now the analogy with the Brownian motion problem becomes apparent. In Einstein's thought experiment, the suspended mirror is free to move in the direction perpendicular to its surface. If the mirror were, for some reason, in motion, and if there were no pressure fluctuations, it would gradually slow down because the reflection on the front side would cause a stronger force than on the back. This force imbalance is analogous to the slowing force, caused by the liquid's viscosity, that acts on a particle suspended in a liquid. However, the pressure fluctuations would not allow it to come to rest. This was Einstein's crucial insight, which led him to the conclusion that fluctuations of heat radiation can be related directly to the material motion of a mirror suspended in a cavity filled with radiation. As a consequence of the incident radiation and the friction force due to radiation pressure, the mirror should exhibit a behavior similar to Brownian motion.

Einstein could show that the radiation pressure variations calculated in the framework of Maxwell's theory, based on the notion of a continuous electromagnetic field, are not sufficient to set the mirror in motion with the amount of energy expected from thermodynamic considerations. Alternately, if one acknowledges that a second type of pressure fluctuation exists, which cannot be derived from Maxwell's theory but is due to the corpuscular nature of the radiation, then the expected motion of the mirror naturally follows.

This argument is not mentioned in the light quantum paper, but in later recollections in which Einstein claimed that he had this idea already in the early 1900s. This is evident in the *Autobiographical Notes* and in a letter to Max von Laue a few years later:

> In 1905 I was already sure that it [Maxwell's theory] led to erroneous fluctuations in radiation pressure and thus to an incorrect Brownian motion of a mirror in Planck's blackbody radiation. In my opinion, one cannot avoid attributing to radiation an objective atomistic structure, which naturally does not fit into the frame of Maxwell's theory.[43]

In 1916, Einstein again established the existence of light quanta in the context of his work on the interaction between atoms and electromagnetic radiation, summarized in his two groundbreaking papers on the quantum theory of emission and absorption of electromagnetic radiation.[44] The absorption of radiation by an atom is proportional to the density of radiation. Atoms emit radiation in a spontaneous random process. Einstein assumed that this process could also be stimulated by the surrounding radiation.

Applying these processes to a system of atoms immersed in a radiation field, he found a simple derivation of Planck's formula. He referred to this in a letter to his friend Michele Besso:

> A brilliant idea dawned on me about radiation absorption and emission; it will interest you. An astonishingly simple derivation, I should say, *the* derivation of Planck's formula. A thoroughly quantized affair.[45]

Einstein's work on the quantum theory of radiation provides significant confirmation (not only as a heuristic idea) of the particle (photon) nature of radiation, with these particles carrying not only energy but also momentum (impulse). In a subsequent letter, Einstein wrote to Besso:

> The result . . . thus obtained is that at each elementary transfer of energy between radiation and matter, the impulse of hv/c is passed on to the molecule. It follows from this that any such elementary process is an *entirely directed* process. Thus light quanta are as good as established.[46]

In 1923 the American physicist Arthur Holly Compton published the results of an experiment involving the scattering of X-rays on electrons, which provided striking evidence for Einstein's hypothesis and convinced most physicists of the reality of light quanta; soon afterwards in 1926 the designation "photons" was introduced.[47] One might think that this would have firmly established the concept of light particles for Einstein and that he would stop reflecting on this idea. On the contrary, he thought about it endlessly throughout his life. In one of his last letters to Besso, he wrote:

> A whole 50 years of deliberate brooding have not brought me closer to the answer to the question "what are light quanta?" Nowadays any fool thinks he knows the answer, but he deceives himself.[48]

f. An Encounter in May—A "Eureka" Moment

Historians of science studying the process that led to the special theory of relativity can only rely on scarce remarks made by Einstein at the time and later recollections in correspondence and in autobiographical texts. This is in contrast to general relativity, where we have eight years of extensive correspondence, drafts of calculations, and intermediate publications.

One episode in this process deserves special attention. We may conclude from later reminiscences that one beautiful day in May 1905, Einstein went to visit his old friend Michele Besso in his apartment.[49] Besso was a colleague at the Bern patent office at the time. The purpose was to discuss once again Einstein's long-standing fascination with the electrodynamics of moving bodies. Although Besso was not a physicist, Einstein valued him highly as a discussion partner. Besso was not afraid to ask seemingly naive questions that could help free them from an intellectual rut.

Let us imagine how this fateful encounter between Einstein and Besso may have taken place, even if no detailed account of it has been recorded. Einstein never tired of explaining his problem over and over again in great detail. Among Einstein's circle of friends in Bern, and also among his fellow students at the Polytechnic in Zurich, it was known that he was on to something big. Only the great breakthrough was missing. Several times already Einstein had thought he was on the verge of solving his crucial problem.

On this day at the end of May 1905, several things occurred differently than usual. Einstein himself admitted that he was about to give up. Still, he made the effort once again to explain the nearly hopeless situation to Besso. Maybe Besso would have an idea. As usual, Besso listened to Einstein's explanations patiently and attentively, even if some technical points went over his head. Again and again, they returned to the behavior of quantities, like electric and magnetic fields, in frames of reference moving relative to one another. As a guiding principle, Einstein could not believe that the relative motion between two uniformly moving observers could be physically perceivable, even when measuring electromagnetic and optical phenomena. For example, consider a system of a magnet and a conducting loop in uniform motion with respect to the other. In classical electrodynamics, it makes a difference whether the magnet is moving with respect to the conductor at rest or vice versa. When the conductor is at rest, the moving magnet produces a magnetic field, which changes according to time and the location of the conductor. According to Faraday's law of induction, the changing magnetic field generates an electric field, which produces a current in the loop. Now suppose that the magnet is at rest and, hence, the magnetic field is static, but the electrons in the conductor are moving in a magnetic field and experience a so-called Lorentz force that produces an electric current in the loop. The current is the same in both cases, but in pre-relativistic physics this is explained by two different physical laws. For Einstein, these two cases represented the same situation observed from different frames of reference. There is one electromagnetic field, but its magnetic and electric components evidently depend on the state of motion (or rest) of the observer. Unlike the established teachings, a comprehensive theory that extends the principle of relativity from mechanics to electromagnetism should give the same explanation for this current, regardless of whether one regards it from the standpoint of the magnet or of the conductor.

For several years, Einstein persistently worked on such a theory without letting the difficulties of finding an alternative to the well-established theory of electromagnetism discourage him. Meanwhile, practically all observations and measurements could be brought into agreement with Lorentz's theory of electromagnetic and optical phenomena. Therefore, this theory undoubtedly played an important role in the discussion between Einstein and Besso on that crucial day in May 1905. Even though Einstein had already many times scrutinized every detail of this theory, it was so technically complex that both Besso and Einstein continued to question its underlying assumptions.

Such questioning was typical of Besso. It was he who, during their time together in Zurich, drew Einstein's attention to the works of Mach who wanted to exclude all concepts from physics that were not supported by direct empirical evidence. Despite the success of Lorentz's theory, it contained concepts that lacked empirical evidence. In particular, there was the obscure concept of the ether and the "deus ex machina" hypothesis of the length contraction experienced by bodies in the direction of their motion through the ether. Lorentz and George Francis Fitzgerald invoked such a notion in order to account for the failure to detect the motion of the earth through the ether.

Einstein and Besso talked and talked. Suddenly Einstein's face lit up, but he remained silent and soon found an excuse to leave. Besso was confused but knew his friend well enough not to take the matter personally. The next day when Einstein again turned to Besso, he did not greet him but only remarked laconically, "Thank you. I have already solved my problem completely."[50] Or, at the very least, this is how it is recorded in Einstein's later account. About five weeks later, on 30 June 1905, Einstein submitted the epochal paper with the title "On the Electrodynamics of Moving Bodies" to the *Annalen der Physik*—and established the special theory of relativity. The paper contains no references, only an acknowledgment to his faithful friend and colleague:

> In conclusion, let me note that my friend and colleague M. Besso steadfastly stood by me in my work on the problem here discussed, and that I am indebted to him for many a valuable suggestion.[51]

This is one way that the story of how Einstein discovered the theory of relativity can be told—with the addition of a few embellishments. Unfortunately, as often is the case in the history of great discoveries, historical records that describe the crucial moment of origin as vividly as this do not exist. However, there is evidence in contemporary documents and later recollections that supports the brief account provided here. Besides the

acknowledgment mentioned above, these include Einstein's indications of the significance of a conversation with Besso a few
weeks before the publication of the relativity paper.[52] This evidence also includes contemporary letters that demonstrate that
the subjects described here indeed played a central role in con-
versations between Einstein and Besso. There is also historical
evidence for Besso's role in Einstein's enthusiasm about Mach.
We can guess what questions were engendered by the discussion
with Besso. They were likely centered around the need for a new
understanding of the meaning of space and time measurements
and the meaning and verifiability of the statement that two
events take place simultaneously. But even if all the details of
such a conversation could be reconstructed, say from the notes
of a housekeeper, what would this kind of account add to the
understanding of a scientific revolution, such as the rise of relativity theory?

In the present book, we try to make the Einsteinian revolution
understandable by placing the known and well-supported biographical details within the context of changes in systems of
knowledge. As we have seen, such systems of knowledge typically
change via slow processes that involve not only scientific knowledge but also other layers of knowledge. Against this background,
the question regarding the origin of relativity not only becomes a
question about the circumstances of Einstein's "eureka" moment
in May 1905, but also a question of how his insights relate to other
layers of knowledge, particularly to the layer that determines our
commonsense understanding of space and time. Furthermore, we
want to show how the breakthrough of 1905 occurred due to the
interaction between the available reservoirs of shared knowledge
of the physics of the time and the unique perspective of one scientist. Whatever shaped Einstein's perspective must certainly have
had a hand in drawing his attention to the borderline problems of
classical physics in the crucial years between 1900 and 1905, described in the previous section.

g. The Origins of Special Relativity—The Electrodynamics of Moving Bodies

Why did Einstein create special relativity in the first place? Its main achievement was an extension of the Galilean-Newtonian relativity principle, which stipulates that the laws of mechanics are the same in all inertial frames of reference that move with constant velocity with respect to each other. Einstein extended this principle to all laws of physics. The classical relativity principle can be illustrated by the mental model of a train (with blocked windows) moving at constant velocity. There is no *mechanical* measurement that the passengers on that train can perform that would tell them if they are at rest or moving with respect to the platform.

Can this relativity principle be extended to all physical phenomena, including electromagnetic phenomena such as light propagation? According to the interpretation of these phenomena prevailing at the time, based on Maxwell's equations, this hardly seemed possible. Light was known to be a wave phenomenon, and such phenomena require the existence of a medium to propagate. As we have pointed out, at the time of the emergence of electromagnetism, this medium was called the "ether." In Lorentz's theory, the ether was assumed to be immobile, constituting a preferred system of reference with respect to which the velocity of light is constant. It is the constant that appeared explicitly in Maxwell's equations. All attempts to detect the existence of ether by experiments failed. Einstein made the bold assumption, incompatible with classical physics, that this velocity is the same in all inertial frames and that the ether does not actually exist, thus extending the relativity principle to all physical phenomena. If the velocity of light were not constant, the laws of electromagnetism would be different in different inertial frames.

Several authors have described Einstein's path to the special theory of relativity in the context of his work, which led to the 1905 papers.[53] In our account of the origin of special relativity, we largely follow the *Autobiographical Notes* as well as our discussion of Einstein's pathway.[54]

Einstein recalls that shortly after 1900, following Planck's work on black-body radiation, he understood that neither mechanics nor electrodynamics could claim total validity except in a limited number of cases, and that new principles and new laws were required. What led him to discover such principles when the giants of physics, like Lorentz, saw what Einstein saw and contemplated the same issues but did not realize that new principles were necessary? They still tried to address the problems within the frameworks of the classical mechanics of Galileo and Newton and the classical electrodynamics of Faraday and Maxwell. One reason for Einstein's different perspective was his broad concern not just with one but with several borderline problems. He was thus aware that Planck's law of black-body radiation posed a serious challenge to the notion of an ether underlying classical electromagnetism. From his work on statistical physics, he knew that such an ether would not allow for a thermal equilibrium of radiation.

Einstein himself gave a partial answer to the aforementioned question, tracing the origin of his success back to a paradox he encountered when he was sixteen years old: "After ten years of reflection such a principle resulted from a paradox upon which I had already hit at the age of sixteen."[55] At that age, young Albert asked himself how a light wave would look to an observer moving alongside this wave at the speed of light. The observer would have to see the oscillating electric and magnetic fields that constitute an electromagnetic wave but are stationary in space. It seemed, however, that such behavior of light never occurs. This thought experiment also raised the question of what speed of light an observer, moving along a light wave with a given velocity, would measure. The answer depended on the underlying model of the ether, the hypothetical medium carrying light waves. In a stationary ether, which is not carried along by the moving system, the speed of light relative to the observer would certainly have to change depending on their state of motion.

It is precisely these changes that the Michelson-Morley experiment was designed to detect but did not find. It is not clear what

Einstein knew specifically about this experiment when writing his paper in 1905. Einstein did not mention the Michelson-Morley experiment explicitly in his first paper on special relativity ("On the Electrodynamics of Moving Bodies"), but he alluded to it, saying that "the failure of attempts to detect a motion of the earth relative to the 'light-medium'" was among the causes which led him to the conclusion "that not only mechanics, but in electrodynamics as well, the phenomena do not have any properties corresponding to the concept of absolute rest."[56] However, from a letter to Mileva, we know that he had read a review article by Wilhelm Wien on numerous experiments testing the motion of the earth with respect to the ether before he started writing the paper.[57]

We have already mentioned, in the previous section, the other puzzle that challenged the young Einstein. He found it curious that a basic phenomenon of electrodynamics, regarding the interaction of electric charges in a conductor with a magnet, is formulated by two different laws depending on the state of motion of the observer. The independence of the interaction between magnet and conductor from the state of the observer would only be an immediate consequence of the principle of relativity in mechanics if this principle was also valid for electrodynamics. But this condition seemed to be excluded because the hypothetical ether, on which classical electrodynamics was based, constituted a preferred system of reference. This borderline problem between electrodynamics and mechanics is mentioned in the introductory remarks of the paper "On the Electrodynamics of Moving Bodies" as one of the incentives for the special theory of relativity.

Einstein does not tell us in the *Autobiographical Notes* what attempts he made to resolve the puzzles that troubled him for so long.[58] In 1905, he realized that the key to the solution lies in the concept of time, which is not simply given but represents a rather complicated conceptual construct, involving relations to other concepts as well as to measuring procedures. This conclusion contradicted the belief, "rooted unrecognized in the unconscious,"[59] about the absolute character of time, but it resonated with his reading of the writings of the philosopher David Hume and the philosopher-scientist Ernst Mach. Throughout his life, Einstein stressed their importance for his thinking leading to the discovery of the theory of relativity. Einstein's early readings of their work made him aware of the delicate relation between fundamental concepts, such as space and time and experience. He admitted that: "It is very possible that without these philosophical studies I would not have arrived at the solution."[60]

Einstein had accepted that Lorentz's theory represented the most viable solution to the problems of electrodynamics. But it was based on the notion of the ether, which he knew was problematic, also on thermodynamic grounds, not admitting for a thermal equilibrium of radiation. On this background, he had to search for an interpretation of the curious auxiliary variables for space and time in a moving reference frame introduced by Lorentz that was not based on the ether. This reflection shifted the entire problem to a different level, from the specifics of electrodynamics to the general framework of kinematics. Einstein thus realized that a new understanding of the meaning of coordinates that describe the location of an event in space and time was necessary. In particular, the methods for measuring a distance in space and the duration of time between two events had to be defined. To this end, he introduced the mental model of measuring rods and clocks and addressed such questions as: How do measuring rods and clocks behave in moving frames? What does it mean to say this event takes place simultaneously with another one, and how does one verify that? In this way, Einstein brought together a mental model of practical knowledge about handling rods and clocks with the theoretical knowledge of electrodynamics.

The discussion of the meaning of time in Einstein's paper "On the Electrodynamics of Moving Bodies" begins with a detailed analysis of the meaning of the statement "the train arrives here at 7 o'clock."[61] A reasonable interpretation of this statement is to say that the small hand of the watch of an observer standing on the platform points at the number seven simultaneously with the arrival of the train. This defines the local time of an event as the time measured by a clock and located at the place of the event, but this definition is not satisfactory when comparing the time of events occurring at different positions.

The analysis of such a comparison requires a careful examination of the meaning of time and its measurement and leads to the conclusion that the basic notion of simultaneity is relative to the reference frame chosen if one requires that the speed of light is the same for all inertial frames. If an observer in one inertial frame of reference determines, through a well-defined method, that two events occur simultaneously, then these two events will not necessarily be simultaneous in another frame of reference moving with constant velocity with respect to the first one. A new interpretation of the concept of simultaneity is required because of the finiteness of the speed of light through which observers receive information about events at distant locations if one requires that the speed of light is to be the same for all observers.

The relative character of time is essential to resolve the paradox implied by the thought experiment of sixteen-year-old Einstein. This paradox is formulated in the *Autobiographical Notes* as the contradiction between the two basic assumptions, the principle of the constancy of the speed of light and the principle of relativity, which states that the laws of physics are the same in all inertial frames. Each of these principles is supported by experience, but, in Newtonian physics, they are mutually incompatible because the relation between the spatial and temporal coordinates describing a specific event in two different inertial frames violates the principle of the constancy of the speed of light.

The fundamental insight that led Einstein to the special theory of relativity was the realization that these two assumptions are compatible if the coordinates describing a specific event in different inertial frames are related by the so-called Lorentz transformations. An event is defined by the three coordinates x, y, and z, defining its position in space, and by the time coordinate t. In another inertial frame, the space and time coordinates are x', y', z', and t'. In Newtonian physics $t = t'$. In the special theory of relativity, t' is a function of x, y, z, and t. The Lorentz transformations are a mathematical expression of the dependence of x', y', z', and t' on x, y, z, and t. They were discovered by Lorentz as the transformations guaranteeing that Maxwell's equations are the same in all inertial frames. The electric and magnetic fields in these equations are functions of the space and time coordinates. In different inertial frames, they assume different values, but they are related by the Lorentz transformations, which ensure that the equations themselves are invariant.

In Lorentz's theory, these transformations ensured that the electrodynamics of moving bodies complied with all measurements that showed that motion with regard to the ether has no observable effects. The transformations thus played an auxiliary role. In contrast, in Einstein's formulation of the special theory of relativity, the Lorentz transformations assume a profoundly different meaning. They are a property of the four-dimensional spacetime continuum. They define the acceptable laws of nature, which are invariant under these transformations. This is the universal principle that Einstein had spent ten years searching for, and it is comparable to the principle of the nonexistence of the "perpetuum mobile" in thermodynamics. Both are restrictive principles for admissible laws and processes in nature.

In his autobiography, Einstein devotes a paragraph to the concept of four-dimensional spacetime, introduced by the mathematician Hermann Minkowski, professor of mathematics at the Federal Technical University in Zurich when Einstein was a student there. Einstein attended several of his courses. In 1908, Minkowski showed that Einstein's special theory of relativity could be understood geometrically as a theory of four-dimensional spacetime. In classical physics, time is absolute and, therefore, there is no advantage in treating "events" described by the four parameters x, y, z, and t as points in four-dimensional spacetime. Instead, we have a three-dimensional space continuum and an independent one-dimensional time continuum. The situation is different for special relativity. Since the time, t', of an event observed from another inertial system depends on both its time and space coordinates in the initial system, this mixing of space and time coordinates makes combining them into a single four-dimensional spacetime convenient.

Minkowski's four-dimensional spacetime is equipped with a "metric" instruction that is employed to measure the distance between two events. The square of this distance is simply the square of the time separation between the two events (multiplied by c^2) minus the square of their spatial separation. This "distance" between two events is invariant when Lorentz transformations are applied between different inertial coordinate systems. It took Einstein some time to appreciate Minkowski's geometric formulation of the theory of special relativity as an interesting and useful contribution. He became convinced of its importance only around 1912, during his search for a relativistic theory of gravitation. We come back to Minkowski's formulation in the following section.

Einstein concludes the discussion of the special theory of relativity in the *Autobiographical Notes* with the far-reaching insights that this theory provided for physics. He argues that the statement, "There is no such thing as simultaneity of distant events,"[62] implies that action between distant points has to be mediated by continuous functions in space (fields) and that material point particles can hardly be conceived as the fundamental concept of the theory. Einstein mentions only briefly what is probably the best-known result of the theory, the equivalence of mass and energy described by the famous equation $E = mc^2$, which eliminates mass as an independent concept.

Biographically, the genesis of special relativity played a very special role. Unlike the other topics of Einstein's miraculous year, it reached back to the earliest scientific ideas of his adolescence, which accompanied him as a leitmotif along his path to physics. For Einstein, grappling with notions of space and time was a drama that unfolded on a timescale of its own, beginning when he was sixteen and continuing even after he completed general relativity at the age of thirty-six.

h. 1900 to 1905—A Panoramic Overview

Einstein's account of his work in the *Autobiographical Notes* on the three themes that led to the 1905 papers highlights the closely interwoven nature of the themes. It is not clear if the order of presentation is related to how his progress on these problems actually evolved. His narrative begins with a critique of mechanics and electrodynamics, described above, followed by attempts to construct a foundational alternative to classical physics. Einstein does not even mention the groundbreaking 1905 papers on light quanta,

Brownian motion, and special relativity, which launched his Co-pernican revolution and which became the pillars of modern physics. Instead, he explores the origins of those achievements, his thought process, and his search for new principles. Throughout the entire text, it is clear that what matters to Einstein is the striv-ing and the struggle, and not the final formulation of successful breakthroughs that brought him universal fame. Just like his work during those years, the discussion of the different topics is a highly interwoven sequence of concepts, ideas, and dilemmas, not di-vided into chapters or sections, providing a panoramic overview of Einstein's miraculous year and the efforts preceding it.

What is interesting about Einstein's various efforts around the turn of the century is not only their results but also the nature of the problems he was speculating about and the consequent influ-ence these efforts had on the further development of his perspec-tive. Most of these problems belong to the category of borderline problems of classical physics, as discussed in section III. Einstein's perspective was characterized by the search for a conceptual basis that could be applied to all areas of physics, which he initially hoped to find with the help of his "interdisciplinary" atomism. From his letters, we know that many of his early pursuits are in-deed based on attempts to use atomistic ideas to explain connec-tions between seemingly different physical properties. For exam-ple, he sought to uncover a connection between the electrical and thermal conductivities of metals, which he traced back to charged mobile particles found within metals.

We have discussed each of the major topics of the 1905 papers separately, but we have also emphasized their shared framework and motivation, which is apparent also in many details of these papers such as his demonstration in the relativity paper of the transformation properties of the energy and frequency of light rays, clearly relevant to Einstein's light quantum hypothesis. This, however, is not mentioned at this point. Let us now point out an-other common feature of these papers. Although they explain a whole range of experimental results, none of them were written with this primary goal in mind. Each article addresses a dilemma in classical physics, raises a fundamental question, or formulates a principle. One of them addresses the duality of wave and particle descriptions of physical systems, another raises the question of observable fluctuations in mechanical systems, and another analyzes the meaning of space and time. In other words, all these papers are deductive in their goal and structure.

In 1919, Einstein published a popular article, "Induction and Deduction in Physics," in an ordinary newspaper (*Berliner Tageblatt*). He argued that great progress in our understanding of the physical world had been achieved through an intuitive postulation of basic laws, from which scientists had derived theoretical conclusions in a logically deductive manner. The comparison of these conclusions with experience supports their validity. This method of developing an empirical scientific discipline is contrary to what seems to be the straightforward, inductive method, where: "Individual facts are selected and grouped together such that their lawful connection becomes clearly apparent."[63] However, Einstein emphasized that a brief review of the evolution of knowledge teaches us that only a small part of the big advances in science can be attributed to an inductive process.

Einstein defined the deductive approach as the task of the physicist: "The supreme task of the physicist is to arrive at those universal elementary laws from which the cosmos can be built up by pure deduction."[64] He had, however, a special understanding of the starting point of such a deductive process. It did not consist in a set of abstract axioms but in the "intuitive grasp of the essentials or a large complex of facts."[65] Years before this statement, while struggling to form a viable understanding of electrodynamics, Einstein had already embraced the deductive approach. As he later recalled, this approach was precipitated by a sense of despair:

Gradually, I despaired of the possibility of discovering the true laws by means of constructive efforts based on known facts. The longer and the more desperately I tried, the more I came to the

conviction that only the discovery of a universal formal principle could lead us to assured results.[66]

Einstein would reach the same conclusion on his road to the theory
of general relativity, which in hindsight he described as follows:

> A theory can be tested by experience but there is no way from
> experience to the construction of a theory. Equations of such
> complexity as are the equations of the gravitational field can be
> found only through the discovery of a logically simple mathe-
> matical condition that determines the equations completely or
> almost completely.[67]

This somewhat different characterization of the starting point of
a deductive process informing a mathematical condition was,
however, colored by another desperate search, that for a unified
field theory of all physics, which he pursued until his death.

i. A Copernican Transformation of Classical Physics

In section II, we described the Galilean revolution as a Copernicus
process. We can now explore whether Einstein's revolutionary
achievements can also be explained within a similar framework. We
have already posed the question of whether Einstein similarly formulated concepts that were implicitly developed for him by the
masters of classical physics. In this sense, Lorentz would be—and
would also not be—the initiator of the theory of relativity; Planck
would be the father of quantum theory; and Boltzmann the origina-
tor of modern statistical mechanics, just as Galileo was both a late
representative of Aristotelianism and a pioneer of classical mechanics. Despite the revolutionary manifestation of Einstein's achievements, several circumstances support the view that the origin of
special relativity, the insight into the quantum nature of radiation,
and the atomistic interpretation of Brownian motion are due to a
similar development, closely connecting the maturation of a traditional framework with transgressing its limits by a shift of perspective. In other words, these revolutionary achievements are to be

understood essentially as reinterpretations of the outermost results at the boundary of classical physics.

Einstein's papers from 1905 appear to cover different phenomenological domains, yet they are interrelated in multiple ways. The hidden connections between these papers, which can be demonstrated, were fairly suppressed by Einstein, not least because they did not achieve, taken together, what Einstein may have initially hoped for: a comprehensive new foundation of physics. These papers were the result of his pursuit of a wide range of physical interests, from the theory of solutions to electrodynamics. They were also undoubtedly the result of an attempt to confront classical physics with a comprehensive plan that uses atomistic ideas and includes new, nonclassical properties to make the connection between previously unconnected neighboring areas of knowledge apparent. Because this attempt eventually failed and Einstein's speculative ideas, such as that of an emission theory of light, reached a dead end, there was reason for him to look to other domains for solutions, even partial ones. In addition, by the end of the nineteenth century, the achievements of the grand masters of physics had already taken into account many of the new experimental findings, such as the measurement of black body radiation or the failure to detect the motion of the earth through the ether. Thus, a simple Kuhnian description of the miraculous year as a paradigm shift emerging from a crisis of normal science triggered by anomalies does not fit this development. The revolutionary papers of 1905 were rather the result of Copernicus processes in which some of the results of classical physics were reinterpreted by a shift of emphasis within the architecture of knowledge.

To conclude, let us point out a remarkable parallel of the Einsteinian revolution and the emergence of classical physics. In both cases, the ideas that paved the way for the revolutions emerged concurrently from different thinkers. In addition to Einstein himself, for the case of statistical mechanics, we refer to Josiah Willard Gibbs; for the light quantum hypothesis to Paul Ehrenfest; for relativity theory to Poincaré; and for Brownian motion to the Polish physicist Marian von Smoluchowski.[68] This shifting conceptual emphasis is often a hallmark of simultaneous discoveries by independent researchers. This is another indication that changes in structural features in a body of knowledge cannot, in general, be attributed to an individual acting alone.

We do not intend to delve more deeply into the topic of simultaneity of discoveries in the history of science but just want to emphasize its symptomatic role, indicating that we are dealing here not with a chain of individual discoveries but with a structural transformation of a knowledge system. However, a few additional remarks in the present context are appropriate. Einstein's papers on statistical physics from 1902 to 1904 originated independently from and roughly simultaneously with Gibbs's foundational papers on the principles of statistical mechanics. Similar conditions led to the formulation of the light quantum hypothesis in 1905. At about the same time, Ehrenfest noted, independently of Einstein, that Planck's treatment of the energy distribution of heat radiation in equilibrium was effectively based on two hypotheses. One of these states that radiative energy is composed of particles of energy, with the energy proportional to the frequency, a hypothesis that corresponds in essence to Einstein's light quantum idea. Whereas Einstein viewed his own hypothesis as revolutionary, for Ehrenfest it was merely a concise and modest interpretation of Planck's theory. For this reason, Ehrenfest's contribution is generally not held in high esteem by historians of science and almost ignored. This is probably because Einstein, unlike Ehrenfest, connected the introduction of the light quantum hypothesis with further physical deductions, leading to an explanation of experimental results, such as those related to the interaction between radiation and matter, in particular the photoelectric effect.

Similar to Ehrenfest's role in the origin of the light quantum hypothesis, Poincaré's part in the history of relativity theory is also controversial. He declared the principle of relativity as one of the central principles of physics. He saw clearly that the simultaneity of spatially separated events was problematic. And he interpreted the Lorentzian local time as the time of moving clocks, synchronized with light signals. Einstein does all of this in his relativity theory. But, in contrast to Einstein, these insights are dispersed among several of Poincaré's papers, and at no place are they gathered to form a coherent theory. However, for our discussion, it is crucial that the central conceptual achievements of relativity are at least indicated in the works of Poincaré and that Poincaré and Einstein reinterpreted results—particularly those of Lorentz—that had been established earlier.

The situation is similar for Brownian motion. In 1906, Smoluchowski submitted an article about the kinetic theory of Brownian motion to the *Annalen der Physik*. His work was inspired by Einstein's papers, but he presented results that were obtained independently. Smoluchowski's arguments differ from Einstein's. But, apart from a numerical factor, his results and his mathematical description of Brownian motion are in essence equivalent to those of Einstein. There are also parallels to some of Einstein's significant intermediate results, particularly in the works of the Australian physicist William Sutherland.[69]

In section II, we argued that Galileo's disciples were able to formulate the basic concepts of classical physics because they did not have to pursue the complex route that led him to his results within the context of preclassical mechanics and did not share his initial conceptual assumptions to the same extent. They interpreted the work of their master from the shifted perspective of his final results and therefore were able to introduce new concepts that were already defined implicitly by these results. We propose that Einstein's conceptual innovations can be understood as the outcome of a comparable structural change in the edifice of classical physics. More precisely, we propose to consider him in this specific case as an "unfaithful" disciple of the masters of classical physics—Boltzmann, Lorentz, and Planck—who created, to use the metaphor by Michel Janssen, the scaffolding upon which Einstein built his arch.[70] In this section, we have thus reconstructed Einstein's process of exploring the limits of classical physics, and have shown that (through a Copernicus process) he conceptually reconfigured the accumulated knowledge as a result of reflecting on its challenging borderline problems and sharpening their inherent paradoxes.

V

The Road to the General Theory of Relativity

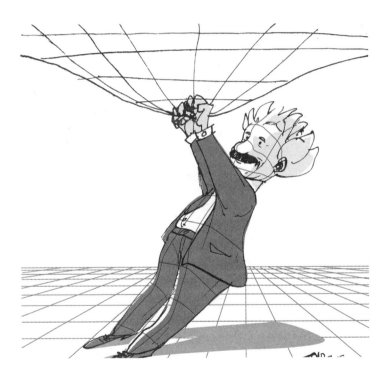

Preview

Einstein's pioneering papers of 1905 were only the beginning of a far-reaching restructuring of the system of knowledge of classical physics. Throughout this process, mental models from intuitive physics, like those associated with space, time, matter, gravity, and radiation, were to lose their fundamental role in the formulation of a physical theory. The new understanding of space and time introduced by the special theory of relativity had to apply to all physical domains. Adapting electromagnetism (which had actually been the scaffolding that special relativity had been built on) to this new framework was not difficult. But the classical law of gravitation presented problems in this respect. A straightforward attempt to include gravitation in the theory of special relativity seemed to imply a violation of Galileo's principle that all bodies fall with the same acceleration, regardless of their mass and constitution. According to classical physics, this proposition follows from the equality of inertial and gravitational mass. Bringing together the special theory of relativity and Newton's theory of gravitation constituted a new borderline problem, and Einstein found an ingenious solution.

In 1907, Einstein realized that the Galileo principle could be preserved if one simulated gravitation through acceleration. This insight led to his "equivalence principle," which states that all physical processes in a uniform and homogeneous gravitational field are equivalent to those occurring in a uniformly accelerated frame of reference without a gravitational field. This "equivalence principle," combined with implications from special relativity, led to the surprising conclusion that the concepts of space and time had to be revised once again. In the course of elaborating his conclusion, Einstein eventually understood in 1912 that space and time, or rather, the spacetime manifold, is characterized by a non-Euclidean geometrical structure. Einstein realized that space and time must therefore lose their function as a fixed stage in which physical processes occur. Space and time are instead determined by the gravitational field, while the gravitational field itself depends on the distribution of the masses in the universe. Thus, Einstein formulated the fundamental idea of the theory of general relativity, a theory that would assume its ultimate form in 1915.

In the search for a field equation for gravitation, Einstein alternated between requirements derived from Newton's theory of gravity and conditions suggested by a mathematical formalism appropriate for the description of curved spacetime, using either of them as the starting point for a specific heuristic strategy. Alternating between these two strategies, he eventually managed to bring together knowledge resources that were crucial for the formulation of a new theory of gravity, albeit initially in a form that is today considered incorrect. This was the *Entwurf* theory, published in 1913 by Einstein and Marcel Grossmann. It did not meet Einstein's expectation, motivated by the equivalence principle, that all reference frames are equivalent. This requirement was called the "general principle of relativity" and assumed to be identical with the mathematical property of "general covariance." For more than two years, Einstein brought up one argument after another to convince himself and the physical community that the *Entwurf* theory was the ultimate theory.

The transition from the *Entwurf* theory to the general theory of relativity was essentially made possible by a physical reinterpretation of a highly developed mathematical formalism. A broader network of knowledge emerged through further elaboration of the *Entwurf* theory, which thus served as the scaffolding for building the final theory of general relativity. And it was only in light of this expanded knowledge that the mathematical assumptions of the new theory of gravitation appeared to be compatible with the existing knowledge of classical physics. Towards the end of 1915, Einstein returned to an approach he had abandoned three years earlier. This seemingly cyclic character of his search process illustrates the central role of reflection in the transformation of a system of knowledge, with the outcome that one and the same result can, depending on the context, take on a different meaning. In its essence, this process of reflection was a typical Copernicus process.

Although formulated in its final form in 1915, the physical interpretation of the field equations continued to be determined by the ambivalent heuristics that had aided their formulation. These heuristics were, in turn, still partially anchored in the knowledge of classical physics. Only further extensions of the theory of general relativity, combined with new astronomical discoveries, revealed that certain heuristic elements were incompatible with the physical meaning that the theory gained through these extensions. This applies particularly to the heuristic role of Mach's principle, according to which matter is supposed to fully determine the structure of spacetime. This one-sided causality eventually proved to be incompatible with the nature of the general theory of relativity. Another heuristic assumption was the equivalence of general covariance and the general principle of relativity, which also turned out to be problematic. The interaction between the technical completion of the theory and its physical interpretation continued to play a central role in the formative years of the new theory and is not finished even today.

It took almost half a century before the theory was sophisticated enough to be applied not only to a limited number of phenomena but in principle to all problems of spacetime physics in the context of astrophysics and modern cosmology. Despite subsequent conceptual transformations of the theory of general relativity and the refutation of some of the heuristic guidelines that had led to its formulation, the new theory was spectacularly confirmed. It predicted the bending of light and gravitational redshift. It could explain the expansion of the universe, the existence and nature of black holes, gravitational lensing, and gravitational waves. None of these phenomena were known when Einstein completed the new theory in 1915.

To conclude this preview, let us emphasize the main message of the present section. General relativity emerged not as a paradigmatic replacement but rather as a reorganization of the established knowledge of classical physics. It owes its origin to a Copernicus process, during which the classical knowledge about gravitation was brought together with special relativity and structured in a new way. This process could only occur after the knowledge that had been accumulated within the framework of a preliminary theory, the *Entwurf* theory, had been sufficiently enriched to serve as a scaffolding that allowed for such a deliberative restructuring. In this sense, Einstein's elaborations between 1913 and 1915 were by no means a wasted effort; they were the prerequisite for incorporating further knowledge resources that proved to be critical for the formulation of the theory of general relativity. These resources included mathematical and astronomical knowledge in particular. Furthermore, contributions to this enhancement of knowledge were made by researchers whose names do not appear in the usual chronicles of the heroes of science. Their contributions either constituted alternative theories that competed with Einstein's approach or offered extensions and critical discussion of this approach, in agreement with Mara Beller's dialogical perspective on the advancement of science.

a. The Challenge of a Relativistic Theory of Gravitation

The 1905 special theory of relativity had established a new understanding of space and time. Additionally, the theory combined the laws of conservation of energy and momentum into a single law and implied that the inertial mass of a closed system is identical to its energy. The consequences of this theory could be conveniently described in the framework of a new mathematical formalism developed by Hermann Minkowski (described in section IV). This formalism combines space and time into one entity—a four-dimensional spacetime—and assigns a geometrical distance between two physical events that occur at two different positions and times.

The special theory of relativity thus posed the challenge to adapt the existing physical knowledge to the new spacetime framework. This was easily accomplished for electromagnetism because Maxwell's electrodynamics had been the inspiration for this new theory. But for gravitation, which is the force of gravity between two masses, it turned out to be a difficult task. Newton's law of gravity assumes an action at a distance without time retardation. This law, in its classical form, was not directly compatible with the spacetime framework of the special theory of relativity, of which one of the consequences was that no causal interaction between two objects can propagate with a speed exceeding that of light in a vacuum. However, this was not the only difficulty.

Gravitational fields have a peculiar property. Unlike the case of an electric or magnetic field, in a gravitational field, bodies of any size or material composition, starting from rest or uniform motion, will move at the same acceleration. This is one of the basic principles of classical physics, established by Galileo in his lifelong studies of falling bodies within the framework of preclassical physics. Within the conceptual framework of Newtonian physics, this principle implies that the *inertial mass* of a body must be always equal to its *gravitational mass*, although, conceptually, the two masses are distinct. The inertial mass determines the acceleration of a body caused by a given force, while the gravitational mass determines the force exerted on a body by the gravitational attraction. The equivalence of these two properties regarding massive bodies was well known in mechanics; its validity had already been demonstrated empirically with great accuracy during Einstein's time, but its significance had not been explored. For reasons to be explained now, only Einstein interpreted it as a basic principle and adopted it as a cornerstone of his general theory of relativity.

The early attempts at formulating a relativistic gravitational theory had to deal with the novel dynamical implications of the special theory of relativity. It turned out that a material body that gains or loses energy also gains or loses inertial mass. But does this change also affect its gravitational mass? This evidently had to be a requirement if Galileo's principle is to remain valid in the relativistic context as well.

There was an obvious way to make classical gravitational theory compatible with the principles of the special theory of relativity, and Einstein was initially thinking in this direction. However, the problem with this obvious generalization was that the resulting theory of gravitation seemed to violate Galileo's principle that all bodies fall with equal acceleration. Einstein realized, in particular, that a body falling vertically from the same height as a horizontally shot projectile would, in this framework, not fall with the same acceleration.

The relation between inertial mass and energy in special relativity, expressed by the formula $E = mc^2$ suggests, on the other hand, that in a relativistic theory of gravitation, the gravitational mass of a physical system should also depend on the energy in a precisely known way so as to maintain Galileo's principle. Contemporary scientists, such as Max Abraham and Gustav Mie, for instance, were quite ready to abandon Galileo's principle in order to obtain a relativistic field theory of gravitation. In contrast, Einstein made the conscious decision to maintain the equality of inertial and gravitational mass as an essential aspect of the new theory. Deviating from this equality would have meant abandoning an important legacy of classical physics which, within its conceptual framework, had, however, only a marginal position and appeared as a mere coincidence.

Initially pursuing the obvious approach of developing a new theory of gravitation with the framework of the special theory of relativity in mind, Einstein concluded:

> It turned out that, within the framework of the program sketched, this simple state of affairs could not at all, or at any rate not in any natural fashion, be represented in a satisfactory way. This convinced me that within the structure of the special theory of relativity there is no niche for a satisfactory theory of gravitation.[1]

In other words, the difficulties in fitting Newton's well-established law of gravity into the framework of the special theory of relativity led Einstein to question once again its concepts of space and time and prompted him to continue the transformation of these concepts with his 1915 theory of general relativity. The equivalence principle suggested to him that a natural formulation of a *general* principle of relativity would read: all frames of reference are equivalent for the description of the laws of nature, whatever their state of motion may be. For Einstein, such a generalization seemed to be an intellectual necessity. In his popular account of *Relativity: The Special and the General Theory*, he writes: "Since the introduction of the special principle of relativity has been justified, every intellect which strives after generalization must feel the temptation to venture the step towards the general principle of relativity."[2]

Motivating such a daring generalization of the special principle of relativity, Einstein could refer to Mach's philosophical critique of Newtonian mechanics. Newtonian mechanics is based on the notion that space is absolute by its nature, has no relation to extraneous objects, and is always the same and immovable, and that there is a distinction between relative and absolute motion. Newton demonstrated this distinction using his famous rotating-bucket thought experiment. This experiment and Mach's reaction to Newton's interpretation of its meaning have been described in section IIIa. The young Einstein accepted Mach's view of mechanics, rejecting the notion of absolute space and absolute motion, and embraced the idea that all classical mechanics should be rewritten in terms of relative motion between bodies.

Einstein noted that Galileo's principle must somehow be related to Mach's view of mechanics. Against this background, he realized that the question of how to maintain Galileo's principle must be answered in the context of a generalization of the principle of relativity. In short, in the conflict between classical mechanics and special relativity embodied by the borderline problem of relativistic theory of gravitation, Einstein decided to keep the equivalence of gravitational and inertial mass and accepted that gravitation lies beyond the scope of special relativity.

b. Einstein's Heuristics—The Equivalence Principle

According to classical mechanics, inertial systems and accelerated systems have a fundamentally different status. Einstein understood well, of course, that there is a difference between uniform and accelerated motion. If a sudden acceleration is applied to a train, a person in a cabin of the train will be subject to a tilt backward or forward. Thus, the mechanical behavior of bodies under such circumstances is different from the behavior in a Galilean (inertial) reference frame. It is then only natural to attribute an absolute physical reality to accelerated motion.

But Einstein, nevertheless, argued that accelerated frames of reference should be admitted on an equal footing with the familiar inertial frames of reference of classical physics and special relativity. If all bodies fall in the same way in a uniform and homogeneous gravitational field, as specified by Galileo's principle, then a falling observer can imagine, at least for a finite time, that they are living in an inertial system. This is true even though they are falling with increasing speed. In fact, they would notice neither their own weight nor any force acting on the bodies that are falling with them, just as if the gravitational field was eliminated by their own accelerated motion. The accelerated frame of the observer, therefore, would be indistinguishable from an inertial system. Conversely, this indistinguishability of accelerated and inertial systems could be converted into a criterion for the validity of Galileo's principle. If the new theory of gravitation were to include this principle, it would have to be a generalized theory of relativity that also admits accelerated frames of reference. In other words, the laws of physics would be required to take the same form in the accelerated frame of reference as they take in the original frame. That in going from one such frame to another, gravitational and inertial forces appear differently, could be likened to the different appearance of electric and magnetic components of the electromagnetic field when going from one reference frame to another in special relativity.

In 1922, Einstein delivered a lecture at the University of Kyoto on "How I Created the Theory of Relativity," in which he recalled an idea that had struck him in 1907 when he was first working on a relativistic theory of gravitation in the context of writing a review article on special relativity:

> I was sitting in a chair in the Patent Office in Bern when all of a sudden I was struck by a thought: "If a person falls freely, he will certainly not feel his own weight." I was startled. This simple thought made a really deep impression on me. My excitement motivated me to develop a new theory of gravity.[3]

Einstein referred to this revelation as the "happiest thought" of his life.[4] The idea led to the conclusion that, under certain conditions, gravitation can be eliminated through the transition to an accelerated frame of reference and to the formulation of his famous "equivalence principle."

Einstein emphasized this analogy between gravitation and acceleration:

In an example worth considering, the gravitational field has a relative existence only in a manner similar to the electric field generated by magneto-electric induction. *Because for an observer in free-fall from the roof of a house there is during the fall*—at least in his immediate vicinity—*no gravitational field.* Namely, if the observer lets go of any bodies, they remain relative to him, in a state of rest or uniform motion, independent of their special chemical or physical nature. The observer, therefore, is justified in interpreting his state as being "at rest."[5]

The "equivalence principle" states that all physical processes in a uniform and homogeneous gravitational field are equivalent to those that occur in a uniformly accelerated frame of reference without a gravitational field. It can be illustrated by the thought experiment of a falling elevator or of an accelerated spaceship in force-free space. An observer in a closed box in outer space, far away from all celestial bodies, will not feel a gravitational field in their vicinity. Suppose that the box is made to move "upward" with constant acceleration. The person in the box has no way to decide if the effects they observe in the box are caused by a uniform acceleration of the box or by a gravitational field exerting a gravitational force in the opposite direction. Two objects released at the same time from the hands of an observer will simultaneously reach the floor. Likewise, the passenger on a train who feels a tilt backward when the train is suddenly accelerated may assume that the train is at rest, but a gravitational field has suddenly been applied to the system.

Einstein's thought experiment, combining simple mental models of motion with implications of special relativity, allowed him as early as 1907 to anticipate crucial insights of his yet to be formulated new theory of gravitation. The bending of light rays in a gravitational field, for instance, could be derived from the argument that the path of a light ray in a vertically accelerated laboratory must be curved due to the superposition of the motion of the laboratory and the horizontal motion of the light. The conclusion that this must also be valid in a gravitational field follows from the equivalence principle and is in agreement with the assumption that energy has not only inertial but also gravitational mass so that light should be subject to attraction by gravity. But light traveling along a curved path must be moving with a variable speed, just as in a transparent medium. Such bending of light rays seemed not to be compatible with a gravitational theory that adheres strictly to the special theory of relativity and its postulate of a constant speed of light. The striking fact that there is such a bending was eventually confirmed experimentally by the observation of the deflection of starlight in the sun's gravitational field during the famous English solar eclipse expedition of 1919. However, the quantitative result turned out to be twice as large as that derived from this simple heuristic reasoning.

Another heuristic insight that could be derived from the relation between inertial and accelerated frames of reference has to do with the nature of time in an accelerating laboratory. The qualitative conclusion, emphasized in the preceding paragraph, that the speed of light in a gravitational field should no longer be assumed to be constant, is also supported by an analysis of time synchronization in an accelerated reference frame. This analysis implies that the notion of time in a gravitational field has to be even more carefully defined than in the special theory of relativity without gravity. One can associate each location in the accelerated frame of reference with an inertial frame that, at that instant, is moving at the same velocity as the accelerated frame. At a later instant, because of the frame's acceleration, one would associate a second inertial frame that would, therefore, be moving at a greater velocity than the first. Because these two inertial frames are in relative motion with respect to each other, there is no agreement between their respective clocks. Events that occur simultaneously in one of the frames of reference will no longer be simultaneous in the other. Therefore, it is no longer possible to refer simply to "the time" of an accelerated reference frame (or of a system with a gravitational field). Einstein infers that the accelerating clocks at different locations along the line of motion run at different rates. He argued that if the acceleration of the frame is upward, the uppermost clocks run at a faster rate. Thus, according to the equivalence principle, this situation cannot be distinguished from that of a laboratory at rest but with a downward directed gravitational field. Hence, Einstein concluded that clocks at positions where the gravitational potential is lower (closer to the source of gravitation) run at a slower rate.

Time can be measured by atomic clocks in which the frequency of the emitted light is equivalent to the frequency of the pendulum of a clock hanging on a wall. The slowing down of such a clock in a gravitational field means that the frequency of the light is reduced. The "color" of light is shifted to the red end of the spectrum of light. This phenomenon is known as the "gravitational redshift." Einstein's daring prediction was verified by terrestrial experiments only in the late 1950s, and is used today together with the time dilatation following from special relativity in satellite-based navigation systems.[6]

The "equivalence principle" thus had far-reaching consequences. Einstein could use different types of inertial forces as test cases for the new theory, for example, those that occur in an elevator and in an accelerating spaceship, as described above. Or he could consider inertial forces that act in a rotating system of reference, such as in Newton's bucket, which will be discussed below. From such test cases, he could draw qualitative conclusions as well as derive requirements for the mathematical apparatus of the new theory. The "equivalence principle" embodied both the idea of a generalization of the relativity principle of accelerated motions and the relative existence of a gravitational field. The idea of a generalization of the relativity principle only makes sense if this relative existence is acknowledged. The "equivalence principle" quickly became the most important heuristic tool for the creation of general relativity.

c. Geometry Enters Physics—First Steps Towards a Field Equation

The qualitative consequences of the "equivalence principle" described above were known to Einstein in 1907 and discussed in his influential review article on the special theory of relativity published that year.[7] A few years later, Einstein explored the mental model of a rotating disk, embodying a rotating reference frame relevant to the heuristics of the bucket experiment. The inclusion of such reference frames presented another conceptual challenge that suggested a change in the concept of space as well.

According to the equivalence principle, an observer on the disk may consider the system as being at rest but located in a peculiar gravitational field. When equipped with standard clocks and measuring rods to conduct space and time measurements within the rotating frame of reference, the observer has to take into account the implications of special relativity. A clock positioned on the rim of the rotating disk and a clock sitting at its center will not tick at the same pace because they exist in reference frames moving with respect to one another. Pursuing the same thought experiment with rods, Einstein discovered further-reaching consequences. For the observer on the rotating disk, the behavior of the standard rods also depends on the place at which they are used. Suppose an observer at the periphery of the rotating disk and moving along with it uses standard rods to measure the circumference of the disk. According to special relativity, these rods are shortened with respect to an observer at rest (Lorentz contraction); therefore, more rods are needed, and the length of the circumference exceeds the result of the same measurement of a nonrotating disk. At the same time, the length of the rods used to measure the diameter is unaffected. Therefore, the ratio of the circumference to the diameter is greater than π. Thus, Euclidean geometry no longer holds in the rotating system.

Einstein and Max Born encountered the challenge posed by rotating frames of reference in 1909 in connection with the special theory of relativity. Paul Ehrenfest had also argued independently that, according to special relativity, a cylinder that is made to rotate about its axis should experience a contraction of its circumference compared to the state at rest, whereas its radius remains unchanged, being perpendicular to the direction of motion.[8] This difficulty became known as the "Ehrenfest paradox" and led to controversial discussions. Most participants in this debate considered this problem to be primarily a problem of the definition of a rigid body. However, Einstein identified the Ehrenfest paradox as a key issue to be addressed in seeking a generalization of the theory of relativity on the basis of the equivalence principle.

In Einstein's thought process, the equivalence principle and the use of elevator and rotating-disk models became subsidiary to a newly formulated heuristic principle, the principle of general relativity. According to this principle, the new theory of gravitation should admit reference systems in arbitrary states of motion, and it should describe the inertial forces occurring therein as the action of a generalized gravitational field. This principle and the conceptual changes implied by the elevator and rotating-disk models played a crucial role in the kind of mathematics necessary for formulating the theory of gravitation. Generalized coordinate systems that can represent frames of reference in arbitrary states of motion had to be admitted. In view of the rotating disk thought experiment, Einstein realized that it would be necessary to go beyond Euclidean geometry, and the desire to include arbitrary systems of reference gave him, in the summer of 1912, the idea to construct the new theory of gravitation using a generalization of the Gaussian theory of curved surfaces. But, first, this theory had to be generalized to the four-dimensional spacetime world of the theory of relativity. Consequently, the distance between two points was determined by a metric represented by a four-by-four symmetric matrix. Mathematicians like Bernhard Riemann, Elwin Christoffel, and Tullio Levi-Civita had provided the necessary groundwork for this generalization by initiating and developing the field of absolute differential geometry. Initially, Einstein was not familiar with these works and had to acquire this new mathematics gradually with help from his friend Marcel Grossmann.

The mental model of motions along curved surfaces familiar from classical physics also led Einstein directly to the formulation of the equation of motion in an arbitrary gravitational field. Consider the motion of an object that is constrained to move without friction along a two-dimensional frictionless curved surface, assuming there are no forces active other than those exerted by the surface itself. It turns out that, irrespective of the starting point and end point on the surface, the path taken by the object will always be the straightest possible. This path is called a geodesic. This is the simplest generalization of a straight line. This idea could immediately be transferred to the case of force-free motion as observed from an arbitrarily accelerated system of reference. Such motion can also be represented as a four-dimensional spacetime geodesic in the curvilinear coordinates used to describe such a system of reference. The equivalence principle suggested that this description of a force-free motion also holds in an arbitrary gravitational field. Curiously, however, the spacetime geodesic trajectory described by a freely moving object turns out to be the path in spacetime along which the spacetime distance is the greatest possible. This is due to the peculiar mathematical properties of the spacetime metric.

The revised description of the gravitational field as the embodiment of geometrical properties of a generalized spacetime continuum meant that gravity was no longer considered to be a force in the sense of Newtonian physics. Indeed, the new theory generalizes Minkowski spacetime in the same way that a curved two-dimensional surface is a generalization of a flat surface. If one does not stray very far from any given point on such a surface, it appears to be flat. In section IVg, we introduced the concept of the metric to generalize the concept of distance. Whereas a flat surface is characterized by a metric that behaves in the same way everywhere on the surface, the geometrical properties of a curved surface must be described by a variable metric. This metric associates different actual distances with a given coordinate difference at different locations on the surface. Thus, for example, on the curved surface of the earth, the angular coordinate difference of one degree of geographic longitude corresponds to a different true distance at the equator than at the arctic circle.

This variable metric turned out to be a suitable representation of the gravitational potential. Thus, the scalar function, which represents the gravitational potential in Newton's theory, is replaced in the theory of general relativity by ten functions of spacetime coordinates, the independent components of the metric, represented by a symmetric four-by-four matrix.

Einstein's next challenge was to find the gravitational field equation, namely, the physical law relating the gravitational potential, or the field derived from it, to its material and non-material sources. Physical laws are typically expressed by mathematical equations between physical entities, which are functions of the position in space and time. They assume different values for observers in different reference frames (coordinate systems). The requirement that the same laws are valid in all reference frames (general covariance) means that even though the two sides of the equation change upon transition from one frame of reference to another, their equality is maintained for all observers. Einstein believed that this covariance represents the physical principle of general relativity, an assumption that turned out to be problematic, as we shall discuss in section Vi. The mathematical quantities involved in these equations are called tensors. The variable metric introduced above is an example of a tensor; it is the basic tensor of the general theory of relativity. We introduce other tensors below when we describe Einstein's search for the gravitational field equations of the general theory of relativity.

d. Einstein's Heuristics—A Plan of Action

Einstein's attempts to construct a relativistic field theory were guided in almost every respect by the model given by Lorentz's theory of electromagnetism. This model represented one of the great successes of nineteenth-century physics and was familiar to contemporary physicists. Unlike the description of interacting particles by forces that act at a distance, the "Lorentz model" is not confined to the interacting particles, but extends to their surroundings. Using a space-filling field, the Lorentz model describes how these surroundings are influenced by the matter considered to be the "source" of the field, and it also describes how this field, in turn, determines the motion of matter. Therefore, a mathematical representation of the physical processes interpreted according to this model necessarily includes two parts:

- an equation of motion, describing the motion of charged particles in a given electromagnetic field;
- a field equation, describing the electromagnetic field generated by its sources: electric charges and currents.

By analogy, the new theory of gravitation would include two parts:

- an equation of motion, describing the motion of particles in a given gravitational field;
- a field equation, describing the gravitational field generated by its sources: matter and energy.

In fact, Newton's law of gravitation can also be brought into this form. The equation of motion follows from Newton's second law, relating force and acceleration. A field equation can then be formulated by relating the classical gravitational potential to the mass distribution via the so-called Poisson equation. Only years after completing his general theory of relativity did Einstein realize that this analogy was not entirely correct. In contrast to electromagnetism, the field equation in general relativity is nonlinear, and both equations are not independent, as the equation of motion can be derived from the field equation. However, when the formulation of this new theory was in its infancy, this separation served as a useful heuristic guideline. Einstein found the equation of motion in the summer of 1912. Finding the field equation posed a greater challenge.

In order to apply the Lorentz model of a field theory to the case of a relativistic theory of gravitation, Einstein needed to first find a suitable mathematical representation of the gravitational potential and its sources, and then—and this proved to be the greatest challenge—to formulate a generalization of the classical Poisson equation for the gravitational potential. We have already mentioned that in the course of Einstein's research, the generalization of the principle of relativity and the unification of gravitation and inertia soon suggested a more complicated entity for the gravitational potential, namely the metric tensor of a four-dimensional curved spacetime. Thus, the same mathematical entity describes the geometrical structure of spacetime and the gravitational potential.

In light of the heuristic guiding role of the Lorentz model, completing a relativistic theory of gravity by a suitable field equation may have seemed like a clearly structured task once the equation of motion and an acceptable representation of the gravitational potential had been established. But finding a field equation was the most difficult challenge Einstein had to face in his struggle to formulate a relativistic theory of gravitation. First, he was confronted with the problem that the representation of the gravitational potential by the metric tensor demanded field equations, not for only a single scalar function but for an object with ten components. He, therefore, quickly realized that he needed the support of a competent mathematician in order to deal with this challenge, as his legendary exclamation illustrates: "Grossmann, you must help me or else I'll go crazy!"[9]

Second, the gravitational field equation that replaced the Poisson equation of classical physics had to be compatible not only with the various insights that Einstein had gained during his earlier work on this problem but also with what was already known about gravitation and its relation to other physical interactions. In particular, it needed to correspond to his new understanding of space and time and incorporate lessons from both classical gravity and special relativity. Einstein had to keep in mind that the effect of the gravitational field under normal circumstances was well known and satisfactorily described by Newton's law of gravity. Therefore, the relativistic field equation for gravitation had to give the same results as Newton's law under the circumstances of weak and static gravitational fields. This demand can be called Einstein's "correspondence principle." Third, clearly, the new field equations had to also be consistent with the basic laws of the conservation of energy and momentum in physical interactions. These laws indeed constitute cornerstones of physical knowledge. This requirement may be called the "conservation principle," for short.

In addition to these established resources of knowledge, Einstein's earlier research, guided by the equivalence principle, yielded several discoveries that had to conform to an acceptable field equation as well. In particular, the insight into the ultimate relation of gravitation and inertia needed to be incorporated. As previously mentioned, this idea was suggested not only by the elevator and rotating-frames models but also generally by the possibility of treating inertial effects in accelerated systems of reference as effects of a so-called generalized gravito-inertial field, in analogy to the electromagnetic field, thereby putting accelerated systems of reference and inertial systems on an equal footing. We follow Einstein's own terminology by calling this heuristic expectation the "generalized relativity principle," extending the basic insight articulated in Einstein's equivalence principle. Thus, Einstein expected that all systems of reference are equally admissible for describing physical processes; the field equations should take the same form when expressed in terms of the potentials present and the coordinates utilized in any system of reference. He believed that a generalized principle of relativity in this sense could be realized by imposing the mathematical demand that the gravitational field equation should maintain its form under as general a coordinate transformation as possible—a demand that can be mathematically expressed by the demand that the field equations be "generally covariant." As we shall see in section Vj below, this turned out only to be a requirement of the mathematical representation of a theory, but at that stage, it led Einstein, together with his other heuristic criteria, in the right direction, given the paramount importance of the equivalence principle for the physical content of the theory.

In summary, Einstein's plan of action was to construct a theory that would satisfy the following principles:

- the correspondence principle;
- the conservation principle;
- the equivalence principle.

In addition, the theory had to be generally covariant, in accor dance with what Einstein understood as the principle of generalized relativity.

e. Between Mathematical and Physical Strategies

As we have seen, the breakthrough of 1912 consisted of recognizing the key role of the four-dimensional variable metric and of the formulation of a general equation of motion in a gravitational field. It was the result of a perfect match between physical knowledge and a mental model of mathematical knowledge, the curved-space model. However, the search for a relativistic field equation demanded a much more complex process of research. This included the systematic evaluation of different candidates for the differential expressions of the metric tensor, analogous to the differential operator on the left-hand side of the electromagnetic field equation. Throughout this process, some of the basic structures of knowledge that dominated Einstein's heuristics and drove his search for a field equation had to be revised. This upending of basic structures of knowledge makes Einstein's well-documented search between 1912 and 1915 an extraordinarily illustrative episode for understanding the transition from classical to modern physics. The course of Einstein's efforts during these years can be described as an interplay between two complementary heuristic strategies: a "physical strategy" and a "mathematical strategy."

Einstein's "physical strategy" in searching for a field equation for gravitation began with an object that was physically plausible in accordance with the correspondence principle, which he subsequently adapted to meet other heuristic requirements, such as the conservation laws and the generalized principle of relativity. More precisely, this strategy consisted of three steps. Einstein started with a field equation that, from the outset, gave the correct law of gravitation in the Newtonian limit and thus satisfied his correspondence principle. He then modified it so as to render the remaining fundamental laws of classical physics valid. These included the principle of conservation of energy and momentum.

The final step was to find the degree of covariance of the resulting equation, thus establishing the degree to which it satisfied a generalized relativity principle.

Einstein also pursued a complementary "mathematical strategy." He could draw on some of the resources offered by the "absolute differential calculus" formulated by Gregorio Ricci-Curbastro and Levi-Civita, who developed the previous work of Riemann, Christoffel, and others into a complete computational scheme. Einstein's interaction with Grossmann, after moving from Prague to Zurich, gave him access to these mathematical methods. This suggested to him new default assumptions on how to build an appropriate differential expression out of the metric tensor to serve as the left-hand side of the required field equation. This expression was not only mathematically well-defined but was also covariant under a large class of coordinate transformations; it therefore offered an immediate implementation of what he saw as a generalized principle of relativity. In other words, this procedure had the advantage of operating from the start with objects that fulfilled a central demand of Einstein's generalized theory of relativity, the requirement that the description is independent of any particular choice for the coordinate system.

Whether such candidates also fulfilled the other physical requirements of a field equation remained to be seen. In particular, the field equation needed to satisfy the conservation and correspondence demands. The main challenge of this procedure, therefore, was to understand the relation of these mathematical objects to the familiar physical concepts. The next step of this procedure was therefore to explore this relation and to possibly manipulate the mathematical expressions in such a way as to recover familiar expressions of physical laws. An acceptable equation had to fulfill both the demand that Newton's theory could be recovered for the special case of a weak static field and the demand that the conservation of energy and momentum was assured. Furthermore, it had to fulfill the condition that the group of admissible coordinate transformations remained wide enough to include those transformations that lead to the special cases of uniform acceleration and uniform rotation of the system of reference.

The process described in the preceding paragraphs, elucidating Einstein's collaboration with Grossmann in the winter of 1912/13, is documented in the so-called Zurich Notebook. This notebook contains dozens of pages of mathematical derivations with very few textual remarks. It documents Einstein's learning of the basic concepts of absolute differential calculus, followed by his search for an appropriate field equation. The notebook contains two important remarks about Grossmann's role in this process. He introduced Einstein to a key mathematical concept, the so-called Riemann tensor, and thereby taught him the language in which the general theory of relativity can be expressed. On another page, Grossmann introduces the so-called Ricci tensor, derived from the Riemann tensor, as a likely object from which to construct a candidate for the gravitational tensor.

However, Einstein and Grossmann soon abandoned the approach based on these tensors. They convinced themselves that in order to achieve the correct Newtonian limit, they had to impose certain restrictions on admissible coordinates. Additional coordinate restrictions were seemingly also required to satisfy the energy and momentum conservation. They explored these conditions and their compatibility with each other as well as with other heuristic requirements and concluded that a theory based on the Riemann tensor was not feasible. This conclusion was revised in 1915 when Einstein realized how the conservation and the correspondence principles were to be understood in the new theory of gravitation, amounting to an important conceptual shift in understanding these principles. Perhaps the most striking evidence of such a shift is that the Zurich Notebook contains, albeit in linear approximation, the correct field equation of general relativity. However, he discarded this because it did not fit into the conceptual framework in which his analysis was rooted at that time.

In his search, Einstein repeatedly alternated between physical requirements derived from Newton's theory of gravity and conditions suggested by a mathematical formalism appropriate for the description of curved spacetime. He hoped that these two strategies would converge. This aspiration did not materialize in the Zurich Notebook.

Against the background of these difficulties, Einstein returned to the physical strategy at the end of the research documented in the Zurich Notebook. Clearly, the vantage point presented by the classical theory of Newton took precedence over the new insights connected with the generalization of the relativity principle. The main result of Einstein's experiments with the mathematical strategy was, paradoxically, a more or less successful execution of the physical strategy, which led him, at the end of the analysis in the Zurich Notebook, to the field equation of what became the core of the so-called *Entwurf* (Outline) theory.

This field equation was, in a sense, a conservative solution to the problem of a relativistic field equation. It primarily satisfied the principles rooted in classical physics, the correspondence principle and the conservation principle. The left-hand side of the field equation of the *Entwurf* theory had exactly the form Einstein expected because one could immediately see how to obtain the Poisson equation of the classical theory of gravitation from it. However, the class of coordinate systems in which the *Entwurf* equation takes on the same form does not satisfy the generalized principle of relativity in the way Einstein imagined. He thus abandoned the condition of general covariance with a heavy heart.

The culmination of the process, documented in the Zurich Notebook, was the publication in 1913, coauthored with Grossmann, of the article "Outline (*Entwurf*) of a Generalized Theory of Relativity and of a Theory of Gravitation." This article consists of two parts: a physical part authored by Einstein and a mathematical part authored by Grossmann. With this publication, Einstein's search for a relativistic theory of gravitation had definitively entered the public stage.

f. The *Entwurf* Theory and Its Consolidation

From a modern perspective, the *Entwurf* theory is incorrect, but at the time Einstein assumed it was the best that could be achieved. Initially, he was not quite satisfied with the result. In a letter to Lorentz, he referred to the lack of general covariance as an "ugly dark spot" of the theory.[10] But later, when Einstein was looking for arguments to defend this deficiency, he came to the conclusion that the restricted covariance of the theory was actually a necessity.

In the summer of 1913, Einstein found an argument—the notorious "hole argument"—claiming that a generally covariant theory is bound to violate causality. In the argument's original formulation, Einstein considered a spacetime filled with matter except in a closed region—the hole. Adopting the apparently plausible assumption that spacetime points can be identified by coordinates, he showed that general covariance implies that a specific matter distribution does not uniquely determine the gravitational field in the hole. He thought that this conclusion was sufficient to reject generally covariant theories. The argument assumes that single points in the continuum can be labeled and ascribed a meaning independently from physical events associated with them. From today's perspective, this argument is based on a false assumption. We quote it here because it played a role in Einstein's reflective process in the transformation of existing knowledge on his road to general relativity, in particular concerning the meaning of coordinates. Only in late 1915 did Einstein realize that this seemingly reasonable argument was untenable because coordinates by themselves have no physical significance in the new theory of gravitation. Einstein learned from discussions with the philosopher Moritz Schlick how to overcome the "hole argument."[11] He realized, in particular, that events in space and time can only be identified by coincidences of real physical processes, such as the encounter of two particles, that is, the crossing of two lines in spacetime describing the motion of two particles. From that point on, Einstein insisted that only such spacetime coincidences "can claim a physical existence."[12]

In 1913, however, it was the erroneous "hole argument" that motivated Einstein to further consolidate the *Entwurf* theory and deal with its "ugly dark spot" in a positive spirit. In a letter to Ludwig Hopf, he wrote

> The fact that the gravitational field equations are not generally covariant, which still bothered me so much some time ago, has proved to be unavoidable; it can easily be proved that a theory with generally covariant equations cannot exist if it is required that the field be mathematically completely determined by the matter.[13]

A few months later he wrote to his friend Michele Besso:

> Now I am completely satisfied and no longer doubt the correctness of the whole system, regardless of whether the observation of the solar eclipse will succeed or not. The logic of the thing is too evident.[14]

However, a nagging question persisted: What was the relation of the *Entwurf* field equation to the mathematical tradition of the absolute differential calculus? This question was connected to the open question about the relation of the *Entwurf* theory to the generalized principle of relativity. Even after this theory had been published, the question about the class of coordinate transformations that preserved the form of the field equation still remained. The defensive arguments Einstein used to justify that it must, in any case, be a restricted group of coordinate transformations were of no immediate help in resolving this question. A breakthrough did not occur until the mathematician Paul Bernays suggested to Einstein and Grossmann in 1913 that they simplify their problem by deducing the field equation from a variational formalism that takes a single function, known as the Lagrangian, as its starting point. When Einstein and Grossmann pursued Bernays's suggestion, energy-momentum conservation emerges as a natural by-product in this formalism. The transformation properties of the Lagrangian could be investigated more easily than those of the field equation itself. Einstein and Grossmann argued that this function was invariant under transformations between coordinate systems specified only by the requirement of energy-momentum conservation. In 1914, they published another joint article in which they showed how the *Entwurf* field equation and energy-momentum conservation can be obtained from the variational formalism.[15] Encouraged by this result, Einstein erroneously concluded that the variational method he used to derive the field equation led uniquely to the *Entwurf* theory.

When Einstein launched the search for a relativistic theory of gravitation, he expected that the new theory would explain two specific physical phenomena. One was the precession of the perihelion of the orbit of planet Mercury. The other was an explanation of the shape of the surface of the liquid in Newton's rotating bucket experiment as a result of interaction with distant matter. To complete the consolidation of the *Entwurf* theory, Einstein and Besso together explored these two phenomena using the *Entwurf* field equation. Their mathematical derivations and numerical calculations fill more than fifty pages of the so-called Einstein-Besso manuscript, about half of them in Einstein's handwriting, the other half in Besso's handwriting. Next to the Zurich Notebook, this is the most important document on Einstein's road to general relativity.[16]

Since the mid-nineteenth century, it has been known that the precession of Mercury's orbit shows a small deviation from the Kepler and Newton laws of planetary motion. This precession, as seen from the sun, consists of a rotation of about 575 arc seconds per century of the elliptic orbit of Mercury. Most of this rotation could be explained by the influence of neighboring planets, but 43 seconds remained unaccounted for. As early as 1907, in a letter to Conrad Habicht, Einstein identified the explanation of this apparent anomaly as one of the goals of a relativistic theory of gravitation. The Einstein-Besso manuscript contains an approximation procedure for solving the *Entwurf* field equation. The calculation of the motion of planet Mercury in the gravitational field of the sun with the help of their procedure results in a rotation of its orbit of 18 seconds per century. At the time, Einstein ignored the disagreement with the expected value and decided not to publish his result. Had he taken this result seriously, he could have dismissed the theory and embarked on the correct route two years earlier. But in this instance, Einstein failed to see the writing on the wall.

The other important calculation in the Einstein-Besso manuscript, which could have led to a similar outcome, had to do with the problem of rotation. In line with Mach's criticism of Newtonian mechanics and the notion of absolute space, Einstein wanted to interpret inertial forces of rotation (centrifugal force and Coriolis force) as generalized gravitational forces. The condition for this is that the metric tensor in a rotating frame of reference is a solution of the *Entwurf* field equation. Einstein convinced himself in 1913 that it is. However, a mistake in this calculation invalidated this conclusion. Einstein realized it only about two years later, in September 1915.

g. The Drama of November 1915— The End of the Beginning

When the shortcomings of the *Entwurf* theory began to appear, Einstein changed his perspective and switched back to the search for the correct field equation, reevaluating the approach that he had dismissed earlier. The suddenness of this change of perspective, by the fall of 1915, was not due to new factual insights, appearing from nowhere, but was generated by reflecting on results accumulated over the previous two years.

In retrospect, Einstein gave three reasons for abandoning the *Entwurf* theory:

- it could not explain Mercury's perihelion rotation;
- it did not allow treating a rotating system of reference as equivalent to a system at rest, and therefore did not satisfy his expectations for a generalized relativity principle, in particular with regard to Mach's interpretation of Newton's bucket experiment;
- the conclusion that the variational procedure led uniquely to the *Entwurf* field equation turned out to be wrong. This dashed the hopes that the mathematical strategy adapted to the *Entwurf* theory would be able to substantiate the uniqueness of this theory.

The *Entwurf* theory nevertheless initially survived all of these blunders. However, the impossibility of uniquely deriving of the *Entwurf* theory from mathematical principles had far-reaching consequences for Einstein's reflection on the results he had achieved. It showed that the adaptation of the mathematical strategy for the *Entwurf* theory did not single out this theory as the only possible one. On the contrary, the mathematical apparatus developed for this purpose turned out to be a tool that could be used more widely than for this single goal. It thus opened up the possibility of examining other candidate field equations and of examining them within the context of the extensive network of conclusions that were developed for the *Entwurf* theory. It was the concurrence of this new possibility with the previously discovered weak points of the *Entwurf* theory that prompted Einstein to give up his attempts to strengthen the latter and to return instead to an exploratory phase, after which he presented the definitive field equations of general relativity to the Prussian Academy on 25 November 1915.

In other words, the lessons that Einstein learned from his preoccupation with the *Entwurf* theory did not contribute to a further solidification of this theory but eventually provided tools that helped him remove the stumbling blocks that had previously prevented him from adopting gravitational field equations based on the Riemann and Ricci tensors. Einstein did not mention the

Entwurf theory in his subsequent writings, neither in the final article on the general theory of relativity nor in his *Autobiographical Notes*, apparently remembering it as wasted time. Historians of science disagree with such a perception of this chapter of Einstein's scientific endeavor. Although the *Entwurf* theory had to be abandoned, it did play an essential role in the evolution of the general theory of relativity. It can be understood as the scaffold on which the present theory was constructed.[17]

The renewed exploratory phase continued for about a month in November 1915, during which Einstein submitted four papers to the Prussian Academy. This short but very intensive chapter of Einstein's scientific odyssey can be described as a dramatic upheaval: the abandonment of a theory that, over the previous three years, Einstein had perceived as the correct and only possible relativistic theory of gravitation, the return to the path he had left three years earlier, and a sprint-like finish to the ultimate general theory of relativity.

Einstein began with a paper, "On the General Theory of Relativity," submitted on 4 November, which brought him back to the mathematical strategy pursued in the Zurich Notebook. He explained his change of perspective in the introductory remarks:

> My efforts in recent years were directed toward basing a general theory of relativity, also for nonuniform motion, upon the supposition of relativity. I believed to have found the only law of gravitation that complies with a reasonably formulated postulate of general relativity . . . I lost trust in the field equations I had derived.[18]

He then recalled regretfully: "I arrived at the demand of general covariance, a demand from which I parted, though with a heavy heart, three years ago when I worked together with my friend Grossmann."[19]

In the 4 November paper, the gravitational field is represented by the so-called Christoffel symbol, which consists of derivatives of the metric tensor. It is constructed in a more complicated way than the corresponding version of the gravitational field in the *Entwurf* theory. The Christoffel symbol is a familiar quantity from the absolute differential calculus; it appears naturally when discussing the main objects of this calculus, the Riemann and Ricci tensors. Up to this point, Einstein had always taken pains to decompose the Christoffel symbol into its components, which are ordinary derivatives of the metric. This is documented by the calculations in his Zurich Notebook. The reason was simply that the Christoffel symbol had no direct physical meaning for Einstein, whereas the derivative of the metric could easily be understood as components of the gravitational field, in analogy to the relation between gravitational field and potential of classical physics. Einstein now referred to the former expression for the gravitational field as a "fateful prejudice."[20] He essentially needed only to insert the new expression for the gravitational field into the mathematical formalism of the *Entwurf* theory to obtain the new field equation. This equation was strikingly similar to one of the equations he had previously analyzed in the Zurich Notebook.

In a letter to Arnold Sommerfeld from 28 November 1915, Einstein wrote:

> The key to this solution was my realization that not [one term with a gradient of the metric] but the related Christoffel symbols ... are to be regarded as the natural expression for the "components" of the gravitational field.[21]

The equation of 4 November (in short, the "November theory") did not, however, implement the general relativity principle completely because it was still bound to a constraint on the admissible coordinate systems. However, this constraint was so slight in comparison with the situation in the *Entwurf* theory that Einstein could view the transition from the latter to the November theory as a breakthrough for the realization of his vision of a generalization of the principle of relativity. When this slight constraint on the admissible coordinate systems was implemented, the variational calculus developed for the *Entwurf* theory yielded the field equation that Einstein published on 4 November 1915 with an apparent feeling of triumph. By adapting the physical arguments used to derive the *Entwurf* theory, he succeeded in reaching a field equation that could be derived by the mathematical strategy, that is, starting from a well-defined object of the absolute differential calculus. Thus, the two strategies had essentially converged. Nevertheless, the tension between the physical and mathematical formalism was not entirely dissipated because the physical meaning of the coordinate restriction that still followed from the conservation principle was not clear.

Only seven days later, Einstein submitted an addendum to the 4 November theory, offering a new interpretation of the theory based on a provocative, albeit unfounded, assumption. In the introduction, he wrote: "I now want to show here that an even more concise and logical structure of the theory can be achieved by introducing an admittedly bold additional hypothesis on the structure of matter."[22] If one assumes that the only sources of gravitation are electromagnetic fields, and thus all matter can ultimately be reduced to the latter, then a field equation based on the Ricci tensor can be formulated without imposing any additional coordinate restrictions. Thus, by temporarily assuming a speculative hypothesis, Einstein moved another step toward the ultimate goal of a generally covariant theory of gravitation.

One week later, on 18 November, Einstein submitted another paper to the Prussian Academy. He applied the method used in the Einstein-Besso manuscript to calculate the perihelion motion of Mercury but now based his calculation on the new field equation. When he got the expected result of 43 seconds per century, he wrote to one of his colleagues that this result caused him physical palpitations.[23] Acknowledging this result, David Hilbert wrote to Einstein:

Cordial congratulations on conquering perihelion motion. If I could calculate as rapidly as you, in my equations the electron would correspondingly have to capitulate, and simultaneously the hydrogen atom would have to produce its note of apology about why it does not radiate.[24]

Einstein did not tell him that only a small change in a calculation previously performed by Besso was necessary to achieve this result.

While working on the November theory, Einstein realized for the first time that coordinate restrictions derived from the correspondence principle (the Newtonian limit) have a very different meaning from the coordinate restrictions imposed by the conservation principle. The choice of a particular coordinate system to satisfy the Newtonian limit is not imposed by the theory itself but is instead a matter of convenience. During the process of calculating the Mercury perihelion precession, Einstein also learned how to interpret the Newtonian limit properly, both insights being part of the conceptual shift that marked this final phase of Einstein's search for the field equation. Taking this limit, the first three diagonal terms of the metric do not reduce to one, as in the Minkowski metric of the special theory of relativity, which was what Einstein expected, given that he assumed this was the way in which his metric theory reduces to Newton's scalar theory with just a single function representing the gravitational potential. However, in the relevant limit, only the fourth term appears in the equation of motion. Thus, the classical Poisson equation of Newtonian physics is obtained within this limit. Einstein had not been aware of this aspect of the Newtonian limit when he wrote the Zurich Notebook. This insight into the nature of the Newtonian limit was ultimately also a result of his exploration of the *Entwurf* theory, thus once more confirming its role as scaffolding. Nevertheless, the conservation principle still imposed restrictions: either a coordinate restriction, as in the first November paper, or a restriction on the structure of matter, as in the second November paper. These were only removed in the fourth and last of Einstein's November papers. All that was required to achieve this goal was to change the way in which the sources of the gravitational field appear on the right-hand side of the gravitational field equation. If the trace of the energy-momentum tensor, that is, the sum of its diagonal components, is appropriately added to the source term, then all the additional conditions become superfluous. In particular, the conservation principle is satisfied as a natural consequence of the modified field equation. This modification only became possible after Einstein learned, from his calculation of the perihelion motion of Mercury, how to interpret the Newtonian limit properly. This was the final step on Einstein's road to the field equation of the general theory of relativity, implemented in his 25 November paper and submitted to the Prussian Academy.

In his later writings, Einstein emphasized, more than once, that his solution to the problem of gravitation was a natural consequence of the mathematical approach based on the Riemann tensor, from which the candidates of the mathematical strategy could be obtained, in particular when he tried to apply the same strategy in his search for a unified field theory. He described the success of November 1915 not as a result of a convergence between the physical and mathematical strategies, which it actually was, but as an exclusive triumph of the latter.[25] Even in the first November paper, Einstein was fascinated by the power of the mathematical formalism: "Nobody who really grasped it can escape from its charm, because it signifies a real triumph of the general differential calculus as founded by GAUSS, RIEMANN, CHRISTOFFEL, RICCI and LEVI-CIVITA."[26]

After 25 November 1915, Einstein was ready to summarize his new theory in a comprehensive article, "The Foundation of the General Theory of Relativity," which was published in 1916. He concluded the introductory remarks by acknowledging the help of his friend: "the mathematician Marcel Grossmann, whose help not only saved me from studying the pertinent mathematical literature, but who also helped me in my search for the field equations of gravitation."[27] The publication of this article marked the end of a convoluted and dramatic intellectual journey that began a decade earlier. It fulfilled Einstein's hopes and rewarded his efforts invested in this enterprise. Indeed, he achieved a generally covariant field theory of gravitation that was mathematically elegant and physically plausible. It also seemed to comply with the heuristic reasoning that had formed the starting point and was inspired by Ernst Mach, whose works Einstein read as a student. There was no room left for Newton's metaphysical concept of absolute space, and all its alleged physical effects, such as inertial forces, could be traced to the effect of matter—or at least so it seemed to Einstein in 1915. But the journey was not over yet.

Why was Einstein's path to the theory of general relativity so involved? Let us briefly summarize what we have discussed so far: The theory of general relativity owes its origin to a Copernicus process, during which preexisting knowledge was structured in a new way. This process could only occur after the knowledge that had been handed down within the framework of classical physics had been sufficiently enriched to provide the means for such a deliberative restructuring. This enrichment took place within the context of the provisional theory of gravitation published by Einstein together with Grossmann in 1913: the *Entwurf* theory. Its elaboration between 1913 and 1915 was by no means a false lead; it was the prerequisite for incorporating knowledge resources that proved to be critical for the formulation of the theory of general relativity. These resources included, in particular, mathematical and astronomical knowledge. Contributions to this enhancement of the stocks of knowledge were also made by researchers—such as Max Abraham, Michele Besso, Gunnar Nordström, or Paul Bernays—whose names do not appear in the usual chronicles of the heroes of the relativity revolution. Their contributions either constituted alternative theories competing with Einstein's approach, or they offered extensions and critical discussion of this approach.

The passage from the *Entwurf* theory to the general theory of relativity was made possible in essence through a physical reinterpretation of a highly developed mathematical formalism. A broader network of knowledge emerged through further elaboration of the *Entwurf* theory. And it was only in light of this expanded knowledge that the mathematical assumptions for the new theory of gravitation appeared to be compatible with the store of knowledge of classical physics. Einstein had himself first formulated these assumptions with Grossmann's help in the Zurich Notebook in the winter of 1912/1913. That he returned in 1915 to an approach he had abandoned three years earlier may seem like the outcome of a comedy of errors. However, this seemingly cyclic character of scientific development illustrates the central role of reflection, with the outcome that one and the same result, depending on the context, can take on a different meaning.

This also applies to the further course of the relativity revolution. The theory of general relativity had not reached its final form when its essential equations were formulated at the end of 1915. The physical interpretation of these equations was, as before, largely determined by the heuristics that aided in their formulation, and these heuristics, in turn, were still partially anchored in the knowledge of classical physics. Only further extensions of the theory of general relativity, combined with new astronomical discoveries, revealed that certain heuristic elements were incompatible with the physical meaning that the theory gained through these extensions. As we discuss in detail below, this applies particularly to the heuristic role of Mach's principle, according to which, matter is supposed to determine space but not the other way around. This one-sided causality eventually proved to be incompatible with the nature of the general theory of relativity.

h. The Role of David Hilbert

When a single figure plays such a distinctive historical role as Einstein did in the emergence of general relativity, it becomes almost unavoidable to tell the story of this emergence in theatrical terms, albeit drama or comedy. The traditional accounts of the history of general relativity thus refer to blunders and breakthroughs, to fatal dilemmas, and the final dawning of truth. The stories characterize this history as a drama of a lonely hero, as a comedy of errors and confusion, or now even as the irresistible rise of a slick opportunist. Dramatic narratives naturally tend to emphasize the achievements of the great heroes and to neglect those of the minor figures; they favor the mysticism of great ideas (or great failures) and usually ignore the long-term development of knowledge. In this form, failures are mentioned primarily to provide the necessary contrast, making the ultimate victory of truth appear even more triumphant. The failures themselves have no intrinsic interest.

As an example of such a dramatic narrative, let us quote from Kip Thorne's fascinating account of recent developments in general relativity. He presents the mathematician David Hilbert as the true hero, who steals the show in the last minute of the drama from the apparently somewhat confused and mathematically incompetent Einstein:

> In autumn 1915, even as Einstein was struggling toward the right law, making mathematical mistake after mistake, Hilbert was mulling over the things he had learned from Einstein's summer visit to Göttingen. While he was on an autumn vacation on the island of Rugen in the Baltic the key idea came to him, and within a few weeks he had the right law—derived not by the arduous trial-and-error path of Einstein, but by an elegant, succinct mathematical route.[28]

Indeed Hilbert presented his famous paper "On the Foundations of Physics (first contribution)," which contains the correct field equation of the theory of general relativity, to the Göttingen Academy on 20 November 1915, that is, five days before Einstein's final paper. Although Hilbert's paper was published only in 1916, many feel he should have been given priority over Einstein for formulating the field equation. Hilbert presented his contribution as emerging from a research program that was entirely his own—the search for an axiomatization of physics as a whole—creating a synthesis of electromagnetism and gravitation. He initially expected that the electron theory of matter would provide the foundation for all of physics. He was therefore attracted to Gustav Mie's theory of matter, a nonlinear generalization of Maxwell's electrodynamics that aimed to overcome the dualism between "ether" and "ponderable matter." Hilbert himself emphasized that his approach had two separate points of departure: Mie's electromagnetic theory of matter, as well as Einstein's attempt to base a theory of gravitation on the representation of the gravitational potential by a four-dimensional metric.

Hilbert's superior mastery of mathematics apparently allowed him to arrive quickly and independently at combined field equations for the electromagnetic and gravitational fields. The use of Mie's ideas initially led Hilbert to a theory that was, from the point of view of the theory of general relativity, restricted to a particular source for the gravitational field: the electromagnetic field. But he is nevertheless regarded by many physicists and historians of science as the first to have established a mathematical framework for general relativity that provides both essential results of the theory, such as the field equations, and a clarification of previously obscure conceptual issues, such as the nature of causality in generally covariant field theories. His contributions to general relativity, although initially inspired by Mie and Einstein, hence appear as a unique and independent achievement. Besides, it was unquestionably Hilbert who did pioneering work in the search for a unified field theory of gravitation and electromagnetism. In view of all these results, established within a very short time, it appears that Hilbert indeed had found a "royal road" to general relativity and beyond. It also appears, as we saw above, that Einstein turned onto this royal road only after much meandering, and even then possibly under the influence of Hilbert, with whom he corresponded in November 1915.

However, detailed research on the origin of the theory of general relativity in the last decades, involving not only the achievements of Einstein but also those of his predecessors and contemporaries, has given rise to doubts about this overly simple story that says the origin of this theory was ultimately a triumph of mathematics. Such doubts emerge when one remembers, as we saw, that Einstein had already in the winter of 1912/1913 formulated the first steps for the correct field equation of gravitation but abandoned them again, not on mathematical but on physical grounds. Therefore there was a reason why Einstein wrote the letter to Arnold Sommerfeld,[29] who was in close contact with Hilbert, expressing his view that the real difficulty did not lie in finding the correct equation. Rather one needed to show that it was compatible with the accepted classical Newtonian description of gravitational fields and with the conservation of energy and momentum.

The doubts that the breakthrough to the theory of general relativity was simply a triumph of mathematics were confirmed when the almost entirely preserved page proofs of Hilbert's article came to light. They even afforded two surprises. For one, the date stamp was 6 December 1915. This is a clear indication that Hilbert did not submit the final version five days before Einstein, as the 20 November publication date would lead one to believe. For another, in some important respects, the theory developed in the proofs differs distinctly from the published version. Even though part of one page of the proofs was apparently later clipped off, this much is clear: before publication Hilbert must have considerably revised the version documented in the proofs. It has now emerged that the physical conceptual basis of the proof version of Hilbert's theory is in many respects more similar to Einstein's *Entwurf* theory than to the theory of general relativity. In particular, as one of the axioms of his theory, Hilbert introduces a restriction on admissible coordinate systems through an energy condition much like what Einstein did in his preliminary theory. Therefore neither theory completely realized the vision of a general relativity theory, and they both still distinguished certain spacetime coordinates by making them satisfy additional physical conditions. Against this background, it now appears unlikely that Hilbert had the key for Einstein's problems in his hand. Rather, it looks very much as if the breakthrough in late 1915 cannot be understood without realizing the crucial role of the *Entwurf* theory as a scaffold for the last steps in formulating the theory of general relativity, and in particular for bringing together physical and mathematical knowledge along the tortuous pathway marked by Einstein's November papers, a pathway that Hilbert apparently followed only after Einstein's breakthrough.

i. The Relativity Revolution Continues—
The Formative Years

In this section, we have reconstructed the complex process through which Einstein's heuristics led to the formulation of the general theory of relativity. In particular, the interplay between Einstein's heuristics and his immediate mathematical results played a key role. Eventually, these results acquired a new physical interpretation, thereby altering the original heuristic. However, this interaction did not end with the concluding paper of November 1915. The tension between Einstein's heuristics and the implications of the new theory also characterized its further evolution until at least 1930, and in some respects this process continues even today.

We refer to the period between 1915 and the early 1930s as the *formative years* of general relativity in which some of the most fundamental consequences of the theory were elaborated, such as its first exact solutions, and in which Einstein's original heuristics was severely challenged. Within a few years, the ideas of the general theory of relativity changed from the esoteric pursuit of an individual into not only concerns of a growing community of scientists and philosophers but also a matter of international public and media attention.

This was the period when Einstein's theory of general relativity was taken up, elaborated, and controversially discussed by the scientific community, including physicists, mathematicians, astronomers, and philosophers. Einstein himself also made further fundamental contributions to the development of his theory, exploring consequences, such as gravitational waves and cosmological solutions, and clarifying concepts, such as the conservation of energy and momentum, and even reinterpreting basic aspects of the theory. For him, the general theory of relativity was an intermediate step toward the unification of gravitation and electromagnetism into one field, a research program initiated by David Hilbert and intensely pursued by other contemporaries, in particular by mathematicians such as Hermann Weyl. Such a unification scheme was expected to account for the basic properties of matter, particularly for the nature of the two known particles at the time— the electron and the proton. A theory of this kind would explain the microscopic properties of elementary particles and the constituents of atoms, and would account for the macroscopic phenomena constituting the fabric of the universe at the same time. These were the goals pursued by Einstein and, particularly in the formative years, by a number of his contemporaries.

Many of the profound conceptual and far-reaching technical consequences of general relativity were, in this initial phase after its creation, still unexplored territory. Even the extent to which the very principles that had formed Einstein's heuristic starting point were actually realized by the theory's definitive formulation was not clear. The formative years thus saw—and this is one of the hallmarks of this period—a comprehensive revision and reinterpretation of these fundamental principles, including the relativity principle itself. In this process of revision, clarification, and reinterpretation, the theory became increasingly independent from the scaffolding elements of classical physics with which Einstein's impressive edifice had been erected. General relativity eventually became an autonomous conceptual framework in its own right. This process was not completed by the end of its formative years, and only came to a certain closure in the late 1950s and early 1960s, a period that has been called the "renaissance of general relativity" (Clifford Will), which we turn to in the next section.

The paradigmatic text of the formative period, reflecting not only Einstein's own efforts but also the engagement of his contemporaries with the theory, is his *The Meaning of Relativity*, based on his lectures at Princeton University in 1921.[30] Einstein returned to the theory of relativity in many later publications, both specialized and popular. He later also expanded *The Meaning of Relativity* with appendices that discussed further developments. But he never made another attempt at such an all-encompassing presentation in which he painstakingly substantiated, explained, and discussed its basic principles and their consequences. The articulation of

Einstein's theory in this text is closer to the present-day understanding of the theory than its presentation in the famous 1915
papers, about which he wrote to Lorentz:

> My series of gravitation papers are a chain of wrong tracks,
> which nevertheless did gradually lead closer to the objective. That
> is why now finally the basic formulas are good, but the deriva-
> tions abominable; this deficiency must still be eliminated.[31]

The "abominable" derivations that marked Einstein's earlier
presentations of his general theory have been elegantly corrected
in *The Meaning of Relativity*.

The exposition of tensor calculus and the discussion of the
metric tensor are simpler and more transparent. But what is more
important is Einstein's treatment of differential geometry in its
physical context. The mathematical framework of his general
theory of relativity emerged from the "absolute differential calculus" formulated by Ricci-Curbastro and Levi-Civita, who developed the previous work of Riemann, Christoffel, and others into
a complete computational scheme. However, in his original formulation of general relativity, Einstein did not systematically introduce non-Euclidean geometry, nor did he interpret his own
theory in terms of differential geometry. When he discussed the
Riemann-Christoffel tensor, for instance, he did not even mention curvature.

The relation of Einstein's theory to differential geometry and its
geometrical interpretation became fully apparent only after the
this theory was established and was not a presupposition for its
formulation. The geometrization of general relativity and the full
understanding of gravity as the curvature of spacetime is a result
of its further development. It was only in the Princeton lectures
that Einstein acknowledged covariant differential operations on
tensors as being best performed by the method introduced by
Levi-Civita, which was based on the notions of "parallel transport"
and "affine connection" and first used in the context of general
relativity by Hermann Weyl, as acknowledged by Einstein. Weyl,

in particular, clarified the geometrical interpretation of the Riemann-Christoffel curvature tensor and related it to the parallel displacement of a vector around a closed loop.

The era of the formative years is itself a major transformation of knowledge and complements the process that started in 1907. In the rest of this section, we describe the main developments that marked this epistemic shift. Here, we confine the scope of the discussion of these developments to what is necessary to prepare for the historiographic analysis of the relativity revolution in the final section of this book.

The formative years were marked by debates about the two main heuristic principles that had guided Einstein on the road to his relativistic theory of gravity: the generalized principle of relativity and Mach's principle. Over the course of these debates, both principles were challenged and substantially modified. The eventual demise of Mach's principle in connection with the rise of relativistic cosmology and the primacy of field theoretical concepts is well known, perhaps less so the problematic character of the general principle of relativity. In the next subsection, we discuss the debate about the general principle of relativity and its consequences. We conclude this section by describing Einstein's road from his ardent efforts to uphold Mach's principle to its abandonment.

j. The Generalized Relativity Principle Revisited

The tension between Einstein's original intentions and the ongoing exploration of the consequences of the new theory became evident when, in 1917, Erich Kretschmann challenged Einstein's interpretation of the meaning of general covariance. Einstein had identified his general principle of relativity with general covariance. Based on the notion that events in space and time can only be identified by coincidences of real physical processes, such as the encounter of two particles (section Vf), Einstein stated in "The Foundation of General Relativity" that: "As all our physical experience can be ultimately reduced to such coincidences, there

is no immediate reason for preferring certain systems of coordinates to others, that is to say, we arrive at the requirement of
general co-variance."[32]

Using the same concept of point-coincidences, Kretschmann
argued that general covariance has no physical meaning and, with
mathematical ingenuity, any spacetime theory, with or without
absolute motion, can be expressed in a generally covariant formulation. He concluded this from the assertion that if

> all physical observations consist in the determination of
> purely topological relations ("coincidences") between objects
> of spatio-temporal perception, from which it follows that no
> coordinate system is privileged by these observations, then
> one is forced to the following conclusion: By means of a
> purely mathematical reformulation of the equations repre-
> senting the theory . . . any physical theory can be brought into
> agreement with any, arbitrary relativity postulate, even the
> most general one.[33]

With this argument, Kretschmann challenged the close link between covariance and the relativity principle.

In 1918, Einstein reacted to Kretschmann's criticism and also
illustrated the problems with implementing a Machian interpretation of general relativity mentioned above. He argued that he
had not previously distinguished between two principles sufficiently, which he now introduced as the principle of relativity
and Mach's principle. Einstein reformulated his understanding
of the underlying principles of the theory of general relativity as
follows:

> a. *Principle of Relativity*. Nature's laws are merely statements
> about temporal-spatial coincidences; therefore, they find their
> only natural expression in generally covariant equations.

> b. *Principle of Equivalence*. Inertia and gravity are phenomena
> identical in nature. From this and from the special theory of
> relativity it follows necessarily that the symmetric "fundamen-

tal tensor" $(g_{\mu\nu})$ determines the metric properties of space, the inertial behavior of bodies in this space, as well as the gravitational effects. We shall call the state of space which is described by this fundamental tensor, the "G-field."

c. *Mach's Principle*. The G-field is completely determined by the masses of the bodies. Since mass and energy are—according to the results of the special theory of relativity—the same, and since energy is formally described by the symmetric energy tensor $(T_{\mu\nu})$, it follows that the G-field is caused and determined by the energy tensor of matter.[34]

The relativity principle is not formulated here, as was the case previously, as the equivalence of all frames of reference. Instead, Einstein states that the only physically meaningful content of a relativistic theory is coincidences of physical events at points in space and time. Since the occurrence of these point coincidences is independent of whether they are described in one or the other coordinate frame, their most appropriate description is by a generally covariant theory. This principle had not been the starting point of Einstein's search for a general relativistic theory of gravitation; it instead constituted a result of his reflection on complications encountered in a long but eventually successful search for such a theory. The formulation of the principle of relativity no longer adheres to the original assumption of a world of isolated bodies distributed in an otherwise empty space whose physical interactions depend only on relative distances and velocities.

Einstein agreed with Kretschmann that this formulation of the relativity principle is not a statement about physical reality but a requirement of the mathematical formulation of the theory, and he even conceded that "every empirical law can be brought into a generally covariant form."[35] In his popular account of the special and general relativity, Einstein argued that the generalization of special relativity was previously described as the quest for incorporating accelerated frames of reference into the theory. Such a description is misleading. Newtonian mechanics and special relativity can also be observed from an accelerated frame of reference, but the laws of physics are then more complicated.

However, Einstein nevertheless attached heuristic value to the principle of relativity, which had proven itself as a heuristic guide in formulating a relativistic theory of gravitation. He claimed that between two formulations of the same theory, one will always favor the simpler one. Later, it was actually possible to formulate simple covariant versions of Newton's theory.[36] But in contrast to general relativity, such a theory presupposes absolute spacetime structures that may act on but are not acted upon by physical processes, which meant that the characteristic feature of Einstein's theory can be best captured by the notion of background independence, in the sense that the theory does not presuppose such absolute spacetime structures.

The equivalence principle was initially formulated to enable the generalization of the relativity principle from uniform to accelerated motion. It was the starting point of the whole theory and led to the generalized principle of relativity. Here the emphasis is on the equivalence of inertia and gravity. In the Princeton lectures, the equivalence principle is formulated in a similar fashion. As he had done many times before, Einstein first introduced a coordinate system K', which is uniformly accelerating with respect to an inertial coordinate system K. Thus: "Relatively to K' all the masses have equal and parallel accelerations; with respect to K' they behave just as if a gravitational field were present and K' were unaccelerated."[37] In this situation,

there is nothing to prevent our conceiving this gravitational field as real, that is, the conception that K' is "at rest" and a gravitational field is present we may consider as equivalent to the conception that only K is an "allowable" system of coordinates and no gravitational field is present. The assumption of the complete physical equivalence of the systems of coordinates, K and K', we call the "principle of equivalence;" this principle is evidently intimately connected with the law of the equality between the inert and the gravitational mass, and sig-nifies an extension of the principle of relativity to co-ordinate systems which are in non-uniform motion relatively to each other. In fact, through this conception we arrive at the unity of the nature of inertia and gravitation.[38]

The last sentence reflects the essence of the formulation of the equivalence principle in Einstein's response to Kretschmann. Ein-stein then offers an almost poetic expression of this point:

The possibility of explaining the numerical equality of inertia and gravitation by the unity of their nature gives to the general theory of relativity, according to my conviction, such a superi-ority over the conceptions of classical mechanics, that all the difficulties encountered must be considered as small in com-parison with this progress.[39]

Einstein initially searched for a theory in which the physical laws would also be the same in accelerated frames of reference. What he actually found was a theory in which gravitation and inertia are recognized as two aspects of the same field.

k. Cosmological Considerations—The Demise of Mach's Principle

After completing his general theory of relativity, Einstein realized its relevance for a description of the universe as a whole. Although none of the modern observations were available, the theory had some definitive implications for the understanding of the struc-ture of the universe. We can see now in hindsight that Einstein's discussion of this subject, his debates with colleagues, and particu-larly his 1917 cosmology paper may appear as the genesis of mod-ern cosmology.

General relativity is today considered the theoretical basis of observational cosmology. But cosmology did not play any role in its genesis. Epistemological considerations, particularly Mach's criticism of Newton's absolute space, were far more important to Einstein's thinking. As we have discussed in section IIIa, he followed Mach's idea to conceive inertial effects occurring in accelerated frames of reference as being due to an interaction with distant masses rather than as a consequence of motion with respect to absolute space. This idea played a key role in Einstein's heuristics. General relativity should explain all inertial effects as being due to such interactions. In his obituary for Mach, Einstein asserted that: "Mach clearly recognized the weak points of classical mechanics, and thus came close to demand a general theory of relativity."[40] Following this line of thought, Einstein's initial reflections on the "cosmological problem" are marked by his struggle to uphold Mach's approach.

In the fall of 1916, Einstein visited Leiden, where he met the Dutch astronomer Willem de Sitter, who—in the midst of the war, which also interrupted scientific communications—played a key role in making the general theory of relativity known outside of Germany. De Sitter became Einstein's principal interlocutor and eventually opponent in the discussion of the allegedly Machian features of general relativity. Since the solutions of the gravitational field equations are determined not only by the mass distribution represented by the right-hand side of the equation but also by boundary conditions, it was unclear whether some trace of absolute space and time was still preserved in these boundary conditions. This question first arose in the discussions between Einstein and de Sitter in Leiden.

When Einstein returned to Berlin, he looked—with his assistant at that time, Jakob Grommer—for a spherically symmetric solution with appropriate boundary conditions that, in accordance with the principle of general relativity, would be independent of the coordinate system. In addition, they required that the resulting metric would have to be time-independent, corresponding to a static universe. De Sitter strongly criticized this approach. In November 1916, he wrote to Einstein: "I have been thinking much about the relativity of inertia and about the distant masses, and the longer I think about it, the more troubling your hypothesis becomes for me."[41]

Einstein responded a few days later:

Now that the covariant field equations have been found, no motive remains to place such great weight on the total relativity of inertia. . . . Which part of the inertia stems from the masses and which part from the boundary conditions depends on the choice of the boundary.[42]

It seems that Einstein relaxed his categorical insistence on the Machian origin of inertia here, but if so, it was not the case for long.

Einstein took a few months to realize that his efforts with Grommer were leading nowhere. After failing to reach a satisfactory solution to the question of boundary conditions in regard to the Machian heuristics, in 1917 he proposed an entirely new way to solve this problem. In his famous article "Cosmological Considerations in the General Theory of Relativity," he claimed: "In a consistent theory of relativity there can be no inertia *relatively to 'space,'* but only an inertia of masses *relatively to one another.*"[43] In his paper, Einstein discussed in detail his initial ideas on the boundary conditions to conclude why they had to be abandoned: "But here it proved that for the system of the fixed stars no boundary conditions of the kind can come into question at all, as was also rightly emphasized by the astronomer de Sitter recently."[44] He then introduced a spacetime that met all his expectations concerning the constitution of the universe, including the explanation of its inertial properties by the distribution of masses acting as sources of the gravitational field. This spacetime describes a spatially closed static universe with a uniform matter distribution. With this solution, Einstein entirely avoided the problem of specifying appropriate boundary conditions—since a closed space does not have a boundary. He believed that this model corresponded to a more or less realistic view of the universe as was known at the time.

However, all of this served him only at the expense of modifying the field equation for which this spacetime was a solution. In fact, as we know from a back-of-the-envelope calculation on a draft letter to the Austrian emperor,[45] the desired cosmological solution formed Einstein's starting point, which then forced him to modify the field equation. This modification consisted of introducing an additional term to the field equation of 1915 that contained a universal constant known as the "cosmological constant" λ. For Einstein, the cosmological constant was a lifesaver for his Machian philosophical conception of a static universe. Contrary to what Einstein wrote in his 1915 formulation of the general theory of relativity, the resulting field equation was not given in the most general form. This additional term does not violate general covariance, preserves the energy-momentum conservation, and essentially represents a small repulsive force acting on a large scale to balance the gravitational forces and make "possible a quasi-static distribution of matter."[46] To justify the introduction of the cosmological constant, Einstein showed, at the beginning of his paper, that, also in Newton's theory of gravitation, an infinite static universe with a finite mass density is possible only by adding a similar constant on the left-hand side of the classical Poisson equation for the gravitational potential.

Shortly after Einstein's "Cosmological Considerations" was published, de Sitter demonstrated that even the modified field equations allow a solution in which there is no matter acting as a source, and that test particles moving in this spacetime do have inertial properties. For Einstein, this discovery was an unpleasant surprise that he found difficult to digest and at first attempted to refute, claiming that in de Sitter's solution, there was a hidden mass concentrated in singularities. In a letter to de Sitter, in addition to claiming the existence of singularities, Einstein remarked:

In my opinion, it would be unsatisfactory if a world without matter were possible. Rather the $g^{\mu\nu}$ field should *be fully determined by matter and not be able to exist without matter.* This is the core of what I mean by "matter conditioning geometry." To me, as long as this requirement had not been fulfilled, the goal of general relativity was not yet completely achieved. This only came about with the λ term.[47]

De Sitter responded to this with a reference to the limited empirical knowledge about the universe then available:

> I must emphatically contest your assumption that the world is mechanically quasi-stationary. We only have a snapshot of the world, and we cannot and must *not* conclude from the fact that we do not see any large changes on this photograph that everything will always remain as at that instant when the picture was taken.[48]

Both Einstein's and de Sitter's cosmological solutions became the subject of intense debate and constituted the principal alternatives that were considered at the time.

Over the course of this debate, Einstein realized that de Sitter's model was free of singularities and that even his modified gravitational field equation admitted solutions without matter. Then, his expectation of a Machian explanation of inertia in the theory of general relativity changed from a requirement imposed on the theory itself to a criterion of acceptability to be applied to specific solutions of the theory, another epistemic shift in the understanding of the physical meaning of the new theory. To specify his modified heuristic expectations, in 1918 Einstein introduced, as we have seen above, what he called "Mach's principle." It stipulated that for solutions that satisfied this principle, the gravitational field must be completely determined by masses occurring on the right-hand side of the field equation in the form of the energy-momentum tensor as the sources of the field. In this way, Einstein translated Mach's original ideas from the language of mechanics to that of field theory. Subsequently, Einstein began to elaborate the field theoretical interpretation more and more at the expense of the mechanical roots of his heuristics.

The last time that Einstein defended, albeit with a certain reservation, his Machian conviction was in his Nobel Prize address in 1923:

Mach's stipulation can be accounted for in the general theory of relativity by regarding the world in spatial terms as finite and self-contained. This hypothesis also makes it possible to assume the mean density of matter in the world as finite, whereas in a spatially infinite (quasi-Euclidian) world it should disappear. It cannot, however, be concealed that to satisfy Mach's postulate in the manner referred to a term with no experimental basis whatsoever must be introduced into the field equations, which term logically is in no way determined by the other terms in the equations. For this reason this solution of the "cosmological problem" will not be completely satisfactory for the time being.[49]

After 1923, Einstein realized that it could not be generally correct that inertial effects can be explained exclusively by the presence of matter in this theory. His attitude toward Mach's ideas changed correspondingly, and the interpretation of the theory of general relativity along the lines of Mach's philosophical critique of classical mechanics ceased to play a significant role in Einstein's research. This shift of interest was caused not least by the reorientation of his research program toward a unified field theory of gravitation and electromagnetism, which had already begun in the late 1910s and pushed questions ultimately rooted in a mechanistic worldview into the background.

Nevertheless, the question of Mach's principle remained open since it was now closely associated with Einstein's cosmological ideas. These largely coincided with the thinking of his contemporaries. In the period between 1917 and 1930, the prevailing debate was about which model of the universe was a better representation of reality. At that time, the question of an expanding universe, raised by Alexander Friedmann in 1922 and by Georges Henri Lemaître in 1927, began to enter the horizon of observational cosmology. In any case, the groundwork had been prepared for a decision about Mach's principle on the basis of astronomical observations.

This decision came with the accumulation of astronomical evidence in favor of an expanding universe, the decisive contribution being the work published in 1929 by the astronomer Edwin Hubble, who was working at the Mount Wilson Observatory in California, supported by Milton L. Humason and extending earlier work by Vesto Slipher. Einstein learned about these results early in 1931 during a stay at the Californian Institute of Technology. Almost immediately after his return to Berlin, Einstein published a paper on the cosmological problem in which he stated that Hubble's results had made his assumption of a static universe untenable. These results could instead be explained by the dynamic solutions of the original field equations and they, therefore, sealed the fate— at least temporarily—of the cosmological constant as well as of Mach's principle. (The cosmological constant would later be resurrected as an important ingredient of modern cosmology.)

Eventually, Einstein quite explicitly rejected his earlier Machian heuristics. In a letter to the physicist Felix Pirani in 1954, he stated that he no longer considered it plausible that the gravitational field should be completely determined by the energy-momentum tensor of matter, as demanded by Mach's principle. Such a determination is possible only if the distribution of matter in spacetime is given first. But this already presupposes knowledge about a given spacetime, which, in turn, demands knowledge about the metric, which is only determined subsequently by the field equation. In the same letter, Einstein expressly rejected Mach's principle:

> But in my opinion one should not speak of Mach's principle at all. It dates back to the time in which one thought that the "ponderable bodies" were the only physically real entities, and that all elements of the theory that are not completely determined by them should be consciously avoided. (I am well aware of the fact that I myself was influenced by this fixed idea for a long time).[50]

The insights that Einstein gathered over decades since first taking steps toward a general principle of relativity under the influence of Mach's critique of mechanics finally made it impossible to bring his original heuristics into accordance with this advancement of knowledge. What we have shown here in detail for the case of Machian heuristics is equally valid for other heuristic elements that accompanied Einstein on his way to the theory of general relativity.

Above, we discussed the modified understanding of the relativity principle, but even the Lorentz model, the basic mental model of a field theory, was called into question by the completion and further evolution of the theory. The relationship between the field equation and equation of motion also appears different in the fully developed theory than in classical field theory because, as it turned out, in the theory of general relativity the equation of motion is not independent of the field equation but rather a consequence of the latter. Similarly, the correspondence principle, which governs the transition to the Newtonian limit, and the conservation principle attain a new meaning in the full theory. Einstein's heuristics has much in common with the famous Wittgenstein ladder, which one has to dispose of after reaching one's goal.

VI

The Einsteinian Revolution as a Transformation of a System of Knowledge

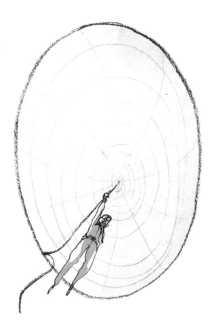

Preview

This book focuses on an understanding of the origins and the dynamics of the conceptual transformation that constitutes the hallmark of the scientific revolution associated with Einstein's name and on its standing within the broader context of the long-term history of science. We have already emphasized that any attempt at understanding this revolution primarily as the outcome of one person's story of discovery will encounter serious difficulties. From the standpoint of a historical theory of knowledge, as outlined in section II, speculations about Einstein's creativity originating in his brain, in his supposedly childlike disposition, in his relationships with women, or in his conviction that imagination and curiosity are more important than knowledge are indeed not very helpful.

Instead, the conditions for this conceptual transformation are only revealed when one takes into account the social, cultural, and intellectual environment that generated the new concepts connected with this revolution. Only in this way does it become clear that Einstein's breakthroughs are connected with the transformation of an entire system of knowledge. To state our position in the most general form: the preservation of knowledge passed down from the dawn of culture is just as important as its metamorphosis through the transformation processes of scientific revolutions. In this final section of our book, we take a closer look at this transformation process, situating it within the wider context of knowledge evolution. Recent work in the history of science, upon which this book is based, has radically changed not only our view of Einstein but also our understanding of the structures of scientific revolutions. Einstein no longer appears as the isolated pioneer of the twentieth century but rather as a scientist who, somewhat paradoxically but in line with the general dynamics of knowledge evolution, helped bring classical physics to its completion and thereby contributed to the shake-up of its foundations.

The first phase of the relativity revolution was clearly not an isolated event but rather the result of exploiting hidden potentials that had accumulated in the highly specialized science of the nineteenth century. As we saw in section IV, the relativity revolution started with the reinterpretation of the Lorentzian theory of electromagnetism, representing a Copernicus process and, therefore, essentially continued the traditions of classical physics, albeit in a different way. The origin of the theory of special relativity was without doubt part of a more general process. This is already evident from Poincaré's contemporary contribution, which displays some striking similarities with Einstein's concerning interpreting the Lorentzian theory. By contrast, the next phase of the relativity revolution, the theory of general relativity, originated largely as the work of a single person who took a stand against the trend of contemporary physics and was supported only by a few outsiders. The point of origin of the theory of general relativity was a commonly accepted problem—the incompatibility of Newton's classical theory of gravity with the theory of special relativity of 1905. But neither Einstein's research path nor the theory that resolved this conflict in November 1915 met the expectations of his contemporaries. Against this background, we discuss the unique, almost paradoxical, features of the Einsteinian revolution that made it so perplexing to current and contemporary observers alike, including Einstein himself: it was not primarily motivated by new empirical results but instead was guided by an ultimately delusive heuristics, and it was based on the knowledge of classical physics, yet gave rise to nonclassical insights incompatible with the framework that Einstein's research was originally based on. We argue that even this unique character of the general relativity revolution can only be understood in the broader context of the long-term history of science. The unique character of general relativity is also reflected by its further development in the one hundred years since its inception. In this period, the theory of general relativity itself went through significant transitions, illustrating that the Einsteinian revolution was indeed no sudden paradigm shift but part of a long-term evolution of knowledge. In conclusion, we present some lessons to be learned from this historical account.

a. A Short History of Physics

In section III we dealt with the knowledge structures of classical physics, which generated in their evolution the problems that were central to the Einsteinian revolution. But several of these structures, changed by this revolution, reach back much further, some of them to the very beginnings of science. So where do we find the roots of this revolution, and what exactly is its place in the long-term evolution of knowledge? To answer these questions, we glance at the long-term history of physics, recapitulating some of the central points elaborated in previous sections.

It should, above all, become evident that the Einsteinian revolution can also be viewed as the end point of the centuries-long evolution of the mechanistic worldview, which itself resulted from a transformation of ancient natural philosophy. Both systems of knowledge, the ancient one and the nineteenth-century worldview of mechanics, include an understanding of the notions of space, time, gravity, matter, and motion that was shaped by mental models of intuitive and practical thinking.

We have already discussed the essential features of Aristotelian physics in section II in the context of the Galilean revolution. The core of the Aristotelian theory of motion is the intuitive motion-implies-force model, implying that there is no motion without a mover in contact with the moving body. Embedding such an intuitive mental model into a theory like Aristotle's natural philosophy puts more restrictive demands on the explanatory potential of the model than does intuitive physics; in particular its articulation within a theoretical framework promotes its universalization, as well as consistency of its use. The failure of this model to identify a mover led to the exclusion of two types of motion from the motion-implies-force model: first, the motion of celestial bodies, which instead is conceived as eternal circular motion; second, the motion of heavy objects falling to the center of the earth, as well as the ascending motion of light objects in the opposite direction, both conceived as the result of an inner tendency of heavy or light bodies to act according to their nature. Aristotle referred to these motions as "natural" motions, which do not require an external cause, as opposed to "violent" motions, which are the subject of his theory of causation of motion by force. For almost two thousand years, these ideas dominated the understanding of what are now considered to be the effects of gravitation.

In the sixteenth century, Copernicus used the long tradition of observational and calculational astronomy as a basis to suggest a new interpretation of celestial events, which brought new order to the knowledge that had been passed down. The heliocentric system of Copernicus called into question not only Aristotle's view of the cosmos as an onion-like layered structure with the earth at its center, but it also challenged the understanding of motion as described above because the fact that the motion of the earth around its axis and around the sun is not felt by its inhabitants required an explanation. In particular the distinction between real and apparent motions became a world-shattering question, whose study ultimately led to the introduction of the modern concept of relativity of motion. It is, in a way, a precursor of Einstein's deliberations concerning an extension of the relativity principle to electrodynamics. Such deliberations led him first to the special theory of relativity and then ultimately to a new cosmological model based on the general theory of relativity. We thus observe a remarkable interaction between mental models of motion and conceptions of the world at large, but also between novel conceptions brought about by scientific abstractions and expectations rooted in the mental models of intuitive and practical thinking.

This tension between novel scientific concepts and intuitive expectations also shaped the development of classical mechanics. Newton's conception of the gravitational force as an action at a distance was criticized by his contemporaries, as well as by later scientists, because it does not represent a type of interaction expected from intuitive physics, that is, an interaction mediated by material contact. Therefore models of gravitational effects were developed that attempted to either undermine or evade this objection. The perplexing properties of inertial motion were another frequently discussed, counterintuitive challenge of Newtonian physics. The bewilderment about a continuous uniform motion, for which no external cause or force could be identified, never quite vanished. This was true whether the motion was terrestrial or celestial, even though the Aristotelian worldview had long ago perished. Newtonian physics was extremely successful in explaining the motion of planets and other heavenly bodies, but it could not silence certain objections, for example, against the rather artificial division of a planet's orbital motion into an inertial component (due to its inner tendency of motion) and an accelerated component (due to the invisible gravity of the sun). In a way, the account of this motion as a force-free motion, determined not by a force but by the geometry of spacetime in general relativity, may be considered as a partial return to an Aristotelian-like conception of natural motion.

During the nineteenth century, more and more concepts that had been reshaped by the science of mechanics found their way into daily life. Concepts like metric space and universal time acquired a practical usage through that century's economic and technological developments. The implementation of standardized measuring systems and the introduction of a global time definition, which grew out of the expansion of the railroad systems, provide illustrations of this process. Other developments challenged the apparent universal validity of these concepts. These include, for example, the discovery of the mathematical possibility of non-Euclidean geometries. As a consequence, the question about the validity of the classical concept of space shifted from the sphere of epistemology as in Kant's philosophy into the sphere of empirical verifiability.

In spite of the rise of new branches of science, as discussed in section III, mechanics remained the common benchmark of science. Initial attempts to explain nonmechanical interactions like heat, electricity, or light by mechanical models even increased its importance. The explanation of heat phenomena was at first based on the notion of a heat substance and then on the idea that heat is nothing but the motion of atoms. James Clerk Maxwell explained electromagnetic phenomena, including light, by means of a mechanical ether. He did so by continuing Michael Faraday's thoughts about electric and magnetic lines of force, and also by building on the tradition of wave optics. With this background, searching for an explanation of gravity by means of this same medium was plausible.

Newton's law of attraction of two masses has the same form as Coulomb's law for the attraction between electrical particles at rest. In either case, the force is inversely proportional to the square of the distance between the particles and proportional in the first case to the product of the masses, in the second case to the product of the charges. It was therefore natural to interpret mass as a kind of "gravitational charge," which causes a disturbance of the surrounding ether and leads to a gravitational field, which then propagates through the ether and thus acts on other gravitational charges. However, attempts to construct a field theory of gravitation following the example of the theory of the electromagnetic field faced nearly insurmountable difficulties; yet the mental model of a field theory, as elaborated by Hendrik A. Lorentz, eventually served Einstein as a heuristic guide in his creation of general relativity.

As knowledge accumulated, designing consistent mental models based on mechanical knowledge became successively more difficult. The models needed to do justice not only to the various applications in the realm of classical physics but also to contemporary chemistry. Ether and atoms had to fulfill increasingly numerous functions in various areas—from optics to heat to gravitation—which eventually were no longer mutually compatible in the framework of classical physics. At the same time, electrodynamics and thermodynamics were separated into independent areas of physics. Their central concepts of "field," "energy," and "entropy" no longer required a mechanical justification. Philosophers and historians of science like Mach saw this as an opportunity to critically review the basic concepts of mechanics itself. As a consequence, a totally new situation had evolved toward the end of the nineteenth century.

Classical physics was thus, as we discussed in section III, divided into three conceptually distinct areas: mechanics, electromagnetism, and thermodynamics. These areas were not only connected with each other by their still common roots in classical notions of space, time, and matter, but were also connected by overlapping, new concepts like that of energy. Moreover, borderline areas developed between these conceptual continents, where problems accumulated and bore the potential of clashes between different conceptual systems. These borderline problems were central subjects of research for Wilhelm Wien, Max Planck, Hendrik A. Lorentz, Ludwig Boltzmann, and others. The masters of classical physics investigated these problems from the viewpoint of their respective specializations, whereas the full potential of the solutions they found became manifest only from a broader perspective that included a critical reflection on the foundations of classical physics.

From the perspective of Einstein's intellectual orientation, the borderline problems of classical physics and their solutions by the masters of classical physics became the starting point for the breakthroughs of his *annus mirabilis*, 1905. We analyzed this process in section IV. Einstein's largely autodidactic study, and the discussions with his friends of the Swiss bohemia of his student days, formed the intellectual laboratory in which these results were transformed into the foundations of a new physics. The substance of Einstein's work was not new but rather was the result of an accumulation of knowledge over centuries; it was his conceptual organization that was new. It developed through reinterpreting and transforming existing knowledge, which we have called a Copernicus process. New concepts of space and time took the place of the concept of ether. A dualism of wave and particle—which was not compatible with the concepts of classical physics—took the place of the wave picture of light. The existence of atoms and their motions was no longer called into question, and their properties could now only be described by means of statistical laws.

A precondition for this revolutionary renewal of physics was certainly the manner in which Einstein was able to retain what was handed down to him. But equally important was a kind of orientation knowledge that permitted him to recognize its boundaries. An important part of Einstein's attitude regarding knowledge was his epistemological awareness of the malleability of its conceptual frameworks and their long-term evolution. This is clearly evident in his reflections on his own achievements. His familiarity with the philosophy and history of science was an important precondition for his breakthroughs of 1905, as well as for his later development of general relativity.

As we saw in section VI, after 1905 he continued to scrutinize the further implications of these breakthroughs. No other scientific contribution is perhaps a more eloquent testimonial for the significance of a philosophically and historically informed perspective than the creation of the theory of general relativity of 1915. As we saw there, it drew on the historical-philosophical critique of Mach for its essential motivations and thus was able to solve the puzzle of gravitation in a surprising new way. Newton's notion of gravitation is modeled after an anthropomorphically inspired concept of force. General relativity explains gravity instead as a curvature of a non-Euclidean spacetime, replacing the notion that space and time constitute a fixed arena on which physical events take place, and thus giving rise to a novel view of the physical world that has no precedent in the evolution of knowledge.

b. The Epistemic Character of the Relativity Revolution

In section V, we outlined the evolution of the general theory of relativity from its inception in 1907 to its final formulation in November 1915, and the subsequent formative years when basic aspects of the theory were clarified and reinterpreted and its immediate consequences explored. In the present section, we have already begun to place the general theory of relativity within the larger framework of the history of science in order to better understand its historical place and unique features. Against this background, it is worthwhile to take a final look at the four essential stages of the decisive period in the genesis of Einstein's theory, the years 1912 to 1915:

- *The tinkering phase* of the fall of 1912 is documented by Einstein's first calculations related to general relativity in the Zurich Notebook. This phase is characterized by an almost complete absence of complex mathematical operations. Nevertheless, by reflecting on his first attempts to formulate a field equation along the lines of his heuristic principles, Einstein managed to build the higher-order structures and a plan of action that would assume strategic importance for his later systematic implementation of these principles. Most notably, he established the physical and the mathematical strategies of his search for the gravitational field equation.

- *The systematic searching phase* lasted from late 1912 to early 1913. It can also be reconstructed from the Zurich Notebook. In this phase, Einstein, together with Marcel Grossmann, systematically examined various candidates, guided by his heuristic principles, alternating between physical and mathematical strategies. Over the course of their efforts, the relative weight of the heuristic principles gradually changed, with the conservation principle emerging as the principal challenge. Paradoxically, the main result of the pursuit of the mathematical strategy was a shift to the physical strategy, leading to a preliminary version of his theory of gravitation. This was the *Entwurf* theory, published in the spring of 1913.

- *The consolidation phase* is documented by Einstein's publications and correspondences between 1913 and mid-1915. During this phase, he elaborated the *Entwurf* theory, essentially following his earlier heuristics but using them with the goal of consolidation rather than exploration. Paradoxically, however, the main result of the consolidation period was the creation of the prerequisites for a renewed search for candidates for the field equations. While trying to use the mathematical strategy to legitimize the *Entwurf* theory, Einstein found that the resulting mathematical formalism did not single out just one theory but gave occasion to reexamine previously excluded candidates. Through this process, the difficulty of implementing the conservation principle was removed. On the basis of the network of results assembled in the meantime, this reexami-

nation could now take the form of a reflective reorganiza
tion of Einstein's earlier achievements.

- *The reflection phase* is documented by the dramatic sequence of Einstein's communications of November 1915. The first communication was a return to a field equation based on the Riemann tensor. It consisted essentially of a reinterpretation of results obtained under the spell of the *Entwurf* theory. The *Entwurf* theory was still conceptually rooted in classical physics. The decisive step in the transition from this theory to the nonclassical theory of relativity was the shift in the physical interpretation of some elements of the formalism created by Einstein. As a consequence of this reinterpretation, Einstein's original heuristic principles also received a new physical interpretation. This transition can be understood as a Copernicus process comparable to the transition from Lorentz's theory to the theory of special relativity. However, in passing from the *Entwurf* theory to the theory of general relativity using the former as scaffolding, Einstein was "his own Lorentz," which also explains the greater isolation in which the second stage of the relativity revolution, the creation of general relativity, took place.

This sequence of steps toward the field equation of general relativity can be understood as an implementation of Einstein's original heuristics in an exploration of the physical and mathematical knowledge resources at his disposal.

Interpreting the genesis of general relativity from the perspective of a historical epistemology of knowledge, which emphasizes the historical change of fundamental categories of knowledge, one must and can furthermore address a number of paradoxical features of this theory, which cannot be resolved within a traditional history of ideas. Indeed, one cannot deal with those challenges without taking into account aspects that are often neglected but crucial: the protracted nature of knowledge development, the complex architecture of knowledge, and the intricate mechanisms

of knowledge dynamics. In the following, we therefore summarize
the role of these aspects by clarifying the unique challenges of
understanding the relativity revolution.

- **The challenge of missing knowledge.** When Einstein
  launched the search for a new theory of gravitation, there
  were practically no known phenomena that could not be
  explained by traditional physics with the exception of the
  Mercury problem for which a "classical" solution, however,
  could not be excluded a priori when Einstein started to
  work on it. How was it then possible to create general
  relativity, which is capable of accounting for a wide range of
  phenomena that were not even known at the time of its
  origin such as gravitational waves or black holes? Most of
  the relevant phenomena were only later discovered over the
  course of several revolutionary developments in observational astronomy. So, to what can we attribute this remarkably precocious character?

An adequate response to these questions is possible only with insights into the long-term development of scientific knowledge.
The astonishing precociousness and stability of general relativity
is based on knowledge accumulated over centuries of physical,
astronomical, and mathematical research. The laws of planetary
motion, such as the curious perihelion advance of Mercury, were
known long before the theory was completed. The same applies
to non-Euclidean geometry and absolute differential calculus, the
mathematical language of general relativity. These tools had been
developed throughout the nineteenth century and had even been
related to astronomical observations by visionary astrophysicists,
like Karl Schwarzschild, well before the advent of relativity.[1]

These resources must all be considered as part of the shared
knowledge available in the early twentieth century to scientists
addressing the problem of gravitation. Their attempts to solve this
problem differed mainly in the perspective from which these
knowledge resources were used or discarded. But even the variety

of individual perspectives may be understood as an aspect of the knowledge system of classical physics, including Einstein's peculiar perspective shaped by the philosophical resources of classical science, allowing a Copernicus process to be engendered in which all of these shared resources were reorganized to constitute a new system of knowledge.

- **The challenge of delusive heuristics.** We have already described the tension between Einstein's heuristics and the final version of the theory. Yet, these heuristics enabled him to formulate the criteria for a gravitational field equation years before he managed to find the right solution. How could this heuristic framework first lead him to a correct mathematical expression in the winter of 1912/1913, while he was working with the Zurich Notebook, and then to the conclusion that it was actually unsound, only to bring him back to precisely the same expression three years later?

The answer to this question also follows naturally from a consideration of the shared knowledge resources available to Einstein, as well as the architecture of this knowledge in terms of the mental models it comprises. As we saw in the previous section, these resources included mental models capable of providing heuristic guidance to his research. In fact, Einstein's search, as we discussed, was guided by a qualitative knowledge structure that was inherited from classical physics. This structure was the mental model of a field theory as embodied in an exemplary way by Lorentz's electron theory.

Einstein's preliminary exploration of a relativistic theory of gravitation in the years 1907 to 1912 had, prior to his search for a field equation documented in the Zurich Notebook, resulted in two default assumptions related to the model of a field equation. He assumed that the field (or rather, the potential that is used in the field equation) was the spacetime metric and that the source of the field was the energy-momentum tensor. However, he did not initially succeed in identifying a satisfactory form of the differential operator that describes how the source produces the field. His difficulty was not that too little was known but rather that too much knowledge had to be taken into account in order to formulate a field equation that complied with the understanding of gravitation as a borderline problem of classical mechanics and field theory.

In short, Einstein's heuristics were determined by the available knowledge of classical physics. This also explains why they were so powerful and, at the same time, so easily limited by the architecture of this knowledge embodied in the mental models of classical physics. The compatibility of the various heuristic requirements could not be easily established a priori but had to be checked by elaborating a mathematical concretization of the Lorentz model, starting from the available default settings and adjusting them, step by step, to the heuristic criteria, thus engendering a process where the architecture of knowledge itself was changed. Einstein's wavering between a physical strategy starting from the correspondence principle and a mathematical strategy starting from the generalized relativity principle can thus be interpreted as a pursuit of alternative and ultimately converging routes for integrating and reorganizing the knowledge of classical physics.

- **The challenge of discontinuous progress.** Einstein's research was undertaken within the preexisting framework of classical and special relativistic physics. But the result of this effort, the general theory of relativity, embodies nonclassical concepts, like the dependence of space and time on physical interactions. These ideas are incompatible with the framework in which this research began. How can this be understood?

The third challenge, that of discontinuous progress, can only be resolved if one takes into account that the development of knowledge is not merely an enhancement of a given structure. It also involves a process of reflection that transforms this structure itself. In the case of Einstein's search for the gravitational field equation, the elaboration of the Lorentz model was guided by the relatively stable higher-order cognitive structures embodied in his heuristic principles: the correspondence principle, the conservation principle, the equivalence principle, and the generalized relativity principle. But Einstein's learning experience was determined not only by the top-down process of assimilation of available knowledge that was guided by these higher-order structures. It was also characterized by a bottom-up process of reflecting on his results, which modified these higher-order structures. This reflection process was based on the experience he had accumulated by concretizing and transforming these very same heuristic principles into an actual physical theory. The interplay between adaptation and accommodation, assimilation to higher-order structures, and their modification based on experience—each mediated by working out the mathematical formalism—was the crucial process that enabled the knowledge dynamics that led to the genesis of general relativity as a nonclassical theory of physics. This was concluded in the *reflection phase* described above as the centerpiece of this Copernicus process.

In addition to these three challenges there is another peculiar feature of the relativity revolution. During its formative years, a deep gulf opened between general relativity and the mainstream of physics. It lasted for almost half a century until general relativity entered the core of physics. One can say that only then was the relativity revolution completed. In this sense, the relativity revolution was indeed a most protracted scientific revolution. Next, we discuss this characteristic feature of the evolution of knowledge.

c. A Long Revolution—From the Mainstream of Physics to Its Periphery and Back

The development of the mathematical formalism of the general theory of relativity reached a first plateau in 1915 (later, the cosmological constant was introduced into the field equation). This was followed by a very active period, to which we referred as "the formative years of general relativity." Einstein already discussed gravitational waves in 1916 and, correcting an error in his first paper on the subject, he arrived in 1918 at what we now call the "quadrupole formula," showing how physical systems emit gravitational waves.[2] After Arthur Eddington's observations of the predicted bending of light in 1919, interest in general relativity grew, attracting more and more scientists to the field.[3] This interest lasted throughout the 1920s and focused on two challenging problems. One was an attempt to combine gravity and electromagnetism into a unified set of field equations. This goal was emphasized by Einstein in his Nobel Prize lecture and undertaken also by others in the early 1920s. From 1925 until the end of his life, Einstein devoted his time and effort almost exclusively to this goal. The other theme of research and debate was the application of the new theory of gravitation to the universe as a whole, precipitated by Einstein's groundbreaking paper from 1917 on this issue. It marked the beginning of relativistic cosmology, boosted by Edwin Hubble's 1929 discovery of the expansion of the universe. Another milestone of that period was the discovery by Karl Schwarzschild of the first exact solution of the gravitational field equations for a spherical mass. This turned out to be the basic model of a black hole, but it took many years until its meaning was fully understood.[4]

Looking back at the period of about fifteen years following the formulation of the general theory of relativity, one could have expected that the major theoretical and empirical achievements of those years would have led to rapid progress, establishing general relativity on a firm physical basis as an active domain in the mainstream of physics. But this is not what happened. Despite this impressive activity, the formative years of general relativity were still marked by an epistemic uncertainty, ranging from the understanding of its mathematical apparatus to the understanding of its physical implications. The correspondence between Einstein, Schwarzschild, Willem de Sitter, Nordström, and others about gravitational waves and approximate solutions illustrates how controversial the connections between the theory and its physical consequences were in those days.

Instead of the anticipated trajectory of progress akin to that of the 1920s, the theory underwent a process of marginalization within the field of physics. The historian of physics Jean Eisenstaedt characterized these years as the "low-water mark period," lasting until the mid-1950s.[5] This characterization applies both to the epistemological and the sociological status of the theory in this period. Concerning its epistemological status, work on the theory was largely characterized by a neo-Newtonian interpretation, which conceived general relativity as providing small corrections to the Newtonian view, albeit with the notable exception of astronomical investigations of the expanding universe, an issue that was, however, mainly treated from a kinematical point of view. Concerning its sociological aspect, many physicists who had been working in this field shifted to other areas of research, specifically to quantum theory. During this period, Einstein's theory generated more interest among mathematicians and philosophers than among physicists.

Throughout the low-water mark period, most physicists considered general relativity as a highly formalistic theory that provided only minor corrections to the Newtonian view. Only a small number of theoretical physicists worked on the theory, as the majority focused on the development of quantum theory, which had much stronger connections with experimental activities and possible technological applications. Other research projects pursued in this period aimed to go beyond general relativity and had, in any case, little connection to empirical investigations. The only empirical domain where general relativity had some impact beyond minor corrections to the Newtonian view was cosmology. But even in cosmology, only certain aspects of general relativity were considered useful in specific contexts. They were not being investigated from the perspective of an extensive research focus with general relativity at its center.

Nevertheless, these disparate research traditions kept the interest in the theory alive until the 1950s, when the theory returned to the mainstream of physics. Clifford Will labeled this period as the "renaissance of general relativity."[6] Its beginnings can be traced to the mid-1950s. This process was accompanied by an epistemic shift eventually leading to the development of an intuitive physical understanding of the intricacies of the theory.[7] We have already elaborated on the role of intuition and heuristics in Einstein's quest for the relativistic theory of gravitation. Physical intuition and the emergence of novel mental models also played a role for the further development of the theory and paved the way for crucial tests of its validity.

Even in the 1950s, physicists still could not agree on whether Schwarzschild's solution described real physical objects, nor on whether gravitational waves were physically real or just an artifact of complicated mathematics. Turning the Schwarzschild solution into a model that could describe the gravitational collapse of a real star, as proposed by J. Robert Oppenheimer and Hartland Snyder in 1939, was a challenging task that was accomplished only during the renaissance of relativity and involved the contributions of many outstanding physicists, including John Archibald Wheeler and Roger Penrose. The existence of gravitational waves carrying energy was gradually accepted by the community, and around 1960 a mental model emerged of the relation between periodic changes in the dimensions of massive objects and gravitational waves emitted, which prompted Joseph Weber and his students to embark on an empirical endeavor to detect such changes.[8] Although a consensus eventually emerged that no gravitational waves were observed in Weber's experiments, his work had a significant impact on the scientific community.

The epistemic developments that marked the renaissance of general relativity were prompted also by organizational developments within the scientific community. Around 1955, a number of research centers focusing on aspects of general relativity were active in different parts of the world. One crucial factor that aided the dynamics of the renaissance was the establishment of the tradition of a long post-doctoral education involving visits to the different centers of general relativity and thus enabling an exchange of knowledge among these centers. Another essential factor was the explicit attempts to build a community to integrate and transform the existing diverse and loosely connected research agendas. One important starting point for this community building was a conference held in 1955 in Bern, the year of Einstein's death. It was organized with the intention to celebrate the fiftieth anniversary of special relativity but was mostly concerned with topics and problems related to general relativity. The Bern conference provided an occasion to recognize links between the existing distinct research traditions and draw consequences from this recognition for future research and collaborations. This recognition led to the organization of further important meetings, such as the Chapel Hill conference in 1957 and the Royaumont conference in 1959, which precipitated a stable and long-lasting tradition of conferences, as well as the creation of international bodies and collaborations.[9] This renewed activity was made possible by the considerable funding for theoretical physics after World War II, by the ability of scientists to cross international borders, and by the physicists themselves, who recognized the potential in establishing a vibrant community interested in the many aspects of Einstein's theory. These activities, together with the astrophysical discoveries of the 1960s, such as quasars and the cosmic microwave background, laid the groundwork for what Kip Thorne has called the "Golden Age" of general relativity in the 1960s and 1970s.[10]

Many of the achievements that had first been made during the formative years had meanwhile been forgotten and had to be rediscovered. There is a remarkable number of results in general relativity that were found twice or even more times, highlighting its fragility as a field and as a tradition. Still, neither the renaissance nor the Golden Age would have been possible without the broad basis for general relativity that was built during the formative years. This basis encompasses the early work of astronomers and mathematicians, the philosophical struggles surrounding its interpretation, the first efforts to integrate Einstein's ideas into the larger field of physics, the first textbooks elaborating the theory, and the attempts to make it accessible to the next generation. All of these achievements made the later flourishing of general relativity possible.

The basic ideas and mathematical equations of general relativity had emerged with Einstein's work early in the twentieth century. As we have extensively discussed, the establishment of the new theory was itself the result of a process of knowledge reorganization in which not only Einstein but a small community of collaborators and competitors were involved. Yet in 1915, when Einstein published the field equation of general relativity, it was not yet a scientific paradigm in the sense that it provided a guiding framework for a community of practitioners. Not only did an epistemic community practicing it not yet exist, the theory itself had not yet been elaborated into a comprehensive system of knowledge broadly applicable to the physical world. Its range of application was initially limited to a few astronomical phenomena, such as the perihelion anomaly of Mercury or the deflection of light in a gravitational field. Many of its conceptual implications remained unexplored, in particular those that were in conflict with the knowledge system of classical physics from which it was built. Only gradually did general relativity emerge as a universally applicable conceptual framework profoundly distinct from classical physics. This development was not an achievement of Einstein but of an emergent community—a veritable thought collective in the sense of Ludwik Fleck. It only came to a preliminary completion in the early 1960s.

With the help of network analysis, we can trace both the epistemic and the social dimensions of such a reorganization process of a knowledge system in greater detail.[11] Social networks shape knowledge systems just as much as knowledge systems may in turn trigger, via social networks, the creation of epistemic communities concerned with this knowledge. The result of such a process of self-organization, in which a new system of knowledge emerges alongside an epistemic community practicing it, may indeed be characterized as a "paradigm" (adopting and modifying the notion introduced by Kuhn) in the sense of a unity of practice and practitioners. The relevant paradigm shift, however, is not to be understood as the product of a sudden and unstructured gestalt switch attributable to a single ingenious scientist, as Kuhn initially believed, but of a protracted reorganization of knowledge that is usually a community effort extending over generations.

d. Einsteinian Revolution as a Transformation of Knowledge—Lessons for the Future

We have coauthored four books on the life and science of Albert Einstein. Each of these books focused on one of Einstein's canonical texts, interpreting them within the broader historical and epistemological context of his own scientific odyssey and developments in the scientific arena of the time. The present book places Einstein's science in a much broader context, interpreting it as an episode in the evolution of human knowledge. First and foremost, we have attempted to relate the Einstein phenomenon to centuries of previous developments as well as to the science of his time, which affected both its contents and its structure.

We have shown that Einstein's scientific achievements, which are often considered paradigmatic examples of a scientific revolution, can actually be better understood as conceptual transformations of systems of knowledge involving long-term processes. The physicist Freeman Dyson has claimed that such transformations play a less-important role in the history of science than those related to instrumental or tool-driven innovations, such as those that have shaped the history of modern astronomy since the invention of the telescope or the new experimental techniques that enabled molecular biology or modern materials science.[12] Such a distinction between tool-driven and conceptual transformations of science is, however, hardly absolute. Einstein emphasized, particularly in his later years, "that the concept is the primary thing. That you have to find the right concept and that the rightness of the concept will reveal itself in . . . the logical simplicity of the theory to which it leads." He quoted from Goethe's *Faust*, when Faust criticized his assistant, whose approach is more like that of an experimental physicist:

"And what she (nature) won't reveal to your spirit, you do not force from her with levers and screws."[13] But, as the Nobel prize winning physicist Rainer Weiss rightly remarked: "If only Goethe could have lived through our centuries and noted the number of beautiful ideas that have fallen away as they did not conform to the way nature showed herself when really asked by experiment."[14] Indeed, beautiful theories can be killed by ugly facts, as John Stachel once put it succinctly; they are not plucked from some platonic heaven but take a long time to reach the maturity that can only be achieved in an ongoing dialogue with nature. A clear example for a beautiful theory killed by an ugly fact in our context is Einstein's abandonment of his theory of the static universe—and of the cosmological constant—enforced by the improvement of observational techniques that enabled Hubble and his collaborators to correlate the distances and redshift of galaxies and thus to provide evidence for the expansion of the universe.

As we have suggested in this book, conceptual changes are also often rooted in changes in practice. Thus, Einstein's science developed within the context of important technological and industrial changes, most notably in the field of electrotechnology but also in the interrelated fields of chemistry and thermodynamics.[15] These fields constituted the material "working worlds" behind Einstein's science and its conceptual transformations.[16] But also later experiments, observations, and measurements played a significant role in the long history of general relativity. This history was thus, at the same time, characterized by experimental and observational progress and by conceptual developments that transformed existing empirical knowledge into a new theoretical framework that only then opened up the possibility for new empirical tests and observations.

Though Einstein's construction of general relativity was a monumental achievement, one should not be deluded into believing that the entire theory as we know it today emerged fully shaped from Einstein's mind in 1915. As we have argued in this book, Einstein's work was only the beginning of the "long relativity revolution."[17]

Nowhere is this more obvious than for the case of gravitational waves. A large gap separates the actual prediction and ultimate discovery of gravitational waves from Einstein's first feeble and *necessarily inconclusive* musings on the subject. As we have argued, it was only after World War II that general relativity gradually became suffused with empirical content, going far beyond the three traditional tests. Only then was the technology sufficiently advanced to test general relativistic effects with great precision, from the terrestrial test of gravitational redshift between 1959 and 1965 to the spectacular direct detection of gravitational waves in 2016.

Daniel Kennefick has masterfully explored the further development of the gravitational wave issue after Einstein,[18] but much remains to be understood of how—through developments in theory, observation, and experiment—general relativity came to be the empirically rich theory we know today. That story begins with and builds on Einstein's work but was not yet, not even implicitly, contained within it. The history of empirical tests of general relativity is, like its conceptual history that is foregrounded here, full of unexpected twists and turns as well as heroic achievements. One such achievement is Robert Dicke's proposal for a systematic program to test general relativity on the background of his development of a viable alternative theory. This story has been told in a contribution to a recent volume entirely dedicated to the empirical tests of general relativity.[19]

Furthermore, Einstein's science emerged within a classical disciplinary organization of science that fostered the development of specialized expert knowledge but not necessarily its integration across disciplinary boundaries. Crossing these boundaries was, in contrast, a hallmark of Einstein's breakthroughs, as we have emphasized. This crossing of boundaries was enabled by his broad overview of physics, his philosophical acumen, his singularly inquisitive mind, his readiness to challenge established views, his community of like-minded friends, and certainly also some fortunate circumstances, such as the scientific knowledge handed down by the masters of classical physics and codified in textbooks making this knowledge available also to someone working at the margins of the academic community. This capability to look beyond the disciplinary confines makes Einstein stand out as a singular figure, both then, among his contemporaries, and now.

Today we often still think in terms of this disciplinary view of science. It is so ingrained that we can hardly imagine how science could ever have functioned without being guided by its criteria and values. Disciplinary structures shape academic education worldwide; they form the basis of much of the institutional organization of science, and they seem to guarantee a competent division of labor within science. But they also create challenges for the integration of fragments of knowledge into a wider perspective.

Einstein did not respect such disciplinary divisions. Here we have shown how his own views and ways of research transcended this rigid structure. For him, such divisions contradicted the very spirit of culture. "Overemphasis of the competitive system and premature specialization on the ground of immediate usefulness, kill the spirit on which all cultural life depends, specialized knowledge included."[20] Nineteenth-century physics itself was divided into subdisciplines. Without Einstein's ability to foster a unifying perspective that traversed their borderlines, he would not have been able to achieve what he accomplished in his miraculous year and his later work.

The division of the world of knowledge into specific disciplines with well-defined borderlines is actually a relatively new development in the history of science, about two hundred years old. Medieval universities were organized around four basic faculties, three of which were used to train professionals—theology cultivated priests, medicine cultivated doctors, and jurisprudence cultivated judges and lawyers. Basic education rested on the seven liberal arts—grammar, rhetoric, dialectics, arithmetic, geometry, astronomy, and music—from which, by the eighteenth century, the faculty of philosophy emerged, covering everything that is today considered basic science, including the humanities and natural sciences. With the expansion of the scope of knowledge, a process of compartmentalization began, reaching its peak in the twentieth century. This process led to the present-day disciplinary organization of science and the consequent assumption that the unity of science can be achieved by the implicit complementarity of the disciplines. But actually, this is not automatically the case; we still pay too little attention to the integration of the specialized pieces of knowledge into a wider perspective, as envisaged by Einstein in his quest for a scientific worldview.

Today, the disciplinary organization of science is in a state of constant flux. New disciplines and subdisciplines continue to emerge alongside conceptual unifications and the merging of scientific domains. Overcoming borderlines is thus still a vital mechanism of innovation in science. One lesson we can learn from the case of Einstein about the present state of science concerns the elements required for such an integration of knowledge to be successful, most notably, the strengthening of the reflective dimension of science that encompasses an understanding of its historical and philosophical dimensions, education that values a broad overview beyond immediate utility, and a sense of community in which the capacity to preserve *and* question knowledge can be cultivated. This also affects the organization of research and teaching at scientific institutions and the policies of funding bodies.

The role of science has, however, changed in more fundamental ways since Einstein's time, which requires an even more profound rethinking of science. We now realize how science has contributed to changing the planet through its contributions to energy use and the introduction of new materials, mobility, and industrial growth. As we mentioned at the end of section III a great acceleration in all parameters of global human society, in which science has played a pivotal role, has catapulted us into a new geological epoch shaped by the planetary impact of humanity, the Anthropocene. At the same time, science has become ever more relevant to solving the problems of our world: from climate change, biodiversity loss, and the challenges of feeding the global population, to treating diseases, to protecting humankind from ecological hazards as well as from its own self-destructive tendencies. It is unclear whether the traditional organization of science is capable of confronting these challenges.

What is clear is that such challenges cannot be addressed by science and technology alone. Every step and every method applied to cope with these issues, both local and global, have to take into account social, economic, and political considerations, as well as cultural and religious traditions. Thus, in addressing these real-world challenges, the natural sciences are inseparable from the humanities and social sciences. One widespread doctrine is that science and moral values are completely separate domains of reflection. Science is about facts, while ethics is about norms and values. But in the context of the Anthropocene, this rigid separation has become problematic because scientific choices tend, ever more, to involve moral decisions, while ethical reflections often require deep reflections on scientific issues. The key role of science in modern warfare, the intervention of science in life processes, and science's role in affecting the health of the planet make evident the interdependence and inseparability of scientific and moral judgments. We live in a time that demands enhanced societal responsibility and an increased public role of science and scientists, a role pioneered by Einstein in his struggle for peace and against nuclear armament.[21]

During Einstein's lifetime, the question of the societal role of science was mostly framed as the responsibility of individual scientists, leaving the subsequent applications of their results as an afterthought. But, this responsibility has now moved into the very heart of science, becoming inseparable from its fundamental quest for knowledge, particularly when it comes to questions of humanity's survival within the Anthropocene and the provision of the knowledge required to ensure that survival. Integrating intellectual resources that might enable answers to these challenges necessitates a massively increased collaboration across traditional borders within and beyond academia, as well as a sense of common responsibility for our life on this planet. Einstein embodied this sense of responsibility in an exemplary way.

We cannot predict where such comprehensive collaboration will lead. Nor could we have predicted how the Einsteinian revolution achieved its new conceptions of space, time, matter, gravitation, and radiation from the perspective of classical physics. But we now know the necessary conditions for a transformation of a system of knowledge to occur. The culture of science must value and promote the process of reflection, the spirit of cooperation, and the moral integrity of science, which are more important than academic prestige and competition. Scientists should be conscious of the mutability of knowledge structures, and they should be provided with the means to actively participate in their transformation, with the aim of preserving the living conditions for humanity. Appreciating how much a single person, like Einstein, achieved in science under difficult conditions for reflection and cooperation across its borderlines, we can view the history of his revolution as an encouragement to contribute to a culture of science appropriate to today's challenges.

e. Supplementary Reading

In the introduction we mentioned a number of books related to our presentation. Here is a broader and more comprehensive list of books relevant to various aspects of the subject matter of this book (some of which are already given in the general list of references).

On Einstein's Life and Work

AEA. Albert Einstein Archives Online. Hebrew University of Jerusalem. http://www
.alberteinstein.info.

Beller, Mara. *Quantum Dialogue: The Making of a Revolution*. Chicago: University of
Chicago Press, 1999.

Beller, Mara, Robert S. Cohen, and Jürgen Renn, eds. *Einstein in Context*. Vol. 6 of
Science in Context. Cambridge: Cambridge University Press, 1993.

Calaprice, Alice, ed. *The New Quotable Einstein*. Rev. ed. Princeton, NJ: Princeton
University Press, 2005.

CPAE. *The Collected Papers of Albert* Einstein: https://einsteinpapers.press.princeton
.edu.

Dongen, Jeroen van. *Einstein's Unification*. Cambridge: Cambridge University Press, 2010.

Einstein, Albert. *Einstein's Annalen Papers: The Complete Collection 1901–1922*. Edited by Jürgen Renn. Berlin: Wiley-VCH, 2005.

Eisenstaedt, Jean. *The Curious History of Relativity: How Einstein's Theory of Gravity Was Lost and Found Again*. Princeton: Princeton University Press, 2006.

Fölsing, Albrecht. *Albert Einstein: A Biography*. Translated by Ewald Osers. New York: Viking, 1997.

Galison, Peter. *Einstein's Clocks, Poincaré's Maps: Empires of Time*. New York: W. W. Norton, 2003.

Galison, Peter L., Gerald Holton, and Silvan S. Schweber, eds. *Einstein for the 21st Century: His Legacy in Science, Art, and Modern Culture*. Princeton: Princeton University Press, 2008.

Hoffmann, Dieter. *Einstein's Berlin: In the Footsteps of a Genius*. Baltimore: Johns Hopkins University Press, 2013.

Howard, Don. *Albert Einstein: Physicist, Philosopher, Humanitarian* (DVD). The Teaching Company, 2008.

Howard, Don, and John Stachel, eds. *Einstein Studies*, 16 Vols. New York: Birkhäuser, 1989–2005.

Illy, József. *The Practical Einstein: Experiments, Patents, Inventions*. Baltimore MD: Johns Hopkins University Press, 2013.

Isaacson, Walter. *Einstein: His Life and Universe*. New York: Simon & Schuster, 2007.

Janssen, Michel, and Christoph Lehner, eds. *The Cambridge Companion to Einstein*. Cambridge: Cambridge University Press, 2014.

Kennefick, Daniel. *Traveling at the Speed of Thought: Einstein and the Quest for Gravitational Waves*. Princeton: Princeton University Press, 2007.

Neffe, Jürgen. *Einstein: A Biography*. New York: Farrar, Straus and Giroux, 2007.

Renn, Jürgen, ed. *The Genesis of General Relativity*, 4 Vols. Boston Studies in the Philosophy of Science, Vol. 250. Dordrecht: Springer, 2007.

Renn, Jürgen, and Robert Schulmann, eds. *Albert Einstein—Mileva Marić: The Love Letters*. Princeton: Princeton University Press, 1992.

Rowe, David, and Robert Schulmann, eds. *Einstein on Politics: His Private Thoughts and Public Stands on Nationalism, Zionism, War, Peace, and the Bomb*. Princeton: Princeton University Press, 2007.

Stachel, John. *Einstein from 'B' to 'Z.'* Vol. 9 of *Einstein Studies*. Boston: Birkhäuser, 2002.

Stachel, John, ed. *Einstein's Miraculous Year: Five Papers That Changed the Face of Physics*. 2nd ed. Princeton: Princeton University Press, 2005.

Staley, Richard. *Einstein's Generation: The Origins of the Relativity Revolution*. Princeton: Princeton University Press, 2008.

Thorne, Kip. *Black Holes & Time Warps: Einstein's Outrageous Legacy*. New York: W. W. Norton, 1994.

Wazeck, Milena. *Einstein's Opponents*. Cambridge: Cambridge University Press, 2013.

Will, Clifford M. *Was Einstein Right? Putting General Relativity to the Test*. New York: Basic Books, 1986.

More Recent Publications

Buchwald, Jed. Z., ed. *Einstein Was Right: The Science and History of Gravitational Waves*. Princeton: Princeton University Press, 2020

Darrigol, Olivier. *Relativity Principles and Theories from Galileo to Einstein*. Oxford: Oxford University Press, 2022.

DeWitt, Cécile M., and Dean Rickles, eds. *The Role of Gravitation in Physics. Report from the 1957 Chapel Hill Conference*. Berlin: Edition Open Access, 2017, https://edition-open-sources.org/sources/5/index.html.

Duncan, Anthony, and Michel Janssen. *Constructing Quantum Mechanics*. Vol. 1, *The Scaffold: 1900–1923*. Oxford: Oxford University Press, 2019.

Duncan, Anthony, and Michel Janssen. *Constructing Quantum Mechanics*. Vol. 2, *The Arch: 1923–1927*. Oxford: Oxford University Press, 2023.

Engler, Fynn Ole, Mathias Iven, and Jürgen Renn, eds. *Albert Einstein / Moritz Schlick: Briefwechsel*. Vol. 754, Philosophische Bibliothek. Hamburg: Meiner, 2022.

Gordin, Michael D. *Einstein in Bohemia*. Princeton: Princeton University Press, 2020.

Janssen, Michel, and Jürgen Renn. *How Einstein Found His Field Equations: Sources and Interpretation*. Cham, Switzerland: Birkhäuser/Springer, 2022.

Kennefick, Daniel. *No Shadow of a Doubt: The 1919 Eclipse That Confirmed Einstein's Theory of Relativity*. Princeton: Princeton University Press, 2019.

Rosenkranz, Ze'ev, ed. *The Travel Diaries of Albert Einstein: The Far East, Palestine, and Spain, 1922–1923*. Princeton: Princeton University Press, 2018.

Rosenkranz, Ze'ev, ed. *The Travel Diaries of Albert Einstein: South America, 1925*. Princeton: Princeton University Press, 2023.

Ryckmann, Thomas. *Einstein*. London: Routledge, 2017.

Stone, Douglas. *Einstein and the Quantum: The Quest of the Valiant Swabian*. Princeton: Princeton University Press, 2016.

On the Renaissance of Relativity

Blum, Alexander S., Domenico Giulini, Roberto Lalli, and Jürgen Renn. "The Renaissance of Einstein's Theory of Gravitation." Special issue, *European Physical Journal H* (2017) 42:95–105.

Blum, Alexander S., Roberto Lalli, and Jürgen Renn, eds. *The Renaissance of General Relativity in Context*. Vol. 16 of *Einstein Studies*. Cham: Switzerland: Birkhäuser/Springer, 2020.

Eisenstaedt, Jean. *The Curious History of Relativity: How Einstein's Theory of Gravity Was Lost and Found Again*. Princeton: Princeton University Press, 2006.

Lalli, Roberto. *Building the General Relativity and Gravitation Community During the Cold War*. SpringerBriefs in History of Science and Technology. Cham, Switzerland: Springer, 2017.

NOTES

Introduction

1. For a detailed analysis of such transformations of knowledge systems from the perspectives of a historical epistemology and an evolutionary theory of knowledge, see Jürgen Renn, *The Evolution of Knowledge: Rethinking Science for the Anthropocene* (Princeton: Princeton University Press, 2020).

2. Thomas Kuhn, *The Structure of Scientific Revolutions* (Chicago: University of Chicago Press, 1962).

3. Jürgen Renn and Robert Rynasiewicz, "Einstein's Copernican Revolution," in *The Cambridge Companion to Einstein*, ed. Michel Janssen and Christoph Lehner (Cambridge: Cambridge University Press, 2014), pp. 38–71.

4. Jürgen Renn, "Einstein as a Disciple of Galileo: A Comparative Study of Concept Development in Physics," special issue, *Einstein in Context*, ed. Mara Beller, Robert S. Cohen and Jürgen Renn, pp. 311–41(Cambridge: Cambridge University Press, 1993).

5. Hanoch Gutfreund and Jürgen Renn, *The Formative Years of Relativity: The History and Meaning of Einstein's Princeton Lectures* (Princeton: Princeton University Press, 2017).

6. See Jean Eisenstaedt, "The Low Water Mark of General Relativity: 1925–1955," in *Einstein and the History of General Relativity*, ed. Don Howard and John Stachel, vol. 1 of *Einstein Studies* (Basel, Switzerland: Birkhäuser, 1989), pp. 277–92; and Jean Eisenstaedt, *The Curious History of Relativity: How Einstein's Theory of Gravity Was Lost and Found Again* (Princeton: Princeton University Press, 2006).

I. The Einstein Phenomenon

1. Kuhn, *Structure of Scientific Revolutions*, p. 12.

2. Albert Einstein, *Autobiographical Notes: A Centennial Edition* (La Salle, IL: Open Court, 1979), p. 5.

3. Einstein, *Autobiographical Notes*, pp. 3, 5; Hanoch Gutfreund and Jürgen Renn, *Einstein on Einstein: Autobiographical and Scientific Reflections* (Princeton: Princton University Press, 2020), p. 157.

4. Albert Einstein, *Matura* Examination (B) French: "My Future Plans," in CPAE 1, Doc. 22.

5. Einstein to Caesar Koch, Summer 1895, in CPAE 1, Doc. 6.

6. Tilman Sauer, "Marcel Grossmann and His Contribution to the General Theory of Relativity," In *Proceedings of the Thirteenth Marcel Grossmann Meeting on General Relativity*, pp. 456–503 (World Scientific, 2015).

7. Jürgen Renn and Robert Schulmann, eds., *Albert Einstein—Mileva Marić: The Love Letters* (Princeton: Princeton University Press, 1992).

8. Michel Janssen and Jürgen Renn, *How Einstein Found His Field Equations: Sources and Interpretation* (Cham, Switzerland: Birkhäuser/Springer, 2022).

9. Einstein to Arnold Sommerfeld, 29 October 1912, in CPAE 5, Doc. 421.

10. Ernst G. Straus, "Reminiscences," in *Albert Einstein, Historical and Cultural Perspectives*, ed. Gerald J. Holton and Yehuda Elkana (Princeton: Princeton University Press, 1982), p. 422.

11. Michel Janssen, Jürgen Renn, John Norton, Tilman Sauer, and John Stachel, *Einstein's Zurich Notebook: Introduction and Source*, vol. 1 of *The Genesis of General Relativity* (Dordt: Springer, 2007); Michel Janssen, Jürgen Renn, John Norton, Tilman Sauer, and John Stachel, *Einstein's Zurich Notebook: Commentary and Essays*, vol. 2 of *The Genesis of General Relativity* (Dordt: Springer, 2007).

12. Einstein, "The Formal Foundation of the General Theory of Relativity," in CPAE 6, Doc. 9.

13. Gerald J. Holton, "Who Was Einstein? Why Is He Still So Alive?," in *Einstein for the 21st Century: His Legacy in Science, Art, and Modern Culture*, ed. Peter L. Galison, Gerald Holton, and Silvan S. Schweber (Princeton: Princeton University Press, 2008), p. 4.

14. Holton, "Who Was Einstein?," p. 4.

15. Einstein to Jakob Laub, 17 May 1909, in CPAE 5, Doc. 160. The history of quantum physics and Einstein's contributions to this history is widely discussed in the literature. For a recent, most comprehensive account, see Anthony Duncan and Michel Janssen, *Constructing Quantum Mechanics*. Vol. 1, *The Scaffold: 1900–1923*; Vol 2. *The Arch: 1923–1927* (Oxford: Oxford University Press, 2019, 2023), see also Douglas Stone, *Einstein and the Quantum: The Quest of the Valiant Swabian* (Princeton: Princeton University Press, 2016).

16. Einstein to Michele Besso, 11 August 1916, in CPAE 8, Doc. 250.

17. Albert Einstein, Boris Podolsky, and Nathan Rosen, "Can Quantum-Mechanical Description of Physical Reality Be Considered Complete?," *Physical Review* (1935) 47:10.

18. Einstein, *Autobiographical Notes*, p. 83.

19. Albert Einstein, "Physics and Reality," in *Ideas and Opinions: Based on "Mein Weltbild,"* ed. Carl Seelig (New York: Bonanza Books, 1954), pp. 290–323, here pp. 315–16.

20. Don Howard, "Time for a Moratorium? Isaacson, Einstein, and the Challenge of Scientific Biography," *Journal of Historical Biography* (2008) 3:124–33, here p. 124.

II. Ideas on Progress and Revolutions in Science

1. Renn and Rynasiewicz, "Einstein's Copernican Revolution," p. 38.

2. Isaac Newton, "Letter from Sir Isaac Newton to Robert Hooke," *Historical Society of Pennsylvania*, https://digitallibrary.hsp.org/index.php/Detail/objects/9792.

3. Michael Friedmann, ed. and trans., *Kant: Metaphysical Foundations of Natural Science* (Cambridge: Cambridge University Press, 2004).

4. Albert Einstein, *The Meaning of Relativity*, 5th ed. (Princeton: Princeton University Press, 1956), p. 2.

5. Gerald J. Holton, *Science and Anti-Science* (Cambridge, MA: Harvard University Press, 1993).

6. This expression is borrowed from Friedrich Nietzsche.

7. Gutfreund and Renn, *Einstein on Einstein*; Gutfreund and Renn, *Formative Years*.

8. Albert Einstein, "Remarks to the Essays Appearing in this Collective Volume," in *Albert Einstein: Philosopher-Scientist*, ed. Paul Arthur Schilpp (La Salle, IL: Open Court; Cambridge: Cambridge University Press, 1949), pp. 683–84.

9. Einstein, *Autobiographical Notes*, p. 13.

10. Albert Einstein, "Remarks on Bertrand Russell's Theory of Knowledge," in *The Philosophy of Bertrand Russell*, ed. Paul Arthur Schilpp (Evanston, IL: Library of Living Philosophers, 1946), p. 279.

11. Einstein, *Autobiographical Notes*, p. 11.

12. Einstein, "Remarks on Bertrand Russell's Theory of Knowledge," p. 287.

13. Einstein, *Autobiographical Notes*, p. 7.

14. Einstein, *Autobiographical Notes*, p. 13.

15. "Alles Begriffliche ist konstruktiv und nicht auf logischem Wege aus dem unmittelbaren Erlebnis ableitbar. Also sind wir im Prinzip auch voellig frei in der Wahl derjenigen Grundbegriffe, auf die wir unsere Darstellung der Welt gruenden. Alles kommt nur darauf an, inwieweit unsere Konstruktion geeignet ist, Ordnung in das anscheinende Chaos der Erlebniswelt hineinzubringen." Albert Einstein, suplementary remarks to *Autobiographical Notes*, unpublished, AEA 2–024.

16. Einstein, "Physics and Reality," p. 292.

17. Einstein, *Autobiographical Notes*, p. 7.

18. Albert Einstein, *Ideas and Opinions: Based on "Mein Weltbild,"* ed. Carl Seelig (New York: Crown, 1954), pp. 25–26.

19. Max Wertheimer, *Productive Thinking* (New York: Harper, 1945), p. 232.

20. Wertheimer, *Productive Thinking*, p. 232.

21. Einstein, "Motives for Research," in CPAE 7, Doc. 7, p. 44.

22. Jeroen van Dongen, *Einstein's Unification* (Cambridge: Cambridge University Press, 2010).

23. Einstein, *Autobiographical Notes*, p. 85.

24. Don Howard, "Einstein and the Development of Twentieth-Century Philosophy of Science," in *The Cambridge Companion to Einstein*, ed. Michel Janssen and Christoph Lehner (Cambridge: Cambridge University Press, 2014), p. 375.

25. Einstein, "Physics and Reality," p. 292.

26. Michel Janssen and Jürgen Renn, "Arch and Scaffold: How Einstein Found His Field Equations," *Physics Today* (2015) 68, no. 11:30–36.

27. Peter Damerow, Gideon Freudenthal, Peter McLaughlin, and Jürgen Renn, *Exploring the Limits of Preclassical Mechanics*, 2nd ed. (New York: Springer-Verlag, 2004); Rivka Feldhay, Jürgen Renn, Matthias Schemmel, and Matteo Valleriani, eds. *Emergence and Expansion of Preclassical Mechanics* (Cham, Switzerland: Springer, 2018).

28. Evangelista Torricelli, *Opera geometrica*, 1644, Florence.

29. See Fynn Ole Engler, Mathias Iven, and Jürgen Renn, eds., *Albert Einstein / Moritz Schlick: Briefwechsel*, vol. 754, Philosophische Bibliothek (Hamburg: Meiner, 2022).

30. Both studies in Boris Hessen, "The Social and Economic Roots of Newton's Principia," in *The Social and Economic Roots of the Scientific Revolution. Texts by Boris Hessen and Henryk Grossmann*, ed. Gideon Freudenthal and Peter McLaughlin, Boston Studies in the Philsophy of Science (Dordt: Springer, 2009).

31. Ludwik Fleck to Moritz Schlick, The Analysis of a Scientific Fact: Outline of a Comparative Epistemology, 5 September 1933, Moritz Schlick Estate, Nord-Holland Archive, inv. No. 100/Fleck-1; Ludwik Fleck, *Genesis and Development of a Scientific Fact*, ed. T. J. Trenn and R. K. Merton (Chicago: University of Chicago Press, 1979), first published in German in 1935 as *Entstehung und Entwicklung einer wissenschaftlichen Tatsache: Einführung in die Lehre vom Denkstil und Denkkollektiv*. See also Fynn Ole Engler and Jürgen Renn, *Gespaltene Vernunft: Vom Ende eines Dialogs zwischen Wissenschaft und Philosophie* (Berlin: Mattes & Seitz, 2018).

32. Ludwik Fleck to Moritz Schlick, 5 September 1933. Cited in Fynn Ole Engler and Jürgen Renn, "Two Encounters," in *Shifting Paradigms: Thomas S. Kuhn and the History of Science*, ed. A. Blum, K. Gavroglu, C. Joas, and J. Renn (Berlin: Edition Open Access, 2016), p. 140–41.

33. Mara Beller, *Quantum Dialogue: The Making of a Revolution* (Chicago: University of Chicago Press, 1999).

34. Beller, *Quantum Dialogue*, p. 301.

35. Beller, *Quantum Dialogue*, p. 306.

36. Albert Einstein, *Relativity: The Special and the General Theory—100th Anniversary Edition*, ed. Hanoch Gutfreund and Jürgen Renn (Princteon: Princeton University Press, 2015), p. 91.

III. The Continents of Classical Physics and the Problems at Their Borders

1. Einstein, *Autobiographical Notes*, p. 19.

2. Einstein, "Physics and Reality," pp. 304–5.

3. Einstein, *Autobiographical Notes*, p. 31.

4. Einstein, *Autobiographical Notes*, p. 23.

5. Einstein, "On the Electrodynamics of Moving Bodies," in CPAE 2, Doc. 23.

6. Einstein, *Autobiographical Notes*, p. 19.

7. Daniel Greenberger, ed., *Compendium of Quantum Physics: Concepts, Experiments, History and Philosophy* (Berlin: Springer, 2009), p. 615.

8. For a historical discussion of the notion of classical physics, see Richard Staley, "Worldviews and Physicists' Experience of Disciplinary Change: On the Uses of 'Classical' Physics," *Studies in History and Philosophy of Science* (2008) Part A 39, no. 3:298–311; see also Richard Staley, *Einstein's Generation: The Origins of the Relativity Revolution* (Chicago: University of Chicago Press, 2008).

9. Max Planck, "The Genesis and Present State of Development of the Quantum Theory, Nobel lecture, 2 June 1920," in *Nobel Lectures: Physics, 1901–1921*, ed. Nobel Foundation (Amsterdam: Elsevier, 1967), p. 407.

10. Max Planck to Einstein, 6 July 1907, in CPAE 5, Doc. 47. Emphasis in original.

IV. Classical Physics Put Back on Its Feet—The Miraculous Year

1. Banesh Hoffmann and Helen Dukas, *Albert Einstein: Creator and Rebel* (London: Hart-Davis, MacGibbon, 1973), p. 12.

2. CPAE 2, Docs. 3, 4, 5. The following discussion of these papers closely follows the account in Gutfreund and Renn, *Einstein on Einstein*, p. 65f.

3. For a discussion of this issue, see Jürgen Renn, "Einstein's Controversy with Drude and the Origin of Statistical Mechanics: A New Glimpse from the 'Love Letters,'" *Archive for History of Exact Sciences* (1997) 51.

4. Einstein, *Autobiographical Notes*, p. 45.

5. Einstein to Mileva Marić, 13[?] September 1900, in CPAE 1, Doc. 75.

6. Einstein to Mileva Marić, 30 April 1901, in CPAE 1, Doc. 102.

7. Einstein to Marcel Grossmann, 6? September 1901, in CPAE 1, Doc. 122.

8. Einstein, *Autobiographical Notes*, p. 19.

9. Albert Einstein, "Kinetic Theory of Thermal Equilibrium and of the Second Law of Thermodynamics," in CPAE 2, Doc. 3, p. 30.

10. See discussion of this point in Martin J. Klein, "Fluctuations and Statistical Physics in Einstein's Early Work," in *Albert Einstein, Historical and Cultural Perspectives*, p. 39.

11. Einstein to Michele Besso, 22? January 1903, in CPAE 5, Doc. 5.

12. Einstein, "On the General Molecular Theory of Heat," in CPAE 2, Doc. 5, p. 77.

13. Einstein to Conrad Habicht, 15 April 1904, in CPAE 5, Doc. 18.

14. Einstein to Conrad Habicht, 18 or 25 May 1905, in CPAE 5, Doc. 27.

15. Einstein, "On a Heuristic Point of View," in CPAE 2, Doc. 14.

16. Einstein, "A New Determination of Molecular Dimensions," PhD dissertation, 1905, in CPAE 2, Doc. 15.

17. Einstein, "On the Movement of Small Particles Suspended in Stationary Liquids Required by the Molecular-Kinetic Theory of Heat," in CPAE 2, Doc. 16.

18. Einstein, "On the Movement of Small Particles," in CPAE 2, Doc. 16.

19. Einstein, "On the Electrodynamics of Moving Bodies," in CPAE 2, Doc. 23.

20. Einstein to Conrad Habicht, 30 June–22 September, 1905, in CPAE 5, Doc. 28.

21. Einstein, "On the Movement of Small Particles," in CPAE 2, Doc. 16.

22. Klein, "Fluctuations and Statistical Physics in Einstein's Early Work," p. 47. Emphasis in original.

23. Einstein to Johannes Stark, 7 December 1907, in CPAE 5, Doc. 66.

24. Einstein, "On the Thermodynamic Theory of the Difference in Potentials between Metals and Fully Dissociated Solutions of their Salts and on an Electrical Method for Investigating Molecular Forces," in CPAE 2, Doc. 2.

25. Einstein, "A New Determination of Molecular Dimensions," in CPAE 2, Doc. 15.

26. Reprinted and discussed in John Stachel, ed., *Einstein's Miraculous Year: Five Papers That Changed the Face of Physics*, 2nd ed. (Princeton: Princeton University Press, 2005), pp. 85–98.

27. Einstein, "On the Movement of Small Particles," in CPAE 2, Doc. 16.

28. Einstein to Jean Perrin, 11 November 1909, in CPAE 5, Doc. 186. On the scientific work of Jean Perrin, see Mary Jo Nye. *Molecular Reality: A Perspective on the Scientific Work of Jean Perrin* (New York: American Elsevier, 1972).

29. Einstein, *Autobiographical Notes*, p. 47.

30. Arnold Sommerfeld, "To Albert Einstein's Seventieth Birthday," in *Albert Einstein: Philosopher-Scientist*, ed. Paul Arthur Schilpp, Library of Living Philosophers (La Salle, IL: Open Court; Cambridge: Cambridge University Press, 1949), p. 105.

31. Max Born, "Einstein's Statistical Theories," in *Albert Einstein: Philosopher-Scientist*, ed. Paul Arthur Schilpp (La Salle, IL: Open Court; Cambridge: Cambridge University Press, 1949), p. 166.

32. Cathode rays are electrons released from the cathode in a vacuum tube.

33. Einstein to Mileva Marić, 28[?] May 1901, in CPAE 1, Doc. 111.

34. Einstein to Mileva Marić, 10 April 1901, in CPAE 1, Doc. 97.

35. Einstein, *Autobiographical Notes*, p. 43.

36. Einstein to Conrad Habicht, 18 or 25 May 1905, in CPAE 5, Doc. 27.

37. Einstein, "On a Heuristic Point of View," in CPAE 2, Doc. 14, p. 86.

38. Einstein, "On a Heuristic Point of View," in CPAE 2, Doc. 14, p. 86.

39. Einstein, "On a Heuristic Point of View," in CPAE 2, Doc. 14, p. 87.

40. Einstein, "On a Heuristic Point of View," in CPAE 2, Doc. 14, p. 97.

41. Robert A. Millikan, "The Electron and the Light-Quant from the Experimental Point of View," Nobel Lecture, 23 May 1924, https://www.nobelprize.org/prizes/physics/1923/millikan/lecture/. Emphasis in original.

42. Einstein, "On the Present State of the Radiation Problem," in CPAE 2, Doc. 56; "On the Development of Our Views Concerning the Nature and Constitution of Radiation," in CPAE 2, Doc. 60.

43. "Aber 1905 wusste ich schon sicher, dass sie zu falschen Schwankungen des Strahlungsdruckes fuehrt und damit zu einer unrichtigen Brown'schen Bewegung eines Spiegels in einem Planck'schen Strahlungs-Hohlraum. Nach meiner Ansicht kommt man nicht darum herum, der Strahlung eine objektive atomistische Struktur zuzuschreiben, die natuerlich nicht in den Rahmen der Maxwell'schen Theorie hinein passt." Einstein to Max von Laue, 17 January 1952, AEA 16–168. See also Einstein, *Autobiographical Notes*, p. 47.

44. Einstein, "Emission and Absorption of Radiation in Quantum Theory," in CPAE 6, Doc. 34; "On the Quantum Theory of Radiation," in CPAE 6, Doc. 38.

45. Einstein to Michele Besso, 11 August 1916, in CPAE 8, Doc. 250. Emphasis in original.

46. Einstein to Michele Besso, 6 September 1916, in CPAE 8, Doc. 254. Emphasis in original.

47. Arthur H. Compton, "A Quantum Theory of the Scattering of X-rays by Light Elements," *Physical Review* (1923) 21, no. 5:483–502, 483.

48. "Die ganzen 50 Jahre bewusster Grübelei haben mich der Antwort der Frage 'Was sind Lichtsystemen' nicht näher gebracht. Heute glaubt zwar jeden Lump, er wisse es, aber er täuscht sich." Einstein to Michele Besso, 12 December 1951, AEA 7–401.

49. Einstein recalls this conversation with Besso in a lecture given at Kyoto University on 14 December 1922, "How I Created the Theory of Relativity," Jun Ishiwara's Notes of Einstein's Lecture at Kyoto University, in CPAE 13, Doc. 399, p. 637.

50. Einstein, "How I Created the Theory of Relativity," p. 637.

51. Einstein, "On the Electrodynamics of Moving Bodies," in CPAE 2, Doc. 23, p. 171.

52. Einstein, "How I Created the Theory of Relativity," p. 637.

53. See for example: Renn and Rynasiewicz, "Einstein's Copernican Revolution"; John Norton, "Einstein's Special Theory of Relativity and the Problems in the Electrodynamics of Moving Bodies That Led Him to It," in *The Cambridge Companion to Einstein*, ed. Michel Janssen and Christoph Lehner (Cambridge: Cambridge University Press, 2014).

54. Gutfreund and Renn, *Einstein on Einstein*, chap. 10.

55. Einstein, *Autobiographical Notes*, p. 49.

56. Einstein, "On the Electrodynamics of Moving Bodies" in CPAE 2, Doc. 23, p. 140.

57. Einstein to Mileva Marić, 28? September 1899, in CPAE 1, Doc. 57; Renn and Schulmann, *Love Letters*.

58. On this point, see for example: Renn and Rynasiewicz, "Einstein's Copernican Revolution," p. 66.

59. Einstein, *Autobiographical Notes*, p. 51; Gutfreund and Renn, *Einstein on Einstein*, p. 171.

60. Einstein to Moritz Schlick, 14 December 1915, in CPAE 8, Doc. 165.

61. Einstein, "On the Electrodynamics of Moving Bodies," in CPAE 2, Doc. 23, p. 141.

62. Einstein, *Autobiographical Notes*, p. 57.

63. Einstein, "Induction and Deduction in Physics," in CPAE 7, Doc. 28, p. 108.

64. Einstein, "Motives for Research," in CPAE 7, Doc. 7, p. 44.

65. Einstein, "Induction and Deduction in Physics," in CPAE 7, Doc. 28, p. 108.

66. Einstein, *Autobiographical Notes*, p. 49.

67. Einstein, *Autobiographical Notes*, p. 85.

68. Paul Ehrenfest, "Über die physikalischen Voraussetzungen der Planck'schen Theorie der irreversiblen Strahlungsvorgange," *Sitzungsberichte der Mathematisch-naturwissenschaftlichen Klasse der Kaiserlichen Akademie der Wissenschaften* (1905) 114, no. 8:1301–14; Josiah Williard Gibbs, *Elementare Grundlagen der Statistischen Mechanik: Entwickelt Besonders im Hinblick auf eine Rationelle Begründung der Thermodynamik* (Leipzig: Barth, 1905); Henri Poincaré, "Sur la Dynamique de L'électron," *Comptes Rendus des Séances de L'académie des Sciences* (1905) 140:1504–8; Marian von Smoluchowski, "Zur Kinetischen Theorie der Brownschen Molekularbewegung und der Suspensionen," *Annalen der Physik* (1906) 21:756–80.

69. Smoluchowski, "Zur Kinetischen Theorie"; William Sutherland, "A Dynamical Theory of Diffusion for Non-Electrolytes and the Molecular Mass of Albumin," *Philosophical Magazine and Journal of Science* (1905) 9:781–85.

70. Janssen and Renn, "Arch and Scaffold"; Duncan and Janssen, *Constructing Quantum Mechanics*, 2 vols.

V. The Road to the General Theory of Relativity

1. Einstein, *Autobiographical Notes*, p. 61.

2. Einstein, *Relativity: The Special and the General Theory—100th Anniversary Edition*, p. 74.

3. Einstein, "How I Created the Theory of Relativity," in CPAE 13, Doc. 399, p. 638.

4. Einstein, "Fundamental Ideas and Methods of the Theory of Relativity, Presented in their Development," in CPAE 7, Doc. 31. p. 136.

5. Einstein, "Fundamental Ideas and Methods," in CPAE 7, Doc. 31. p. 136. Emphasis in original.

6. Clifford M. Will, *Was Einstein Right? Putting General Relativity to the Test* (New York: Basic Books, 1986); Clifford M. Will and Nicolás Yunes, *Is Einstein Still Right? Black Holes, Gravitational Waves, and the Quest to Verify Einstein's Greatest Creation* (Oxford: Oxford University Press, 2020).

7. Einstein, "On the Relativity Principle and the Conclusions Drawn from it," in CPAE 2, Doc. 47.

8. Paul Ehrenfest, "Gleichförmige Rotation starrer Körper und Relativitätstheorie," *Physikalische Zeitschrift* (1909) 10:918; John Stachel, "Einstein and the Rigidly Rotating Disk," in *General Relativity and Gravitation: One Hundred Years after the Birth of Albert Einstein*, ed. Alan Held, 1–15 (New York: Plenum, 1980).

9. "Großmann, Du mußt mir helfen, sonst werd' ich verrückt!" Cited in Louis Kollross, "Erinnerungen eines Kommilitonen," in *Helle Zeiten—Dunkle Zeiten: In Memoriam Albert Einstein*, ed. Carl Seelig (Zurich: Europa Verlag, 1955), p. 27.

10. Einstein to Hendrik A. Lorentz, 16 August 1913, in CPAE 5, Doc. 470, p. 353.

11. Engler, Iven, and Renn, eds., *Albert Einstein / Moritz Schlick*.

12. Einstein, *Relativity: The Special and the General Theory—100th Anniversary Edition*, p. 111.

13. Einstein to Ludwig Hopf, 2 November 1913, in CPAE 5, Doc. 480, p. 358.

14. Einstein to Michele Besso, 10 March 1914, in CPAE 5, Doc. 514, p. 382.

15. Einstein and Marcel Grossmann, "Covariance Properties of the Field Equations of the Theory of Gravitation Based on the Generalized Theory of Relativity," in CPAE 6, Doc. 2.

16. Michel Janssen and Jürgen Renn, "Einstein and the Perihelion Motion of Mercury," *arXiv*, arXiv:2111.11238, 2021.

17. Janssen and Renn, "Arch and Scaffold"; Duncan and Janssen, *Constructing Quantum Mechanics*, 2 vols.

18. Einstein, "On the General Theory of Relativity," in CPAE 6, Doc. 21, p. 98.

19. Einstein, "On the General Theory of Relativity," in CPAE 6, Doc. 21, p. 98.

20. Einstein, "On the General Theory of Relativity," in CPAE 6, Doc. 21, p. 102.

21. Einstein to Arnold Sommerfeld, 28 November 1915, in CPAE 8, Doc. 153. Cited in Janssen and Renn, *How Einstein Found His Field Equations*, p. 41.

22. Einstein, "On the General Theory of Relativity (Addendum)," in CPAE 6, Doc. 22, p. 108.

23. "Toen hij in 1915 de seculaire beweging van het perihelium van Mercurius berekend had, en zag dat de uitkomst klopte met de onverklaarde rest der astronomen, toen, zei hij mij later, kreeg hij er fysieke hartkloppingen van." Adriaan

Fokker, "Albert Einstein. 14 Maart 1878–18 April 1955," *Nederlands Tijdschrift voor Natuurkunde* (1955) 21:125–29, p. 1\\\\

24. David Hilbert to Einstein, 19 November 1915, in CPAE 8, Doc. 149, p. 149.

25. Dongen, *Einstein's Unification.*

26. Einstein, "On the General Theory of Relativity," in CPAE 6, Doc. 21, p. 98. The names are capitalized in the original publication.

27. Einstein, "The Foundation of General Theory of Relativity," in CPAE 6, Doc. 30, p. 146.

28. Kip S. Thorne, *Black Holes & Time Warps: Einstein's Outrageous Legacy* (New York: W. W. Norton, 1994), p. 117.

29. Einstein to Arnold Sommerfeld, 9 December 1915, in CPAE 8, Doc 161.

30. Gutfreund and Renn, *Formative Years.*

31. Einstein to Hendrik A. Lorentz, 17 January 1916, in CPAE 8, Doc. 183, p. 179.

32. Einstein, "The Foundation of General Relativity," in CPAE 6, Doc. 30, p. 154.

33. Erich Kretschmann, "Über den Physikalischen Sinn der Relativitätspostulate, A. Einsteins neue und seine ursprüngliche Relativitätstheorie," *Annalen der Physik* 358 (1918); translated in John Norton, "Did Einstein Stumble? The Debate over General Covariance," in *Reflections on Spacetime: Foundations, Philosophy, History*, ed. U. Majer and H.-J. Schmidt (Dordt: Kluwer Academic, 1995), p. 228.

34. Einstein "On the Foundations of the General Theory of Relativity," in CPAE 7, Doc. 4, pp. 33–34.

35. Einstein, "On the Foundations of the General Theory of Relativity," in CPAE 7, Doc. 4, p. 34.

36. Élie Cartan, "Sur les varietes a connexion affine et la theorie de la relativitee generalisee (premiere partie)," *Annales scientific de l'E.N.S.* (1923) 3:325–412.

37. Einstein, *Meaning of Relativity*, p. 57.

38. Einstein, *Meaning of Relativity*, pp. 57–58. Cited in Gutfreund and Renn, *Formative Years*, pp. 38–39, 217–18.

39. Einstein, *Meaning of Relativity*, p. 58.

40. Einstein, "Ernst Mach," in CPAE 6, Doc. 29, p. 144.

41. Willem de Sitter to Einstein, 1 November 1916, in CPAE 8, Doc. 272.

42. Einstein to Willem de Sitter, 4 November 1916, in CPAE 8, Doc. 273.

43. Einstein, "Cosmological Considerations in the General Theory of Relativity," in CPAE 6, Doc. 43, p. 424. Emphasis in original.

44. Einstein, "Cosmological Considerations," in CPAE 6, Doc. 43, p. 425.

45. Einstein to Emperor Karl I, 1917, AEA 91–157. See Gutfreund and Renn, *Formative Years*, pp. 72–74.

46. Einstein, "Cosmological Considerations," in CPAE 6, Doc. 43, p. 432.

47. Einstein to Willem de Sitter, 24 March 1917, in CPAE 8, Doc. 317, p. 309. Emphasis in original.

48. Willem de Sitter to Einstein, 1 April 1917, in CPAE 8, Doc. 321, p. 313. Emphasis in original.

49. Albert Einstein, "Fundamental Ideas and Problems of the Theory of Relativity," in *Les Prix Nobel en 1921–1922*, ed. C. G. Santesson (Stockholm: Nobel Foundation, 1923), p. 489.

50. "Von dem Mach'schen Prinzip aber sollte man nach meiner Meinung überhaupt nicht mehr sprechen. Es stammt aus der Zeit, in der man dachte, dass die 'ponderabeln Körper' das einzige physikalisch Reale seien, und dass alle nicht durch sie völlig bestimmten Elemente in der Theorie wohl bewusst vermieden werden sollten. (Ich bin mir der Tatsache wohl bewusst, dass auch ich lange Zeit durch diese fixe Idee beeinflusst war)." Einstein to Felix Pirani, 2 February 1954, AEA 17–447.

VI. The Einsteinian Revolution as a Transformation of a System of Knowledge

1. Matthias Schemmel, "The Continuity between Classical and Relativistic Cosmology in the Work of Karl Schwarzschild," in *Gravitation in the Twilight of Classical Physics: The Promise of Mathematics*, ed. Jürgen Renn and Matthias Schemmel, 155–181, vol. 4 of *The Genesis of General Relativity* (Dordt: Springer, 2007).

2. Daniel Kennefick, *Traveling at the Speed of Thought: Einstein and the Quest for Gravitational Waves* (Princeton: Princeton University Press, 2007).

3. Daniel Kennefick, *No Shadow of a Doubt: The 1919 Eclipse That Confirmed Einstein's Theory of Relativity* (Princeton: Princeton University Press, 2019).

4. Jean Eisenstaedt, "The Early Interpretation of the Schwarzschild Solution," in *Einstein and the History of General Relativity*, ed. Don Howard and John Stachel, 1–213 (Boston: Birkhäuser, 1989); "De L'influence de la Gravitation sur la Propagation de la Lumière en Théorie Newtonienne: L'archéologie des Trous Noirs," *Archive for History of Exact Sciences* (1991) 42:315–86.

5. Eisenstaedt, "Low Water Mark of General Relativity."

6. See Will, *Was Einstein Right?*, pp. 3–18.

7. Bernard Schutz, "Intuition in Einsteinian Physics," in *Teaching Einsteinian Physics in Schools: An Essential Guide for Teachers in Training and Practice*, ed. M. Kersting and D. Blair (Oxford: Routledge 2021).

8. Joseph Weber, "Evidence for Discovery of Gravitational Radiation," *Physical Review Letters* (1969) 22:1320–24. For historical discussion, see Alexander S. Blum, Roberto Lalli, and Jürgen Renn, "Gravitational Waves and the Long Relativity Revolution," *Nature Astronomy* (2018) 2:534–43, p. 540.

9. Jean Charles Marcel Jacquot, *Les Théâtres D'asie: Études de Jeannine Auboyer [and Others] . . . Réunies et Présentées par Jean Jacquot [Proceedings of the Conférences*

du *Théâtres des Nations, 1958–1959, and of the Journeées D'herétudes de Royaumont, 28 May–1 June 1959]* (Paris: Government Publication, 1961); Cécile M. DeWitt and Dean Rickles, eds., *The Role of Gravitation in Physics: Report from the 1957 Chapel Hill Conference.* (Berlin: Edition Open Access, 2017).

10. Thorne, *Black Holes & Time Warps.*

11. Alexander S. Blum, Domenico Giulini, Roberto Lalli, and Jürgen Renn, "The Renaissance of Einstein's Theory of Gravitation," special issue, *The European Physical Journal H* (2017) 42:95–105; Blum, Lalli, and Renn, "Gravitational Waves and the Long Relativity evolution"; Roberto Lalli, Riaz Howey, and Dirk Wintergrün, "The Socio-Epistemic Networks of General Relativity, 1925–1970," in *The Renaissance of General Relativity in Context,* ed. Alexander S. Blum, Roberto Lalli, and Jürgen Renn, 15–84 (Cham, Switzerland: Birkhäuser/Springer, 2020).

12. Freeman J. Dyson, *The Sun, the Genome and the Internet: Tools of Scientific Revolutions.* (Oxford: Oxford University Press, 1999).

13. Reminiscences of Einstein's Assistant Ernst Straus, in "Working with Einstein," Symposium in Memoriam, Princeton, 1979, AEA 94–860.

14. Personal communication.

15. Angelo Baracca, *Scientific Developments Connected with the Second Industrial Revolution. A. Baracca, S. Ruffo, and A. Russo, Scienza e Industria 1848–1915, 41 years later* (Preprint 508: Max Planck Institute for the History of Science, 2021).

16. Jon Agar, *Science in the Twentieth Century and Beyond* (Cambridge: Polity Press, 2012).

17. See Blum, Lalli, and Renn, "Gravitational Waves and the Long Relativity Revolution," pp. 1–10.

18. Kennefick, *Traveling at the Speed of Thought.*

19. Alexander Blum, Roberto Lalli, Jürgen Renn, "Brans-Dicke Theory and the Empirical Renaissance of General Relativity," in *One Hundred Years of Testing Einstein,* ed. Brian C. Odom and Daniel Kennefick (Cambridge MA: MIT Press, forthcoming 2024).

20. Albert Einstein, "Education for Independent Thought," *New York Times,* October 5, 1952.

21. David Rowe and Robert Schulmann, eds., *Einstein on Politics: His Private Thoughts and Public Stands on Nationalism, Zionism, War, Peace, and the Bomb* (Princeton: Princeton University Press, 2007); Albert Einstein, "Atomic War or Peace," *The Atlantic,* November 1947.

REFERENCES

AEA. Albert Einstein Archives Online. Hebrew University of Jerusalem. http://www.alberteinstein.info.

Agar, Jon. *Science in the Twentieth Century and Beyond*. Cambridge: Polity Press, 2012.

Baracca, Angelo. *Scientific Developments Connected with the Second Industrial Revolution. A. Baracca, S. Ruffo, and A. Russo, Scienza e Industria 1848–1915, 41 Years Later*. Preprint 508: Max Planck Institute for the History of Science, 2021. https://www.mpiwg-berlin.mpg.de/preprint/scientific-developments-connected-second-industrial-revolution-baracca-s-ruffo-and-russo.

Beller, Mara. *Quantum Dialogue: The Making of a Revolution*. Chicago: University of Chicago Press, 1999.

Blackwood, Michael, dir. *Working with Einstein*. New York: Michael Blackwood Productions, 1979.

Blum, Alexander S., Domenico Giulini, Roberto Lalli, and Jürgen Renn, eds. "The Renaissance of Einstein's Theory of Gravitation." Special issue, *European Physical Journal H* (2017) 42:95–105.

Blum, Alexander S., Roberto Lalli, Jürgen Renn. "Brans-Dicke Theory and the Empirical Renaissance of General Relativity." In *One Hundred Years of Testing Einstein*, eds. Brian C. Odom and Daniel Kennefick. Cambridge MA: MIT Press, forthcoming 2024.

Blum, Alexander S., Roberto Lalli, and Jürgen Renn. "Gravitational Waves and the Long Relativity Revolution." *Nature Astronomy* (2018) 2:534–43.

Blum, Alexander S., Roberto Lalli, and Jürgen Renn, eds. *The Renaissance of General Relativity in Context*. Vol. 16 of *Einstein Studies*. Cham, Switzerland: Birkhäuser/Springer, 2020.

Born, Max. "Einstein's Statistical Theories." In *Albert Einstein: Philosopher-Scientist*, edited by Paul Arthur Schilpp. La Salle, IL: Open Court; Cambridge: Cambridge University Press, 1949.

Cartan, Élie. "Sur les varietes a connexion affine et la theorie de la relativitee generalisee (premiere partie)." *Annales scientific de l'E.N.S.* (1923) 3:325–412.

Compton, Arthur H. "A Quantum Theory of the Scattering of X-rays by Light Elements." *Physical Review* (1923) 21, no. 5:483–502, 483.

CPAE. The Collected Papers of Albert Einstein, online edition, https://einsteinpapers .press.princeton.edu/.

CPAE 1. *The Collected Papers of Albert Einstein*. Vol. 1, *The Early Years, 1879–1902*, English translation supplement. Princeton: Princeton University Press, 1987, https://einsteinpapers.press.princeton.edu/vol1-trans/.

CPAE 2. *The Collected Papers of Albert Einstein*. Vol. 2, *The Swiss Years: Writings, 1900– 1909*, English translation Supplement. Princeton: Princeton University Press, 1990, https://einsteinpapers.press.princeton.edu/vol2-trans/.

CPAE 5. *The Collected Papers of Albert Einstein*. Vol. 5, *The Swiss Years: Correspondence, 1902–1914*, English translation supplement. Princeton: Princeton University Press, 1995, https://einsteinpapers.press.princeton.edu/vol5-trans/.

CPAE 6. *The Collected Papers of Albert Einstein*. Vol. 6, *The Berlin Years: Writings, 1914–1917*, English translation supplement. Princeton: Princeton University Press, 1997, https://einsteinpapers.press.princeton.edu/vol6-trans/.

CPAE 7. *The Collected Papers of Albert Einstein*. Vol. 7, *The Berlin Years: Writings, 1918–1921*. Princeton: Princeton University Press, 2002, https://einsteinpapers .press.princeton.edu/vol7-doc/.

CPAE 7. *The Collected Papers of Albert Einstein*. Vol. 7, *The Berlin Years: Writings, 1918–1921*, English translation supplement. Princeton: Princeton University Press, 2002, https://einsteinpapers.press.princeton.edu/vol7-trans/.

CPAE 8. *The Collected Papers of Albert Einstein*. Vol. 8, *Writings & Correspondence 1914–1918*, English translation supplement. Princeton: Princeton University Press, 1998, https://einsteinpapers.press.princeton.edu/vol8-trans/.

CPAE 13. *The Collected Papers of Albert Einstein*. Vol. 13, *The Berlin Years: Writings & Correspondence January 1922–March 1923*. Princeton: Princeton University Press, 2013, https://einsteinpapers.press.princeton.edu/vol13-doc/.

Damerow, Peter, Gideon Freudenthal, Peter McLaughlin, and Jürgen Renn. *Exploring the Limits of Preclassical Mechanics*. 2nd ed. New York: Springer-Verlag, 2004.

DeWitt, Cécile M., and Dean Rickles, eds. *The Role of Gravitation in Physics. Report from the 1957 Chapel Hill Conference*. Berlin: Edition Open Access, 2017, https:// edition-open-sources.org/sources/5/index.html.

Dongen, Jeroen van. *Einstein's Unification*. Cambridge: Cambridge University Press, 2010.

Duncan, Anthony, and Michel Janssen. *Constructing Quantum Mechanics*. Vol. 1, *The Scaffold: 1900–1923*. Oxford: Oxford University Press, 2019.

Duncan, Anthony, and Michel Janssen. *Constructing Quantum Mechanics*. Vol. 2, *The Arch: 1923–1927*. Oxford: Oxford University Press, 2023.

Dyson, Freeman J. *The Sun, the Genome and the Internet: Tools of Scientific Revolutions*. Oxford: Oxford University Press, 1999.

Ehrenfest, Paul. "Gleichförmige Rotation starrer Körper und Relativitätstheorie," *Physikalische Zeitschrift* (1909) 10:918.

Ehrenfest, Paul. "Über die Physikalischen Voraussetzungen der Planck'schen Theorie der Irreversiblen Strahlungsvorgange," *Sitzungsberichte der Mathematisch-naturwissenschaftlichen Klasse der Kaiserlichen Akademie der Wissenschaften* (1905) 114:1301–14.

Einstein, Albert. *Autobiographical Notes: A Centennial Edition.* La Salle, IL: Open Court, 1979.

Einstein, Albert. "Education for Independent Thought." *New York Times*, October 5, 1952.

Einstein, Albert. "Fundamental Ideas and Problems of the Theory of Relativity." In *Les Prix Nobel En 1921–1922*, edited by C. G. Santesson, 482–90. Stockholm: Nobel Foundation, 1923.

Einstein, Albert. *Ideas and Opinions: Based on "Mein Weltbild."* Edited by Carl Seelig. New York: Crown, 1954.

Einstein, Albert. *The Meaning of Relativity.* 5th ed. Princeton: Princeton University Press, 1956.

Einstein, Albert. "Physics and Reality." In *Ideas and Opinions: Based on "Mein Weltbild,"* edited by Carl Seelig, 290–323. New York: Bonanza Books, 1954.

Einstein, Albert. *Relativity: The Special and the General Theory—100th Anniversary Edition.* With commentaries and background material by Hanoch Gutfreund and Jürgen Renn. Princeton: Princeton University Press, 2015.

Einstein, Albert. "Remarks on Bertrand Russell's Theory of Knowledge." In *The Philosophy of Bertrand Russell*, edited by Paul Arthur Schilpp, 279–91. Evanston, IL: Library of Living Philosophers, 1946.

Einstein, Albert. "Remarks to the Essays Appearing in This Collective Volume." In *Albert Einstein: Philosopher-Scientist*, edited by Paul Arthur Schilpp, 663–88. La Salle, IL: Open Court; Cambridge: Cambridge University Press 1949.

Einstein, Albert, and Max Born. "Einstein an Max Born, 3. März 1947." In *Albert Einstein Und Max Born, Briefwechsel 1916–1955.* Munich: Nymphenburger, 1991.

Einstein, Albert, Boris Podolsky, and Nathan Rosen. "Can Quantum-Mechanical Description of Physical Reality Be Considered Complete?" *Physical Review* (1935) 47 no. 10:777–80.

Eisenstaedt, Jean. *The Curious History of Relativity: How Einstein's Theory of Gravity Was Lost and Found Again.* Princeton: Princeton University Press, 2006.

Eisenstaedt, Jean. "De L'influence de la Gravitation sur la Propagation de la Lumière en Théorie Newtonienne: L'archéologie des Trous Noirs." *Archive for History of Exact Sciences* (1991) 42:315–86.

Eisenstaedt, Jean. "The Low Water Mark of General Relativity: 1925–1955." In *Einstein and the History of General Relativity*, edited by Don Howard and John Stachel, vol. 1 of *Einstein Studies*, 277–92. Basel, Switzerland: Birkhäuser, 1989.

Engler, Fynn Ole, Mathias Iven, and Jürgen Renn, eds. *Albert Einstein / Moritz Schlick: Briefwechsel.* Vol. 754, Philosophische Bibliothek. Hamburg: Meiner, 2022.

Engler, Fynn Ole, and Jürgen Renn. *Gespaltene Vernunft: Vom Ende eines Dialogs zwischen Wissenschaft und Philosophie.* Berlin: Mattes & Seitz, 2018.

Engler, Fynn Ole, and Jürgen Renn. "Two Encounters." In *Shifting Paradigms: Thomas S. Kuhn and the History of Science,* ed. A. Blum, K. Gavroglu, C. Joas, and J. Renn. Berlin: Edition Open Access, 2016.

Feldhay, Rivka, Jürgen Renn, Matthias Schemmel, and Matteo Valleriani, eds. *Emergence and Expansion of Preclassical Mechanics.* Cham, Switzerland: Springer, 2018.

Feyerabend, Paul. *Against Method.* 4th ed. New York: Verso Books, 2010.

Fleck, Ludwik. *Genesis and Development of a Scientific Fact.* Edited by T. J. Trenn and R. K. Merton. Chicago: Chicago University Press, [1935] 1979.

Fokker, Adriaan. "Albert Einstein. 14 Maart 1878–18 April 1955, " *Nederlands Tijdschrift voor Natuurkunde* (1955) 21:125–29.

Friedmann, Michael, ed. and trans. *Kant: Metaphysical Foundations of Natural Science.* Cambridge: Cambridge University Press, 2004.

Greenberger, Daniel, ed. *Compendium of Quantum Physics: Concepts, Experiments, History and Philosophy.* Berlin: Springer, 2009.

Gutfreund, Hanoch, and Jürgen Renn. *Einstein on Einstein: Autobiographical and Scientific Reflections.* Princeton: Princeton University Press, 2020.

Gutfreund, Hanoch, and Jürgen Renn. *The Formative Years of Relativity: The History and Meaning of Einstein's Princeton Lectures.* Princeton: Princeton University Press, 2017.

Gutfreund, Hanoch, and Jürgen Renn. *The Road to Relativity: The History and Meaning of Einstein's "The Foundation of General Relativity".* Princeton: Princeton University Press, 2015.

Hessen, Boris. "The Social and Economic Roots of Newton's *Principia.*" In *The Social and Economic Roots of the Scientific Revolution. Texts by Boris Hessen and Henryk Grossmann,* edited by Gideon Freudenthal and Peter McLaughlin. Boston Studies in the Philsophy of Science. Dordt: Springer, 2009.

Hoffmann, Banesh, and Helen Dukas. *Albert Einstein: Creator and Rebel.* London: Hart-Davis, MacGibbon, 1973.

Holton, Gerald J. *Science and Anti-Science.* Cambridge, MA: Harvard University Press, 1993.

Holton, Gerald J. "Who Was Einstein? Why Is He Still So Alive?" In *Einstein for the 21st Century: His Legacy in Science, Art, and Modern Culture,* edited by Peter L. Galison, Gerald Holton, and Silvan S. Schweber. Princeton: Princeton University Press, 2008.

Howard, Don. "Einstein and the Development of Twentieth-Century Philosophy of Science." In *The Cambridge Companion to Einstein,* edited by Michel Janssen and Christoph Lehner, 354–76. Cambridge: Cambridge University Press, 2014.

Howard, Don. "Time for a Moratorium? Isaacson, Einstein, and the Challenge of Scientific Biography." *Journal of Historical Biography* (2008) 3:124–33.

Jacquot, Jean Charles Marcel. *Les Théâtres D'asie. Études de Jeannine Auboyer [and Others] . . . Réunies et Présentées par Jean Jacquot [Proceedings of the Conférences du Théâtres des Nations, 1958–1959, and of the Journeées D'herétudes de Royaumont, 28 May–1 June 1959].* Paris: Government Publication, 1961.

Janssen, Michel, and Jürgen Renn. "Arch and Scaffold: How Einstein Found His Field Equations." *Physics Today* (2015) 68, no. 11:30–36.

Janssen, Michel, and Jürgen Renn. *How Einstein Found His Field Equations: Sources and Interpretation.* Cham, Switzerland: Birkhäuser/Springer, 2022.

Janssen, Michel, Jürgen Renn, John Norton, Tilman Sauer, and John Stachel. *The Genesis of General Relativity.* Vol. 1, *Einstein's Zurich Notebook: Introduction and Source.* Dordt: Springer, 2007.

Janssen, Michel, Jürgen Renn, John Norton, Tilman Sauer, and John Stachel. *The Genesis of General Relativity.* Vol. 2, *Einstein's Zurich Notebook: Commentary and Essays.* Dordt: Springer, 2007.

Kennefick, Daniel. *No Shadow of a Doubt: The 1919 Eclipse That Confirmed Einstein's Theory of Relativity.* Princeton: Princeton University Press, 2019.

Kennefick, Daniel. *Traveling at the Speed of Thought: Einstein and the Quest for Gravitational Waves.* Princeton: Princeton University Press, 2007.

Klein, Martin J. "Fluctuations and Statistical Physics in Einstein's Early Work." In *Albert Einstein, Historical and Cultural Perspectives: The Centennial Symposium in Jerusalem,* edited by Gerald J. Holton and Yehuda Elkana, 39–58. Princeton: Princeton University Press, 1982.

Kollross, Louis. "Erinnerungen eines Kommilitonen." In *Helle Zeiten—Dunkle Zeiten: In Memoriam Albert Einstein,* edited by Carl Seelig, 17–31. Zurich: Europa Verlag, 1955.

Kretschmann, Erich. "Über den Physikalischen Sinn der Relativitätspostulate, A. Einsteins Neue Und Seine Ursprüngliche Relativitätstheorie." *Annalen der Physik* (1918) 358:575–614.

Kuhn, Thomas. *The Structure of Scientific Revolutions.* Chicago: University of Chicago Press, 1962.

Lalli, Roberto. *Building the General Relativity and Gravitation Community During the Cold War.* SpringerBriefs in History of Science and Technology. Cham, Switzerland: Springer, 2017.

Millikan, Robert A. "The Electron and the Light-quant from the Experimental Point of View." Nobel Lecture, 23 May 1924, https://www.nobelprize.org/prizes/physics/1923/millikan/lecture/.

Norton, John. "Did Einstein Stumble? The Debate over General Covariance." In *Reflections on Spacetime: Foundations, Philosophy, History,* edited by U. Majer and H.-J. Schmidt, 103–25. Dordt: Kluwer Academic Publishers, 1995.

Norton, John. "Einstein's Special Theory of Relativity and the Problems in the Electrodynamics of Moving Bodies That Led Him to It." In *The Cambridge Companion to Einstein*, edited by Michel Janssen and Christoph Lehner. Cambridge: Cambridge University Press, 2014.

Nye, Mary Jo. *Molecular Reality: A Perspective on the Scientific Work of Jean Perrin.* New York: American Elsevier, 1972.

Planck, Max. "The Genesis and Present State of Development of the Quantum Theory. Nobel Lecture, 2 June 1920." In *Nobel Lectures: Physics, 1901–1921*, edited by Nobel Foundation. Amsterdam: Elsevier, 1967.

Poincaré, Henri. "Sur la Dynamique de L'électron." *Comptes rendus des Séances de L'académie des Sciences* (1905) 140:1504–8.

Regge, Tullio, and John A. Wheeler. "Stability of a Schwarzschild Singularity." *Physical Review* (1957) 108:1063–69.

Renn, Jürgen. "Einstein as a Disciple of Galileo: A Comparative Study of Concept Development in Physics." Special issue, *Einstein in Context*, edited by Mara Beller, Robert S. Cohen, and Jürgen Renn, 311–41 (Cambridge: Cambridge University Press, 1993).

Renn, Jürgen. "Einstein's Controversy with Drude and the Origin of Statistical Mechanics: A New Glimpse from the 'Love Letters.'" *Archive for History of Exact Sciences* (1997) 51:315–54.

Renn, Jürgen. *The Evolution of Knowledge: Rethinking Science for the Anthropocene.* Princeton: Princeton University Press, 2020.

Renn, Jürgen, and Robert Rynasiewicz. "Einstein's Copernican Revolution." In *The Cambridge Companion to Einstein*, edited by Michel Janssen and Christoph Lehner, 38–71. Cambridge: Cambridge University Press, 2014.

Renn, Jürgen, and Robert Schulmann, eds. *Albert Einstein—Mileva Marić: The Love Letters.* Princeton: Princeton University Press, 1992.

Rosenkranz, Ze'ev, ed. *Einstein Before Israel: Zionist Icon or Iconoclast?* Princeton: Princeton University Press, 2011.

Rosenkranz, Ze'ev, ed. *The Travel Diaries of Albert Einstein: The Far East, Palestine, and Spain, 1922–1923.* Princeton: Princeton University Press, 2018.

Rosenkranz, Ze'ev, ed. *The Travel Diaries of Albert Einstein: South America, 1925.* Princeton: Princeton University Press, 2023.

Rowe, David, and Robert Schulmann, eds. *Einstein on Politics: His Private Thoughts and Public Stands on Nationalism, Zionism, War, Peace, and the Bomb.* Princeton: Princeton University Press, 2007.

Sauer, Tilman. "Marcel Grossmann and His Contribution to the General Theory of Relativity." In *Proceedings of the Thirteenth Marcel Grossmann Meeting on General Relativity*, 456–503. World Scientific, 2015.

Schemmel, Matthias. "The Continuity Between Classical and Relativistic Cosmology in the Work of Karl Schwarzschild." In *Gravitation in the Twilight of Classi-*

cal Physics: The Promise of Mathematics, edited by Jürgen Renn and Matthias Schemmel, 155–181, vol. 4 of The Genesis of General Relativity. Dordt: Springer, 2007.

Schutz, Bernard. "Intuition in Einsteinian Physics." In Teaching Einsteinian Physics in Schools: An Essential Guide for Teachers in Training and Practice, edited by Magdalena Kersting and David Blair. Oxford: Routledge, 2021.

Smoluchowski, Marian von. "Zur Kinetischen Theorie der Brownschen Molekularbewegung und der Suspensionen." Annalen der Physik (1906) 21:756–80.

Sommerfeld, Arnold. "To Albert Einstein's Seventieth Birthday." In Albert Einstein: Philosopher-Scientist, edited by Paul Arthur Schilpp. Library of Living Philosophers. La Salle, IL: Open Court; Cambridge: Cambridge University Press, 1949.

Stachel, John. "Einstein and the Rigidly Rotating Disk." In General Relativity and Gravitation: One Hundred Years after the Birth of Albert Einstein, edited by Alan Held, 1–15. New York: Plenum, 1980.

Stachel, John, ed. Einstein's Miraculous Year: Five Papers That Changed the Face of Physics. 2nd ed. Princeton: Princeton University Press, 2005.

Staley, Richard. Einstein's Generation: The Origins of the Relativity Revolution (Chicago: University of Chicago Press, 2008).

Staley, Richard. "Worldviews and Physicists' Experience of Disciplinary Change: On the Uses of 'Classical' Physics." Studies in History and Philosophy of Science (2008) Part A, 39, no. 3:298–311.

Straus, Ernst G. "Reminiscences." In Albert Einstein, Historical and Cultural Perspectives, edited by Gerald J. Holton and Yehuda Elkana, 417–24. Princeton: Princeton University Press, 1982.

Stone, Douglas. Einstein and the Quantum: The Quest of the Valiant Swabian. Princeton: Princeton University Press, 2016.

Sutherland, William. "A Dynamical Theory of Diffusion for Non-Electrolytes and the Molecular Mass of Albumin." Philosophical Magazine and Journal of Science (1905) 9:781–85.

Thorne, Kip. Black Holes & Time Warps: Einstein's Outrageous Legacy. New York: W. W. Norton, 1994.

Torricelli, Evangelista. Opera Geometrica. Florence: Typis Amatoris Masse & Laurentii de Landis, 1644.

Weber, Joseph. "Evidence for Discovery of Gravitational Radiation." Physical Review Letters (1969) 22:1320–24.

Wertheimer, Max. Productive Thinking. New York: Harper, 1945.

Will, Clifford M. Was Einstein Right? Putting General Relativity to the Test. New York: Basic Books, 1986.

Will, Clifford M., and Nicolás Yunes. Is Einstein Still Right? Black Holes, Gravitational Waves, and the Quest to Verify Einstein's Greatest Creation. Oxford: Oxford University Press, 2020.

INDEX

A NOTE ON THE TYPE

This book has been composed in Arno, an Old-style serif typeface in the classic Venetian tradition, designed by Robert Slimbach at Adobe.